Child and Adolescent Psychiatry

Robert Goodman PhD, FRCPsych, MRCP

Professor of Brain and Behavioural Medicine, Institute of Psychiatry, King's College, London

Stephen Scott BSc, FRCP, FRCPsych

Professor of Child Health and Behaviour, Department of Child & Adolescent Psychiatry, Institute of Psychiatry, King's College, London

THIRD EDITION

FOREWORD BY PROFESSOR SIR MICHAEL RUTTER FRS

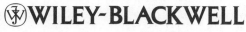

WILEY-BLACKWELL

A John Wiley & Sons, Ltd., Publication

Library of Congress Cataloging-in-Publication Data

Goodman, Robert, MRCPsych.
  Child and adolescent psychiatry / Robert Goodman and Stephen Scott. – 3rd ed.
     p. ; cm.
  Rev. ed. of: Child psychiatry / Robert Goodman and Stephen Scott. 2nd ed. Oxford, UK : Blackwell, 2005.
  Includes bibliographical references and index.
  ISBN 978-1-119-97968-5 (pbk.)
  I. Scott, Stephen, MRCPsych. II. Goodman, Robert, MRCPsych. Child psychiatry. III. Title.
  [DNLM: 1. Mental Disorders. 2. Adolescent. 3. Child. WS 350]
  618.92'89–dc23

                                                              2012011738

A catalogue record for this book is available from the British Library.

Wiley also publishes its books in a variety of electronic formats. Some content that appears in print may not be available in electronic books.

Cover photos courtesy of Stephen Scott, Catherine Lincoln and iStockphoto.com

Set in 9.5/12pt Meridien by Aptara Inc., New Delhi, India
Printed in Singapore by Ho Printing Singapore Pte Ltd

1   2012

Contents

Companion website

The book is accompanied by a companion resources site:

goodmanchildpsychiatry.com

with self-assessment material for each chapter.

Foreword to First Edition

There is nothing quite like this gem of a book, which provides much the best introduction to child psychiatry that has been written. It is succinct, very easy to read, and immensely practical in the guidance it provides on conceptual issues, on diagnosis and on treatment. Most introductory text-books achieve accessibility for practitioners at the cost of a lack of scientific rigour and questioning; this splendid volume shows well that this price need not be paid. It is thoroughly up to date in its distillation of research findings and it conveys, with both interest and clarity, how modern clinical work is being shaped by the products of scientific investigation. Quite appropriately, the details of the research are not described, but the spirit of scientific inquiry pervades the whole of the book. References to a well-selected, short list of key review papers and chapters are provided, so that readers may both extend their understanding and also assess the evidence for themselves. The account given here, however, does a remarkably good job of selecting from an immense literature the research findings that are of greatest clinical relevance now. I would be surprised if reading this book does not stimulate most people to read further. Equally, I am sure that they will be astonished to discover how little that is important has not already been well covered in this volume. Quite a feat!

Both the authors are experienced clinicians and their wealth of practical knowledge, together with their 'feel' for clinical issues and for patients' needs, comes through on every page. All the major varieties of mental disorders are covered but the approach taken is distinctive in four main respects. To begin with, the book provides very helpful guidance on the details of *how* to do what is needed. This is as evident in the first chapter on assessment as in those dealing with different forms of treatment. Indeed, the description of how clinicians need to think about the questions in-volved in assessment is masterly despite (or perhaps because of) its brevity. Second, there is a particularly insightful description of the different kinds of risk and protective factors and of how they might operate. Third, the discussion of clinical issues involves an explicitly developmental focus with an accompanying consideration of just how overt disorders relate to the variations in normal development. Finally, the book is skilfully organised to be most helpful to those preparing for professional examinations (with a useful list of 200 multiple choice questions). Remarkably, it achieves this organisation without the drawback of unwarranted dogmatism that mars so many introductory texts. My only regret is that I did not write this excellent book!

Professor Sir Michael Rutter
Honorary Director
MRC Child Psychiatry Unit, Institute of Psychiatry

Foreword to Third Edition

This splendid new third edition retains all the strengths of its prede-
cessors and it not only brings things up to date but it broadens the
coverage through additional material on adolescence. The timing of the
book coincides with a period during which DSM-5 and ICD-11, the new
classifications from the American Psychiatric Association and the World
Health Organisation, are currently being finalised. Nevertheless, it is very
much to the authors' credit that they have finessed this very skillfully by
presenting issues, concepts, findings and clinical matters in a way that
deals with the big issues without getting bogged down in the details. As
with the two previous editions, there is a very skilful integration of science
and clinical practice. The main target audience is certainly clinicians but
researchers, too, will find that there is much to learn here on areas of
research that are a bit outside of their own interest.

The book is also very interesting to read. It is a bit like watching one
of David Attenborough's marvellous TV programmes – you never feel
lectured at, your interest is engaged throughout, but in the course of that
engagement you actually learn a lot. Readers will not find here dogmatic
assertions that are not supported by evidence. The suggested readings at
the end of each chapter provide an easy way for readers to find out more
of the detail if they wish but the book already contains an immense
amount. There is no better book for those who want an accessible introduction to child and adolescent psychiatry as a whole, or as a means
of keeping up to date with relevant scientific understanding and clinical
practice.

Professor Sir Michael Rutter
Honorary Director
MRC Child Psychiatry Unit, Institute of Psychiatry

Preface

Aware that this is often our readers' only book on the subject, we have aimed to get straight to the heart of child and adolescent psychiatry. Our goal has been to be brief, clear, practical, thoughtful, up-to-date, scientifically accurate, clinically sound, and relevant for examinations. We have been very encouraged by the exceptionally positive response to the first and second editions from trainees and senior colleagues from a variety of disciplines. We have renamed the book – it is now *Child and Adolescent Psychiatry* rather than just *Child Psychiatry*. The previous editions also covered adolescents as well as children, but we have strengthened the adolescent component, with new chapters on mania, schizophrenia, eating disorders and substance abuse. We have also thoroughly updated all the existing chapters.

The chapters are grouped into four Parts: Part 1, an introductory section on assessment, classification and epidemiology; Part 2, a section covering each of the main specific disorders and presentations; Part 3, a section on the major risk factors predisposing to child and adolescent psychiatric disorders; and, finally, Part 4, a section on the main methods of treatment. Each chapter presents the key facts, concepts and growing points in the area, drawing on clinical experience as well as the latest research findings.

It has been our good fortune to work alongside a diverse and talented group of clinicians and researchers at one of the world's leading centres of child and adolescent psychiatry. We hope we have communicated some of the excitement of being at the 'cutting edge' of a discipline that is increasingly benefiting from advances in subjects as varied as developmental psychology, neurobiology, genetics, social anthropology, linguistics and ethology. As practising clinicians, we have also been keen to make this a book about working with children and families, as well as theory. Because successful practitioners need to master techniques as well as concepts, we have included plenty of 'how to' tips on assessment and treatment.

To make the book read as easily as possible, we have not interrupted the text with references. Instead, each chapter ends with suggestions for further reading, providing convenient entry points into the current literature. In many instances, we recommend one or more chapters from the fifth edition of Rutter *et al.*'s *Child and Adolescent Psychiatry* – an outstanding source of detailed information and further references. We also suggest a mixture of recent journal articles and books.

The book has been written with several groups of readers in mind. Trainees in psychiatry, paediatrics and general practice should find it useful as an accessible introduction to the subject when they are first working with troubled children and adolescents; as a continuing source of practical and conceptual guidance when assessing and treating individual children and adolescents with unfamiliar disorders; and as a comprehensive textbook when preparing for professional examinations. Trainees from other disciplines (psychology, nursing, social work and education) should find this book meets their needs when working with troubled children and adolescents, and also helps them to understand psychiatric perspectives on problems that often require inter-disciplinary working. Finally, for established professionals in many fields, this book should be an easy way to keep abreast of current thinking, and a convenient source book for preparing teaching sessions and for reference.

Readers can access a special dedicated website (GoodmanScottchild psychiatry.com) with over 200 multiple choice questions (MCQs) on child and adolescent mental health – plus the answers, of course. These are designed for trainees approaching professional examinations as well as for other readers who enjoy quizzes as a way of consolidating their knowledge. Our MCQs are modelled on Membership questions set by the various Royal Colleges, particularly emphasising the examiners' favourite topics.

This book has been greatly strengthened by the comments and suggestions of many colleagues and trainees from a range of disciplines; we are extremely grateful to them all. We are keen to go on improving this book and look to you, our readers, for help. Please do write to us telling us what you liked and what needs changing. What should be cut and what should be expanded? How could we make the book more useful to you? We hope that your advice to us will benefit future readers and, through them, troubled children and their families.

Robert Goodman and Stephen Scott
London

PART 1
Assessment, Classification and Epidemiology

CHAPTER 1

Assessment

Performing a thorough psychiatric assessment of a child or adolescent can all too easily become a long and dreary list of topics to be covered and observations to be made – turning the occasion into an aversive experience for all concerned. It is far better to start with a clear idea of the goals and then pursue them flexibly. Ends and means are different: this first part of the chapter deals with ends; the second half of the chapter deals with means, providing some 'how to' tips with suggestions about the order in which to ask things.

Five key questions

During an assessment you need to engage the family and lay the foundations for treatment while focusing on five key questions, given in the following list, and remembered by the mnemonic SIRSE. There is a lot to be said for carrying out a comprehensive assessment on the first visit, provided this does not result in such a pressured interview that it puts the family off coming again. As long as you are able to engage the family, it is not a disaster if the assessment is incomplete after the first session provided you recognise the gaps and fill them in during subsequent sessions. Indeed, all assessments should be seen as provisional, generating working hypotheses that have to be updated and corrected over the entire course of your contact with the family. Just as it is a mistake to launch into treatment without an adequate assessment, it is also a mistake to forget that your assessment may need to be revised during the course of treatment. Consider the need for a reassessment if treatment does not work.

Symptoms	What sort of problem is it?
Impact	How much distress or impairment does it cause?
Risks	What factors have initiated and maintained the problem?
Strengths	What assets are there to work with?
Explanatory model	What beliefs and expectations do the family bring with them?

Child and Adolescent Psychiatry, Third Edition. Robert Goodman and Stephen Scott.
© 2012 Robert Goodman and Stephen Scott. Published 2012 by John Wiley & Sons, Ltd.

Though child and adolescent psychiatrists and their colleagues may be involved in many types of assessment, these five key questions will be relevant in nearly all cases, albeit with variations in emphasis and approach. Most of the rest of this chapter focuses on an approach that seeks, where possible, to explain the presenting complaint in terms of the child or adolescent having one or more disorders – leading on to a fuller formulation involving aetiology, prognosis and treatment. For some referrals, however, it may be more appropriate to focus on parenting difficulties or problems of the family system as a whole rather than on the problems of the presenting individual.

Symptoms

Most of the psychiatric syndromes that affect children and adolescents involve combinations of symptoms (and signs) from four main areas: emotions, behaviour, development and relationships. As with any rule of thumb, there are exceptions, most notably schizophrenia and anorexia nervosa. The four domains of symptoms are:

1 emotional symptoms
2 behavioural problems
3 developmental delays
4 relationship difficulties.

The *emotional symptoms* of interest to child and adolescent psychiatrists will be very familiar to most mental health trainees. As with adults, it is appropriate to enquire about anxieties and fears (and also about any resultant avoidance). Ask, too, about misery and, if relevant, about associated depressive features including worthlessness, hopelessness, self-harm, inability to take pleasure in activities that are usually enjoyable (anhedonia), poor appetite, sleep disturbance and lack of energy. Classical symptoms of obsessive-compulsive disorder can be present in young children, even preschoolers. One difference in emphasis from adult psychiatry is the need to enquire rather more carefully about 'somatic equivalents' of emotional symptoms, for example, Monday morning tummy aches may be far more evident than the underlying anxiety about school or separation.

Parental reports are the primary source of information on the emotional symptoms of young children, with self-reports becoming increasingly important for older children and adolescents. Somewhat surprisingly, parents and their children often disagree with one another about the presence or absence of emotional symptoms. When faced with discrepant reports, it is sometimes straightforward to decide who to believe. Perhaps the parents have described in convincing detail a string of incidents in which their child's fear of dogs has resulted in panics or aborted outings, while the child's own claim never to be scared of anything seems to be due to a mixture of bravado and a desire to get the interview over with as soon as possible. Alternatively, an adolescent's own account may make it clear that she experiences a level of anxiety that interferes with her sleep and concentration even though her parents are unaware of this because she does not confide in them and spends much of her time in her room. In other instances, it is harder to know who to believe – and perhaps it is more sensible to accept that there are multiple perspectives rather than one single truth.

The *behavioural problems* that dominate much of child and adolescent psychiatric practice are less familiar territory for most mental health trainees since adults with comparable symptoms are more likely to appear in courts than clinics. Enquiry should focus on three main domains of behaviour: defiant behaviour, often associated with irritability and temper outbursts; aggression and destructiveness; and antisocial behaviours such as stealing, fire setting and substance abuse. Reports from parents and teachers are likely to be the main source of information on behavioural problems, though children and adolescents sometimes tell you about misdeeds that their parents or teachers do not know about. There is only limited value in asking children and adolescents about their defiant behaviours since they, like adults, often find it hard to recognise when they are being unreasonable, disruptive or irritable, however good they may be at recognising these traits in others.

Evaluating *developmental delay* can be particularly hard for new trainees who do not have children of their own or a background in child health. Development complicates what, in adults, would be a simple assessment. Consider a physical analogy. An adult height of 1 metre is small, whereas a childhood height of 1 metre may be small, average or large; it obviously depends on the age of the child and, unless you have a growth chart handy, you could easily fail to spot children who were unusually small or tall for their age. The same problem is even more pronounced in the psychological domain. What are you going to make of an attention span of five minutes at different ages? Are you missing children whose speech is immature or excessively grown up for their age? How long should a 5-year-old sit still without fidgeting? In the absence of good published norms, you will mostly have to rely on experienced colleagues until you 'get your eye in'. Remember, too, that experienced parents or teachers are rarely concerned without good reason.

The areas of development that are of particular relevance to child and adolescent psychiatry are: attention and activity regulation; speech and language; play; motor skills; bladder and bowel control; and scholastic attainments, particularly in reading, spelling and mathematics. When judging current levels of functioning, you will be able to draw on direct observations of the child or adolescent as well as reports from parents and teachers. Asking parents about developmental milestones can tell you about their child's previous developmental trajectory.

Assessing children's and adolescents' *difficulties in social relatedness* is another taxing task, partly because relationships change with development. In addition, it is not always clear whether children's problems getting on with other people reflect primarily on them or on the other people. For example, if a child with cerebral palsy is unable to make or keep friends, how far might this reflect the child's lack of social skills, and how far might it reflect the prejudice of other children?

The most striking impairments in relatedness are seen in the autistic disorders, generally taking one of three forms: (1) an aloof indifference to other people as people; (2) a passive acceptance of interactions when others take the initiative and tell them what to do; and (3) an awkward and rather unempathic social interest that tends to put others off because of its gaucheness. Disinhibition and lack of reserve with strangers are prominent in some autistic, hyperactivity and attachment disorders, and may also be seen in mania and after severe bilateral head injury. The disinhibition may be accompanied by a pestering, importuning style. In small doses, some of these traits can seem quite charming. For example, after a few minutes acquaintance, you may judge a boy to be delightfully frank or open or eccentric. However, this sort of charm generally palls with longer acquaintance and the history usually makes it clear that his manner soon becomes very wearing for all those in regular contact with him.

Some children and adolescents have difficulty relating to most social partners, whether young or old, strangers or friends. Other children and adolescents have problems with specific types of social relationship, for example, with attachment or friendship relationships. The problems may even be specific to one important social partner. Thus, most children and adolescents are specifically attached to a relatively small number of key people, and the quality of their attachment (secure, resistant, aloof, disorganised) may vary, depending on which of these key people they are relating to. For example, the attachment may be insecure with the main caregiver but secure with the other caregivers (see Chapter 32). Similar specificity can be seen in sibling relationships.

You can gather information on a child or adolescent's social relationships from several sources. Observing the family interactions in the waiting room or consulting room can be very helpful. See how the child or adolescent relates to you during the physical and mental state examinations. If your assessment follows a fairly standardised pattern, it is all the more striking that one child is shy and monosyllabic throughout while another child of the same age greets you as a best friend and wants to climb onto your lap. Also note what might in other circumstances be called the counter-transference, for example, did you find them irritating? Does the interview leave you feeling exhausted? These are often valuable clues to the feelings that this individual evokes in many other people. Direct observation is supplemented by the history. Parents can often tell you a lot about their child's relationships from the early years onwards. It can also be helpful to get a teacher's report on peer relationships at school, but remember that teachers are not always aware of peer problems, even when these are fairly substantial, particularly if teachers do not usually supervise the playground.

Most patients have symptoms from more than one domain

Only a minority of the children and adolescents attending child mental health services have symptoms restricted to just one domain, but such individuals do exist. Thus you may see pure emotional symptoms in generalised anxiety disorder, pure behavioural symptoms in socialised conduct disorder, and pure relationship difficulties in disinhibited attachment disorder. Pure developmental delays, such as primary enuresis, receptive language disorder or specific reading disorder are not usually seen by child and adolescent psychiatrists in the absence of other symptoms. However, children presenting with ADHD may seem to have fairly pure delays in the development of attention and activity control.

Most of the children and adolescents seen by psychiatrists have symptoms from two or more domains. For example, individuals with conduct disorder also commonly have emotional symptoms, peer problems, and developmental delays, such as specific reading disorder or hyperactivity (see Box 1.1).

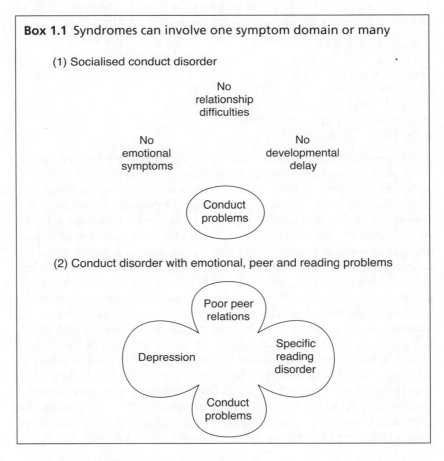

Box 1.1 Syndromes can involve one symptom domain or many

(1) Socialised conduct disorder

No relationship difficulties

No emotional symptoms

No developmental delay

Conduct problems

(2) Conduct disorder with emotional, peer and reading problems

Poor peer relations

Depression

Specific reading disorder

Conduct problems

Autism provides another illustration of symptoms in multiple domains. The core symptoms of autism span two domains, with characteristic patterns of relationship problems and developmental delays (as well as developmental deviance and rigidity). In addition, autistic individuals commonly display some behavioural problems, such as marked temper tantrums, and some emotional problems, such as unusual phobias.

Impact

Nearly all children and adolescents have fears, worries, periods of sadness and times when they misbehave, fidget or fail to concentrate. When do these sorts of symptoms represent a disorder rather than a normal variant? In general, you should only diagnose a disorder if the symptoms are having a substantial impact. DSM-III criteria for psychiatric disorders did not include the need for impact, and the result of that omission is illustrated by a study that found that half of a large representative sample of Puerto Rican children had a psychiatric disorder. This is a ridiculously high rate, and most of these children were not considered 'cases' on clinical grounds. This has since been rectified: DSM-IV and the research diagnostic criteria of ICD-10 generally include impact criteria. Impact is judged from:

1 Social impairment
   (a) family life
   (b) classroom learning
   (c) friendships
   (d) leisure activities.
2 Distress for the child or adolescent.
3 Perhaps by disruption for others.

The main measure of impact should be whether the symptoms result in significant social impairment, substantially compromising the child or adolescent's ability to fulfil normal role expectations in everyday life. The main areas of everyday life to consider are family life, class work, friendships and leisure activities, though interference with paid work or physical health is sometimes relevant. Two subsidiary measures of impact are also important: distress for the child or adolescent; and disruption for others. Like their adult counterparts, children and adolescents who are anxious or depressed can sometimes fulfil normal role expectations while experiencing considerable inner anguish. Equally, behavioural problems can sometimes lead to substantial disruption for others without resulting in much apparent distress or social impairment for the child or adolescent. For example, the parents of children with severe physical or intellectual problems are sometimes remarkably stoical in the face of marked defiance, tantrums, and destructiveness – suffering themselves, but making sure that the child does not 'pay for it'. In these instances, it may be clinically sensible to diagnose a disorder as present, and treat it, even though the individual is not really socially impaired by the symptoms. Is this a slippery slope to labelling all 'deviants' as psychiatrically ill? We hope not.

Risk factors

Why does the individual you are assessing have his or her particular constellation of psychiatric problems? Though the world is full of people who think they do know the cause of particular psychiatric disorders (dietary allergy, lack of discipline, bad genes, poor teaching, hypothalamic damage, unresolved infantile conflicts, etc.), the identification of a single cause for a psychiatric disorder is rarely scientifically justifiable. There are exceptions. Thus, it seems reasonable to say that the compulsive self-biting behaviour in Lesch-Nyhan Syndrome (which can lead to affected children severing their own fingers and extensively damaging their lips and tongue) is caused by a specific genetic deficit resulting in complete deficiency of one of the enzymes involved in purine metabolism. The presence of this inborn error of metabolism seems to guarantee the characteristic behaviour, irrespective of other genetic or environmental factors.

By comparison, most of the 'causes' in child and adolescent psychiatry are best thought of as risk factors that increase the likelihood of a particular disorder without guaranteeing that it will occur. Thus, although exposure to a high level of parental conflict is a risk factor for conduct disorder, many of the children and adolescents who are exposed to marital conflict do not develop conduct disorder. Perhaps we need to explain psychiatric disorders in terms of particular combinations or sequences of risk factors. One such scheme invokes three types of risk factors: predisposing, precipitating and perpetuating factors. The window has a hole in it because the glass was particularly thin and brittle (the predisposing factors), it was hit by a piece of gravel (the precipitating factor), and no one has subsequently replaced the broken pane (the perpetuating factor). A child who has always been rather clingy and has never had many friends (the predisposing factors) refuses to return to school after a row with a friend and a few days off sick with a cold (the precipitating factors). His parents are so worried about his level of distress that they feel it would be harmful to force him to return to school, but every day off makes it harder for him to go back since he falls further behind with his schoolwork and his former playmates find new people to play with (the perpetuating factors). The presence of a disorder can be explained in terms of:

- predisposing factors
- precipitating factors
- perpetuating factors

  and the absence of

- protective factors.

Even if you do train yourself to think in terms of multiple interacting causes, you will still need to remember how incomplete our present knowledge is. Our current understanding of aetiology will probably look ridiculously simplistic or misguided in a hundred years time (or much sooner). It often helps to admit this to parents: dogmatic insistence that you know the whole truth about causation may be less well received than the more defensible claim that you probably know enough about causation to provide some useful pointers to treatment.

In gearing your assessment to look for, or ask about, known risk factors, you will have to cover many areas. The traditional focus on family factors is partly justified since our family provides us with our genes and an important part of our environment. Thus, a family history of Tourette syndrome could be of genetic relevance, while a history of parental friction could be of environmental relevance, and a history of parental mental illness could have genetic or environmental consequences. Most children and adolescents inhabit three rather different social worlds: family, school and peer culture. Do not confine your interest in environmental factors to the social world of the family – school factors, such as scapegoating by a teacher and peer factors, such as bullying, may be at least as important. Also ask about adverse life events and more chronic social adversities. Physical and psychological examinations may also unearth previously unrecognised risk factors for psychiatric problems. For example, an adequate history and physical examination may suggest a dementing disorder, mild cerebral palsy, complex seizures or fetal alcohol syndrome – warranting referral to a specialist for a more definitive view. Psychometric assessment can detect low IQ and specific learning problems – risk factors for various psychiatric problems that may, sadly, have gone undetected in school.

Strengths

If you asked only about symptoms, impact and risk factors, your focus would be almost exclusively negative, dwelling on what is wrong with this individual and this family. It is also important to establish what is right about this individual and family. Identifying protective factors may make it clearer why this individual has a mild rather than a severe disorder. It may also be possible to identify protective factors that apply to siblings, but not to the referred individual, that help to explain why only one child in this family has developed a disorder. Relevant protective factors include a sense of worth stemming from being good at something, a close supportive relationship with an adult, and an easy temperament.

Your treatment plan needs to build on the strengths of the individual and the family – and also on the strengths of the school and wider social network. Though the aim of treatment is determined by what is wrong, the choice of treatment often depends on what is right. You should design the treatment to harness the strengths in the child or adolescent, such as the ability to make friends or respond to praise, and the strengths in the parents, such as an openness to trying new approaches in the family.

If you dwell exclusively on negatives, the family may leave the assessment feeling emotionally battered – and be correspondingly less willing to return. We live in a society that generally blames parents for their children's problems. If a child has a tantrum in the supermarket, most of the bystanders will look reproachfully rather than sympathetically at the accompanying parent. Parents stand accused, and often feel uncertain in their own minds whether they are to blame or not. On the one hand, they are likely to share society's view that parents cause their children's problems and most parents can identify many ways in which their child rearing has been less than perfect. On the other hand, most of the parents you see in clinic will also feel that they are neither better nor worse than many other parents whose children seem fine.

Many parents are frightened that you will judge them 'guilty as charged' and may be defensive and prickly in anticipation of this. One of your key tasks is to convey that you see them not as fundamentally deficient people but as individuals who, like the rest of us, have strengths as well as weaknesses. An interview presents plenty of opportunities for registering in a non-patronising way the positive things parents and their children do. If parents come to feel that you are not judging them, they are much more likely to accept the treatment plan you recommend, including suggestions for change on their part. If you ally yourself with a child against the parents (which is a common temptation for beginners), you will probably only succeed in redoubling the parents' criticisms of the child and discouraging the family from returning to the clinic.

When you meet parents who seem to have particularly glaring weaknesses, it is vital that you put even more effort into identifying their strengths. This is not to say that you should be blind to their difficulties with parenting (these difficulties may need to be the focus of treatment or even the grounds for initiating care proceedings), but you need to remember (for your own sake as well as theirs) that these parents have their own strengths, often despite harrowing personal backgrounds of their own. Parents have usually put a great deal of effort into parenting. Though successful parents may put in more effort, they also generally get much more back from their children, so failing parents may be putting in more effort per unit reward than successful parents!

It is sometimes helpful to identify the presenting problem as the opposite side of the coin to a valuable strength. For example, a strong-willed child who is seen at the clinic because of defiant and disruptive behaviour at home and at school may also show an impressive determination to succeed in the face of adversity. Similarly, a sensitive child who is prey to all manner of anxieties may show admirable empathy and consideration for others. In each case, identifying a trait as both good and bad rather than as entirely bad may make the trait easier to live with. In addition, the therapeutic task is redefined: it is not to abolish the trait (which is likely to be impossible anyway) but only to reduce the trait's troublesome consequences.

The family's explanatory model

The way we construe a child or adolescent's emotional and behavioural difficulties will depend on our cultural and professional backgrounds. This book draws on a set of explanatory models derived from empirically orientated child and adolescent psychiatry. Other professionals, such as social workers, educational psychologists or psychotherapists, may apply a different set of *explanatory models*, leading to radically different formulations even if they see the same child and family. It is easy to forget that colleagues from other disciplines have different explanatory models – an oversight that can severely hamper communication. The same can be said of communication between professionals and families, since professionals are often unaware that families may have distinctive explanatory models of their own, assuming instead that all right-thinking members of the public hold similar, albeit less detailed, views to their own.

Little is yet known about the range of explanatory models that influence the ways in which families from different social and cultural backgrounds think about their children's emotional and behavioural difficulties. Nevertheless, it is clear that members of the public often have complex explanatory models that differ substantially from those of doctors and other professionals – as regards aetiology, phenomenology, pathophysiology, natural history and treatment. In other words, families come to clinics with expectations that may differ radically from your own. You should not guess a family's views on the basis of your stereotypes about their class and culture; the only sensible way to find out what they believe is to ask them open-ended questions and listen carefully to their replies.

After you have asked the family about the presenting complaint, it flows naturally to enquire what they make of the problem; what they think it is due to; and how they think it might be investigated or treated. Some families will look puzzled and say that they don't know, that's for you to tell them. Many others will tell you things you could not easily have guessed. You may learn, for example, that the parents of a child with poor concentration fear he has a brain tumour, or think he needs a brain scan, or believe that you will be able to cure the symptoms with hypnosis. If you had not asked them, they might never have told you and they might have gone away disappointed, never to return again. It is also worth asking the parents whether other important people, including grandparents, friends, neighbours, teachers, have expressed strong opinions about causation, investigation or treatment. A child's mother may tell you, for instance, that her mother-in-law has been very insistent that the child's problems have arisen because the mother has always worked and has not spent enough time with her child.

Knowing about people's explanatory models gives you a chance at the end of the assessment to present your views in the way that will be most relevant to them. You can explain that the symptoms are not at all like those of a brain tumour; that a scan would not alter management; and that although you are not a trained hypnotist, even a professional hypnotist would be unlikely to be of much help in this instance. You can also mention that the quality of the day care that they have arranged for their child gives no reason for concern, and that there is no scientific basis for blaming ADHD on working mothers when the quality of alternative care is good. You can say, too, that you would be very happy to discuss this further with the child's grandmother if the family want you to. Some families hold to their explanatory models with great tenacity, but most families are willing to update their explanatory models if you take the time to present the facts. At the end of a careful assessment in which the family may have invested considerable hope, it would be a great shame if failure to explore the family's explanatory models left you and them at cross-purposes and mutually dissatisfied.

Some 'how to' tips

What means will you employ to answer the five key questions and engage the family? There are no hard and fast rules to suit all clinics, all clinicians, all families and all presenting complaints. This is where good clinical supervision is particularly helpful. Sitting in on assessments carried out by a range of senior colleagues can be very instructive. The rest of the chapter is taken up with a variety of 'how to' suggestions that are guides rather than fixed recipes.

How to: take the history from parents

As a trained clinical interviewer, you should not simply be a speaking questionnaire. If you only want the parents' answers to a fixed series of predetermined questions, a questionnaire would be quicker and easier for them to complete, unless they are poor readers. One style of interviewing, which is known as 'fully structured' or 'respondent-based' interviewing, amounts to little more than a verbally administered questionnaire. The wording of questions is predetermined, and the style of questioning is 'closed', calling for a limited range of possible responses: often a yes/no answer, or a rating of frequency, duration or severity. Questionnaires and fully structured interviews are widely used as research and clinical tools, since they are quick, cheap and easy to administer in a standardised fashion. Their main limitation is that the parents' answers sometimes tell you more about the parents' beliefs (or misunderstandings of the terms used) than about the child or adolescent being described.

A different style of interviewing, known as 'semi-structured' or 'interviewer-based', can help you get beyond the parents' views to the observations on which they are basing their views. The interviewer is expected to ask whatever questions are required to elicit from parents the information needed for the interviewer to decide whether a particular symptom (or impairment or risk factor) is present or not. In order to do this, the interviewer will often need to use 'open' questions that offer the parents the chance to make a wide range of possible responses. Obtaining detailed descriptions of recent instances of the behaviour in question is usually very helpful.

An example may make this clearer. One of the questions in a questionnaire or fully structured interview might be 'Does your child have concentration problems?' If the parents answered 'Yes', you would still not know whether the child's concentration was objectively poor or whether the parents were setting unrealistically high standards (or had misunderstood the question). A semi-structured approach would use a mixture of open and closed prompts to get the parents to describe, using recent examples, how long the child has been able to persist with specific activities without switching from one thing to another: playing alone, playing with friends, watching television, looking at a book, and so on. You could then make up your own mind from this evidence whether the child's concentration at home was age-appropriate or not.

Similar methods can be used to explore irritability, fearfulness or any other reported area of problems. It is also sometimes relevant to explore why parents are not concerned. For instance, if teachers report major problems with concentration but parents do not, it is important to explore whether the child really does concentrate adequately when out of school, or whether the parents simply have unusually low expectations.

Semi-structured interviewing is a valuable technique but you do have to be careful not to overdo it or the interview will go on for hours! One option is to use questionnaires or fully structured interviews to get an overall view and then use semi-structured interviewing to obtain more details about the most relevant aspects of the case. Finding the time to get parents to describe their child's typical day, perhaps yesterday, can often be a particularly illuminating window, not only on symptoms and any resultant impairment but also on family life, child-rearing tactics and expressed emotion.

Here is one possible scheme for taking a history from parents:

1 *Presenting complaint*
   - When did it begin? When was he last completely well or not doing it? How does it show itself? How often? When? Always get specific examples rather than accept general statements. What is going on just before it happens? After? How do you respond? What's the result? What effect is it having on the rest of the family? Why are you coming about it now?
   - Review of other symptoms: emotions, behaviour, attention and activity, somatic:
       - sleeping, eating, bladder and bowels, pains, tics.
2 *Current functioning*
   - Typical day's activities: dressing and eating, play and leisure, going to bed, sleeping. Does this vary much at the weekend? How involved are the parents involved with this child?
   - Social relationships:
       - Friends: Got any? What exactly do they do together? Do they go to one another's homes? How often? Shy? Able to take turns? Leader or follower? Sexuality?
   - Adults: How does the child get on with each parent? With other carers? How do they feel about the child? Any good times? When?
       - Siblings: Who does he or she spend time with? Like? Dislike? Jealous?
3 *Family history*
   - Composition: draw a family tree (a 'genogram'). Ask a few details about each relative, including medical and psychiatric problems. For members of the immediate family, record age, occupation, what they are like.
   - Relationships: how do the parents get on together? Do they support each other? What are their expectations of this child? What were their own childhoods like? Do they agree on rules and how discipline should be applied? Arguments? How do the children get on together?

Who is close to whom? Who gets into most trouble? Who least? How are they treated differently?

• Circumstances: housing, debt. Have circumstances changed recently? Has there been contact with social services?

4 *Personal history*

• Birth and infancy: planned and wanted? What sort of baby was he or she? Milestones – were these earlier or later than siblings or friend's baby?

• Schools: names and dates. Difficulties in classroom, playground or small groups? Academic functioning: their position in class, whether they are under-achieving, whether they are receiving, or ought to be receiving, special help. Social functioning: friends, type of play.

• Physical health: fits and faints, illnesses, hospital or psychiatric contact.

How to: see the child or adolescent alone

Do not rush into difficult topics – it is obviously best to engage with the individual first by focusing initially on pleasant and neutral topics or activities. Equally, do not become so focused on making the interview fun that you avoid difficult topics entirely (though you may want to postpone some difficult topics for a second interview).

• Children under 5: observe play, play too, chat, use fewer directed questions.

• Over-5s: you should both sit down. It is often helpful to ask the child to do a drawing. Chat and use directed questioning.

What to cover

1 This is a useful opportunity to observe:

(a) *Activity and attention*. Is there a lot of squirming and fidgeting? Does he or she keep getting out of the chair and wandering about? Is it hard to get him or her to persist in a task? Is he or she easily distracted by extraneous stimuli?

(b) *Quality of social interaction*. Does he or she show too much or too little anxiety about coming with you initially? Is he or she interested in social interaction? Does he or she make good eye contact? Does he or she talk *with* you or *at* you? Is he or she inappropriately friendly, over-familiar or cheeky? What feelings does the interaction evoke in you?

(c) *Developmental level*. Consider the complexity of language, ideas, drawing and play.

2 Ask what he or she likes doing and discuss this, be it watching or playing sport, talking with friends, playing video games, cooking or whatever. This will help promote engagement and demonstrate that you are a human being!

3 You can enquire about emotional symptoms. It is not unusual for older children and adolescents to be experiencing considerable anxiety or misery without their parents being aware of this. You generally need to ask directly about obsessions and compulsions – children and adolescents are often ashamed to admit to such 'mad' symptoms. Much the same applies to symptoms of post-traumatic stress disorder.

4 Ask about friends, teasing and bullying; the individual's account may differ significantly from the parents' and teachers' accounts.

5 It is often worth asking a general question about undisclosed abuse or traumas. 'Sometimes nasty or frightening things happen to people, and they find it difficult to tell anyone about it. Has anything like that ever happened to you?' Sometimes it is also necessary to ask about abuse more directly.

6 Find out what the child or adolescent makes of his or her biography and current life situation. What account can he or she give of the problems that led to referral? In a first interview you will only be able to explore a few themes, but this will often be useful. It is sometimes helpful to ask for a blow-by-blow description of a typical day, or for a detailed account of the last episode of 'problem behaviour'. 'What happens when you are naughty?', 'How does mummy react when you do that?' It is often revealing to get a child's view of potentially significant life events such as the death of an uncle or grandparent (even if the parents have previously told you that the child was unaffected).

7 The assessment may lead on to direct work, so it is also your first opportunity to engage the child or adolescent. At the very least, the interview should allay any fears that seeing a professional is bound to be unpleasant. Some parents have used referral to the clinic as a threat. As a result, children may fear that they will be told off, taken into care, admitted to the ward, or have painful things done to them. Remember to explain what will happen and allay fears whenever possible.

How to: observe the family as a whole

Are the parents supervising the children and setting limits if necessary? How sensitive and supportive are the parents if their child shows signs of anxiety or distress? How much warmth and criticism do the parents express about this child? (NB: warmth and criticism are independent, not the opposite sides of the same coin.)

Is there overt friction between parents? Do they countermand or back one another up? Who does the talking? Do they notice if they disagree? If so, do they reach a consensus?

How do siblings relate to one another? Do the parents treat the children differently from one another? Are there particular alignments within the family? For example, a mother's child, or a father's child, or father and son 'ganging up against' mother?

What is the relationship between children and parents? Possibilities include exploring from a secure base, interrupting their conversation, ignoring or challenging their requests, and watching them at a distance.

If toys are present in the room, are they used? What can you note about the form of play? Is it imaginative? What developmental level does it suggest? Are there any notable themes in the content of the play (for example, sexualised doll play)? Beware of overhasty interpretation of brief episodes of play.

How to: obtain information from teachers

Behaviour in school is often markedly different from behaviour at home. Although parents can often tell you if teachers have relayed any complaints or concerns about their child, it is best to get the information first hand from the school if at all possible, provided parents are willing to agree to you contacting the school. Having identified someone to contact, you can write and ask for their comments and a copy of a recent school report. It is often helpful for the teacher to complete a brief behavioural screening questionnaire such as the Strengths and Difficulties Questionnaire (www.sdqinfo.org). Since teachers have considerable experience of what to expect of children of any given age, their views are generally accurate. Whereas parents' answers to questionnaires often need to be explored through semi-structured interviewing, it is usually appropriate to take teachers' answers at face value. It is sometimes helpful, though, to get back to the teacher by phone to explore one or two particular issues in greater depth. Though teachers are generally excellent observers, they may miss or misconstrue some symptoms. In a busy classroom, disruptive behaviours are generally a lot more obvious than emotional symptoms. Consequently, teachers may miss anxiety or depression unless these have resulted in a dramatic decrease in the quality or quantity of the child's work. Subdued children may even seem better behaved than before. Thus, in one study, the rate of problems reported by teachers on a standardised questionnaire went down in the aftermath of a disaster.

Recognising the symptoms of ADHD in the classroom can also pose problems when a pupil has learning difficulties or dislikes academic work. Imagine how any child would behave if placed in a class taught in a language they did not understand – they, too, might well appear distracted or wander round the room at any excuse! What you really want to know to make a diagnosis of ADHD is whether the individual is restless and inattentive when engaged in tasks that are within their capabilities and that interest them. Sadly, some children and adolescents are never engaged in any such tasks at school. Finally, as noted earlier, teachers are sometimes unaware of problems in peer relationships because a pupil who seems to be getting on with classmates in class may be isolated or victimised in the playground without teachers necessarily spotting this.

When a pupil is reported to have marked problems in school, it is often very useful to go to the school and observe that individual both in the classroom and playground. Much may be learned, say, from observing a high level of restless, inattentive and impulsive behaviour in the classroom and playground, even though he or she had been fairly well controlled with you and other adults in the clinic; or from discovering that the child is constantly being told off by a highly critical teacher with limited classroom-management skills.

How to: do a physical examination

Systematic observation of a child or adolescent's physical features and skills is an essential part of a complete psychiatric assessment. You are primarily looking for:

1 Evidence of a physical disorder that definitely or probably affects the brain. Recognising that there is a 'hardware fault' is important – characterising the type of disorder is less important, provided the child is referred to an expert. Relevant evidence includes abnormal neurological signs, dysmorphic features, and cutaneous stigmata of a neurocutaneous syndrome.
2 Signs of neglect or abuse. Observing, weighing and measuring the child, and plotting the values on an appropriate growth chart, can provide evidence of injury and growth failure.

Medical trainees should not discard their hard-won medical skills; if the child or adolescent is present at the assessment, you should always set aside some time for observing them with a 'medical hat' on. Even if you never lay hands (or tendon hammer or stethoscope) on them, there is much that you can learn just by looking at their face, hands, gait and play. So, during the time you see them (in the waiting room, in the family interview, or in the individual interview), take some time off from thinking about family relationships or psychiatric symptoms and consciously concentrate on physical features. Are there dysmorphic features? If you do not spot these fairly rapidly, you will be so used to the way they look that you will probably never notice. Do they have a neurological syndrome? Are they peering at things or straining after sounds? Are there any visible bruises, burns, bites or other possible signs of abuse?

Which children and adolescents need neurological examinations?

Ideally you should examine everyone, if only to practise your technique and learn the range of normal variation. If time constraints prevent this, you should at least examine anyone who has one or more of the following features:

1 history of seizures or regression;
2 developmental delay or intellectual disability;
3 abnormal gait;
4 not using both hands well, for example, when playing;
5 dysmorphic features;
6 skin signs of a neurocutaneous disorder;
7 other suspicious features, for example, speech difficulties.

A basic neurological examination

Though some items will be impossible with very young children, aim to include the following in your neurological examination:

1 Measure head circumference and plot it on a chart.
2 Get them to walk, run, hop and walk along a line on the floor as if it was a tightrope.

3 Observe them standing with feet together, arms outstretched, eyes closed.
4 Check eye, face, and tongue movements.
5 Move and shake all four limbs (as part of a game) to assess tone.
6 Test strength: pyramidal weakness is most evident from testing abduction at shoulder, extension at wrist, abduction of fingers, and dorsiflexion of ankle and big toe.
7 Test reflexes.
8 Test coordination: getting them to touch your finger, touch their own nose, touch your finger, and so on; touch their thumb to each finger in turn; tap their finger rapidly, pretend they are playing a piano; put the cap on a pen; or thread a bead.

If you find an abnormality (and asymmetries are often easier to detect than bilateral changes), this probably needs further evaluation by a paediatrician or paediatric neurologist. Similarly, if you suspect visual or hearing problems, it is essential to refer to an appropriate clinic.

Congenital syndromes

There are hundreds of these, only some of which have known chromosomal, genetic or environmental causes. When should you suspect one? The best clues are dysmorphic features, such as unusual-looking facial features or fingers, and extreme values for height, weight and head circumference (below the 3rd or above the 97th centile). Look carefully for unusual features whenever an intellectual disability is present. Three examples are:

1 *Fragile X syndrome*. Probably the most common cause of inherited intellectual disability. Although once said to affect about 1 in 1,000 births, more recent estimates based on DNA analysis suggest that the rate may be closer to 1 in 5,000. It affects both males and females, though the degree of intellectual impairment tends to be greater in males. Physical characteristics are highly variable, but may include a long face, prominent ears, wide jaw, hyper-extensible joints and large testes after puberty. Equally, physical appearance may be normal. Fragile X is associated with gaze avoidance, social anxiety and hyperactivity, but the link with autism remains controversial. It is due to an excess of trinucleotide repeats at a specific site on the long arm of the X chromosome and may be detected by direct DNA analysis.
2 *Fetal alcohol syndrome*. Affects up to 1 in 300 births. May cause up to 10% of mild intellectual disability. Height, weight and head circumference are low from birth onwards. Short palpebral fissures, hypoplastic philtrum. Associated with hyperactivity.
3 *Sotos syndrome* ('Cerebral gigantism'). Sporadic. Excessive height, head circumference and bone age, particularly when young. High forehead with frontal bossing, prominent jaw, widely spaced eyes with a downwards slant. Clumsy. Most have mild or borderline intellectual disability. Associated with hyperactivity and autistic problems.

The neurocutaneous disorders

These disorders involve characteristic combinations of brain and skin abnormalities (reflecting their shared ectodermal origins). Recognising the skin signs allows you to infer a 'hardware' defect. The commonest three neurocutaneous syndromes are:

1 *Tuberous sclerosis* is an autosomal dominant disorder with variable penetrance and expression. It is often a new mutation. Skin lesions include: hypo-pigmented leaf-shaped patches from birth, best seen with UV light (Woods light); the adenoma sebaceum butterfly rash on face, rarely evident before two years, but present in half by five years; a rough irregular 'shagreen' patch over lumbar area; and lumps (periungual fibromata) in and around finger and toe nails. There is a high rate of severe intellectual disability, infantile spasms, and other seizures. Autistic and ADHD features are common in affected individuals, particularly if they have had infantile spasms.
2 *Neurofibromatosis-1* is transmitted as an autosomal dominant with variable expression. Skin lesions include *café au lait* patches that increase in size and number with age (so that by adulthood the presence of over five patches of over 1.5 cm diameter is highly suggestive); axillary freckling; and cutaneous and subcutaneous nodules in the distribution of cutaneous nerves appearing in later childhood. Various neuropsychiatric manifestations are reported but unconfirmed.
3 *Sturge-Weber syndrome* is usually sporadic. There is a port-wine naevus from birth, involving the forehead and variable amounts of the lower face. It is usually unilateral but can be bilateral. The ipsilateral hemisphere is affected, resulting in seizures, hemiplegia, and generalised intellectual disability, plus variable neuropsychiatric features.

Putting it all together: the formulation

Having carried out your full assessment, you are in a position (with advice from other team members as appropriate) to generate a formulation that will crystallise your views on the situation, inform your feedback to the family and referrer, and guide your subsequent management. The elements of a formulation include:

1 *A socio-demographic summary*, for example, Amy is a 7-year-old girl who lives with her mother, stepfather and younger half-brother in a one-bedroom rented flat in Newtown.
2 *The clinical presentation*, for example, John has always been overactive, inattentive and impulsive, and these symptoms have become more apparent and have made more of a difference to his life since starting school.
3 *Diagnosis*. Sometimes this is simple, for example, John meets the full diagnostic criteria for attention-deficit/hyperactivity disorder (ADHD), or for both ADHD and oppositional defiant disorder. On other occasions, matters are more complicated. Perhaps John's symptoms could

be explained by several alternative diagnoses, and you then need to review the evidence for and against each possibility before reaching a conclusion on the likely diagnosis (or diagnoses), or suggesting further assessments or investigations that will clarify the picture. Or perhaps John has elements of several different disorders but does not meet the full criteria for any of them – you may need to recognise that he falls between the cracks of the current diagnostic systems. Or maybe Amy's distress about teasing at school, overcrowding at home and rows between her mother and stepfather warrant recognition and help, but do not warrant a diagnosis.

4 *Causation*, for example, Alan developed obsessive compulsive disorder and tics following a streptococcal infection, probably mediated by an auto-immune response; or Jane's post-traumatic stress disorder followed sexual abuse by a babysitter; or Michael's disruptive behaviour may reflect the combination of constitutional vulnerability linked to his fetal alcohol syndrome, and suboptimal parenting linked to his mother's continuing alcohol problems and depression.

5 *Management plan*, including specific psychological or pharmacological treatments, as well as psycho-educational work with the individual, family and school. The plan should build on the individual's and family's strengths, and boost these still further.

6 *Predicted outcome*, for example, Sarah's specific phobia of dentists is likely to resolve with a brief course of behavioural therapy, and will probably not recur; Roger's conduct disorder is likely to persist, carrying a high long-term price for him and society, unless he receives appropriate intensive treatment such as multi-systemic therapy.

It is not easy to produce a formulation that is accurate, brief and useful – the best way to learn is by practising the skill and getting constructive feedback from more experienced colleagues.

Subject review

Baird G, Gringras P. (2008) Physical examination and medical investigation. *In*: Rutter M *et al.* (eds) *Rutter's Child and Adolescent Psychiatry*, 5th edn. Wiley-Blackwell, Chichester, pp. 317–335.

Le Couteur A, Gardner F. (2008) Use of structured interviews and observational methods in clinical settings. *In*: Rutter M *et al.* (eds) *Rutter's Child and Adolescent Psychiatry*, 5th edn. Wiley-Blackwell, Chichester, pp. 271–288.

Taylor E, Rutter M. (2008) Clinical assessment and diagnostic formulation. *In*: Rutter M *et al.* (eds) *Rutter's Child and Adolescent Psychiatry*, 5th edn. Wiley-Blackwell, Chichester, pp. 42–57.

Further reading

Jones DPH. (2003) *Communicating with Vulnerable Children: A Guide for Practitioners*. Gaskell, London.

CHAPTER 2
Classification

The underlying principles guiding diagnostic groupings

Making it useful

Classification should facilitate communication among clinicians and researchers rather than be a 'train spotting' exercise conducted for its own sake. Classifying a child or adolescent's disorder should be more than a mere 'naming of parts'; it should provide helpful pointers to: aetiology; associated problems (thereby directing further enquiries and investigations); choice of treatment; and prognosis. In general, it is possible to use the same classification for all these purposes. Occasionally, however, it is necessary to use different classifications for different purposes. For example, clinicians will generally want to classify schizophrenia and schizotypal personality disorder separately since they have very different implications for treatment and prognosis. For a genetic researcher, however, it may make more sense to combine the two into a category of 'schizophrenia spectrum disorder'.

How do we decide whether a diagnostic scheme is following nature or imposing arbitrary divisions, whether it is 'carving nature at the joints' or hacking blindly through bones? To start with, a diagnostic category is unlikely to be useful unless individuals with that diagnosis differ significantly from individuals with other diagnoses. These differences must extend well beyond the defining characteristics of the diagnostic group. In the case of conduct disorder, for example, we need to know that individuals with conduct disorder differ on average from individuals with other psychiatric disorders not just in having more conduct problems (which is simply a consequence of the definitions used) but in other respects as well, for example, sex ratio, age of onset, socio-economic status, or association with academic problems. Furthermore, at least some of the validating features that distinguish different diagnoses should be clinically relevant. Thus, if individuals with two diagnoses differ only in sex ratio and socio-economic status, the two diagnoses should be merged rather than kept separate. Demographic variables are certainly worth examining, but some of the

Child and Adolescent Psychiatry, Third Edition. Robert Goodman and Stephen Scott.
© 2012 Robert Goodman and Stephen Scott. Published 2012 by John Wiley & Sons, Ltd.

differences between diagnostic groups should be more immediately relevant to aetiology, associated problems, treatment response, or prognosis.

It is possible to have satisfactory diagnostic categories but an unsatisfactory overall classification. This is true when too many cases fail to meet the criteria for any category, or have to be fitted into 'atypical' or 'miscellaneous' categories. An ideal classification is as valid and as comprehensive as possible, but these two aims sometimes pull in opposite directions.

Phenomenology above all

The classification of psychopathology at all ages has increasingly focused on the presenting features of each disorder rather than on the supposed aetiology or pathogenesis. When disorders are defined in this way, it is possible to study aetiology and pathogenesis with an open mind. Diagnostic categories based on pathogenesis, such as 'minimal brain damage' or 'reactive psychosis', have generally impeded rather than facilitated clinical and research progress. Although most child and adolescent psychiatric disorders are currently defined on the basis of phenomenology alone, a few disorders such as 'reactive attachment disorder' and 'post-traumatic stress disorder' are defined both in terms of phenomenology and the presumed cause.

Dimensions or categories?

Many sorts of psychopathology seem to be extreme values on a continuum that extends into the normal range, with many children and adolescents exhibiting lesser degrees of the same features. Imposing a cut-off between normality and abnormality is sometimes an arbitrary but convenient way of converting a dimension into a category. To take an example from general medicine, blood pressure is continuously distributed, with progressively higher blood pressures leading to progressively higher rates of stroke and heart disease. Keeping blood pressure as a dimension retains more information than imposing a cut-off that fairly arbitrarily divides individuals into those with normal blood pressure and those with 'hypertension' – and yet a simple dichotomy has the potential advantage of feeding directly into a straightforward action plan for busy practitioners: treat those who are hypertensive and leave individuals with normal blood pressure alone. On the other hand, a single dichotomy based on a single cut-off may oversimplify the options. For example, it may be a good idea to titrate the intervention more flexibly, for example, advising simple dietary or lifestyle changes at borderline blood pressures and adding in medication at higher values. Because similar issues apply in mental health, the architects of DSM 5 and ICD 11 are wrestling with how to create hybrid schemes that will retain the simplicity of diagnostic categories alongside the flexibility of dimensional scores.

While dichotomising dimensions is sometimes arbitrary, there are instances where individuals with extreme values are genuinely a case apart. There are three possible indications of discontinuities between normal and extreme values. First, the distribution may be bimodal, for example, with a subsidiary hump in the tail of the main distribution (as for severe intellectual disability). Second, there may be a threshold effect. In the case of behavioural inhibition, for example, marked inhibition as a toddler predicts continuing shyness, whereas moderate inhibition has no such predictive value. Finally, individuals with extreme and less extreme values on some particular scale may differ qualitatively in other important respects. Thus, mild intellectual disability is often associated with social disadvantage and is not commonly associated with neurological abnormalities, whereas severe intellectual disability is less commonly associated with social disadvantage and much more often associated with neurological abnormalities.

Dimensional and categorical classifications of the same phenomenon are sometimes both valuable, but for different purposes. Blood cholesterol provides a convenient example. There is a dose–response relationship between cholesterol level and the risk of ischaemic heart disease, with most of the attributable risk in the population being due to the large number of individuals with 'high normal' values rather than to the small number of individuals with extremely high values. In this respect, high cholesterol is best treated as a dimensional rather than a categorical disorder. At the same time, individuals with extremely high levels of cholesterol are a distinctive category from an aetiological point of view, having a Mendelian rather than a multifactorial-polygenic disorder.

Identifying dimensions and categories

Multivariate statistical techniques now exist to help identify dimensions and categories of disorder. Though complex in detail, the general principles underlying factor analyses and cluster analyses are relatively easy to understand without having to go into the mathematics (see Boxes 2.1

Box 2.1 A do-it-yourself factor analysis

Look at the following list of measures that could be made on a sample of adults. Group these measures in such a way that they correspond to two dimensions:

- Height
- Shoe size
- Size of vocabulary
- Ability to complete puzzles
- Shoulder-to-elbow length
- Skill at mental arithmetic

You will have had no difficulty in grouping height, shoe size and shoulder-to-elbow length as highly correlated measures that tap an underlying dimension that could be labelled 'linear growth'. The remaining three measures are also highly correlated with one another and tap the underlying dimension we normally label 'intelligence'. The two dimensions are almost independent – you do not expect much of a correlation between the two groups of variables, for example, between height and size of vocabulary. Congratulations – you have carried out a factor analysis using your intuitive knowledge of correlated and uncorrelated measures to identify the underlying dimensions.

and 2.2). Factor analyses are used to identify dimensions while cluster analyses identify categories. Whereas factor analyses classify attributes of an individual, cluster analyses classify the individuals themselves.

Box 2.2 A do-it-yourself cluster analysis

Look at the next list of different animals and divide them into groups:

- Tortoise
- Duck-billed platypus
- Cat
- Snail
- Dolphin
- Crocodile
- Mouse
- Giant squid

As you attempted to do so, you will probably have identified some of the key features and limitations of a cluster analysis. First, you may have noticed that how you grouped the animals depended on which features you concentrated on. If you had focused on measures of size and habitat, you might have grouped dolphins, crocodiles and giant squid together as large aquatic animals, and snails and mice together as small terrestrial animals. If, however, you concentrated on morphological and physiological measures, you would have generated a more typically zoological taxonomy, for example, generating a mollusc grouping comprised of snails and giant squid. A second notable feature of cluster analysis is that the method does not tell you how many groups to identify. For instance, you could have gone for a 'two group' solution (for example, mollusc v. vertebrate) or a 'three group' solution (for example, mollusc v. reptile v. mammal). You have to decide for yourself what degree of lumping or splitting is most appropriate (which depends on what use you plan to make of the classification). Finally, the case of the duck-billed platypus, with its mixture of reptilian and mammalian features, is a reminder that some individuals fall midway between neighbouring categories – it is somewhat arbitrary whether they are assigned to one of the neighbouring categories or to a category of their own.

Pervasive or situational?

For hyperactivity problems, and perhaps for other types of problem too, diagnostic schemes increasingly emphasise the distinction between pervasive and situational disorders. Pervasive disorders are evident in a wide variety of everyday settings (for example, at home and at school), whereas situational disorders are only evident in a restricted range of settings (for example, at home but not at school). Pervasiveness suggests that constitutional factors are paramount, while situational specificity suggests that it is more important to establish what is special about that particular environment (or that particular informant).

Unfortunately, the term 'pervasive' is used in two very different ways in classifications of child and adolescent psychiatric disorders. Pervasive hyperactivity or pervasive misery refers to problems that are present in a range of different settings. In the term 'pervasive developmental disorder', however, 'pervasive' refers primarily to the fact that multiple domains of development are affected by autistic spectrum disorders (in contrast to the specific developmental disorders affecting just one domain of development, for example, reading or speech). This is confusing since both sorts of developmental disorder (pervasive and specific) are pervasive in the sense of being present in a range of different settings.

Classifying disordered individuals or disordered families?

Aiming to find a diagnosis for the 'identified patient' might be focusing attention on the wrong organisational level, for example, on one family member rather than on the family system as a whole. Conversely, family therapists might be making the opposite error in their formulations. Multiaxial diagnostic systems potentially provide the best of both worlds since they can record abnormalities at both the individual and the family level. Unfortunately, there is no widely accepted and well-validated system for classifying disordered families.

Diagnostic groupings: current practice

ICD-10 and DSM-IV

There are two main classifications in current use: the International Classification of Diseases (ICD) of the World Health Organization, and the Diagnostic and Statistical Manual (DSM) of the American Psychiatric Association. There used to be many differences between the two schemes but they have converged on very similar classifications (ICD-10 and DSM-IV). It is worth noting that ICD-10 comes as a clinical version that provides clinical descriptions and somewhat impressionistic diagnostic guidelines for each disorder, and as a research version that provides more clearly defined diagnostic criteria, often identical to those used by DSM-IV. This agreement owes at least as much to improved international collaboration as to increased scientific knowledge. Fashion continues to be important in classification and there are likely to be minor and major revisions of the schemes for many years yet. Our current ideas are like early maps of largely unexplored territory – better than nothing, provided you do not take the details too seriously.

Operationalised diagnoses: pluses and minuses

DSM-IV and the research version of ICD-10 both provide operationalised diagnostic criteria for many disorders. For each of these disorders, there are clear criteria that must be fulfilled before the diagnosis can be made. The main advantage of this approach is that different clinicians and researchers are more likely to be referring to similar conditions when they use a particular diagnostic label. There are disadvantages, however. The DSM and ICD criteria can come to seem like Holy Writ, making it easy to forget that the criteria are often built on very shaky foundations. They have become a straitjacket as well as an aid for clinicians and researchers. Furthermore, many children and adolescents who clearly do have psychiatric disorders (since they have symptoms that result in substantial distress, disruption or social impairment) fail to meet the full criteria for an operationalised diagnosis and have to be given one of the 'not otherwise specified' labels. Most of these individuals have *sub-threshold* or *undifferentiated* syndromes. Individuals with sub-threshold syndromes have some of the features of operationalised disorders, but not enough to reach the diagnostic threshold. For example, many children have pronounced autistic features, but fall short of the full criteria for autism. Undifferentiated syndromes involve a mixture of symptoms from different operationalised disorders but do not meet the full criteria for any one of them. For instance, children with a mixture of worries, fears, misery and somatic complaints may clearly have some sort of emotional disorder even though they do not meet all the criteria for generalised anxiety disorder, specific phobia, major depression or any other operationalised diagnosis. Yet other children fall between the cracks of the current schemes, having constellations of problems that have not yet been recognised; the mapping of child and adolescent psychiatric disorders still has a long way to go.

The main diagnostic groupings

Three broad diagnostic groupings are particularly relevant to child and adolescent psychiatrists (see Table 2.1). The *emotional disorders* are also sometimes described as internalising disorders, dating back to the notion that 'stresses' could be turned inwards (internalised), leading to worries, fears, misery, stomach-aches, etc. *Externalising disorders* likewise derive their name from the notion that 'stresses' can alternatively be turned outwards (externalised), resulting in disruptive, defiant, aggressive or antisocial behaviours that impinge on others. The *developmental disorders* are a heterogeneous group characterised by delays or abnormalities in the development of functions that normally unfold in a predictable sequence

Table 2.1 The three main diagnostic groupings

Emotional disorders	Externalising disorders	Developmental disorders
Anxiety disorders	Conduct disorder	Speech/language delay
Phobias	Oppositional-defiant disorder	Reading delay
Depression	Attention-deficit/hyperactivity disorder (ADHD)	Autistic disorders
Obsessive-compulsive disorder		Intellectual disability
Some somatisation		Enuresis and encopresis

as a result of biological maturation. The partition of developmental disorders between different disciplines has largely been determined by history and convenience. Conventionally, some developmental disorders, most notably the autistic disorders, are considered primary psychiatric disorders. Enuresis is sometimes considered a psychiatric problem, though there is little justification for this practice (see Chapter 18). Most developmental disorders are not generally considered psychiatric disorders in themselves, though they are often risk factors for psychiatric disorders (which is why they are covered in this book in Part 3 on risk factors)

The dividing line between the three main groupings is not always clear-cut. ADHD, for example, is usually grouped in the externalising disorders, though it could equally be considered a developmental disorder, particularly affecting the development of attention and activity control. Similarly, depression is grouped with the emotional disorders even though the dominant symptom in children and adolescents is sometimes irritability, which is commonly a symptom of externalising disorders.

Opinions differ on the extent to which it is helpful to subdivide the main groupings. Until about 20 years ago, for example, few clinicians saw much merit in subdividing the emotional disorders into different subgroups, and ICD-9 offered little opportunity to do so. Then the pendulum swung from lumping to splitting, with both ICD-10 and DSM-IV offering a multitude of emotional disorder. The pendulum may swing back again since splitting has probably gone too far, with too many children and adolescents meeting the criteria for multiple closely related disorders.

The swing of the pendulum has also been evident in the extent to which children are regarded as being 'little adults' as far as diagnosis is concerned. There are two polar views of childhood: one view holds that children are radically different from adults, rather like tadpoles and frogs; the other view holds that children and adults are fundamentally similar. As far as psychiatric classification goes, the 'tadpole and frog' view used to dominate, but seems to be waning. For emotional disorders, adult-type diagnoses such as dysthymia or generalised anxiety disorder are used where possible. At the same time, there is an increasing recognition that developmental disorders and disruptive behavioural disorders often persist into adult life. Thus a picture of separate child and adult disorders seems to be in decline. Instead, most disorders are seen as conditions that can occur across the lifespan, with the recognition that the characteristic symptoms may vary at different ages, and so too should the diagnostic criteria. For example, the criteria for ADHD recognise that affected adults experience less fidgeting and rushing around than when they were children, but experience more of an inner sense of restlessness instead. Likewise, modified criteria for post-traumatic stress disorder (PTSD) in very young children recognise that a continuing preoccupation with the trauma may be shown in their pattern of play rather than in what they say.

Finally, it is important to remember that the psychiatric disorders affecting children and adolescents are not limited to the three main groupings. There are inevitably disorders that do not fit into the neat tripartite

Table 2.2 The multi-axial schemes of ICD-10 and DSM-IV

ICD-10 axis	DSM-IV axis	What this axis covers
1	I	Psychiatric disorder, for example, separation anxiety disorder
2	I	Specific delays in development, for example, reading disorder
3	II	Intellectual level, for example, mild intellectual disability
4	III	Medical conditions, for example, epilepsy
5	IV	Psychosocial adversity, for example, institutional upbringing
6	V	Adaptive functioning, for example, serious social disability

classification set out in Table 2.1: early-onset schizophrenia, anorexia nervosa, disinhibited attachment disorder, Tourette syndrome, and many others. In addition, child mental health professionals may spend much of their time on tasks that do not necessarily involve a psychiatric disorder. This is often the case, for example, when assessing dysfunctional families, juvenile offenders, or the victims of abuse.

Multiaxial diagnosis

Diagnostic labels are a useful aid to clinical and research work, allowing similar cases to be grouped together. Sometimes, however, being forced to settle on just one label is too restricting. Should this patient be labelled as having autism or an intellectual disability? Often it will be essential to record both. This idea has been taken further in the multiaxial assessment that is an optional part of DSM-IV, and by the multiaxial version of ICD-10. In these multiaxial schemes, each axis reflects one important aspect of a child or adolescent's presentation (see Table 2.2).

Though many people would regard five or six axes as rather too much of a good thing, the scheme does have advantages. For instance, it is not necessary to decide whether a child has conduct disorder, specific reading disorder or intellectual disability; if the child has all three, each can be coded. Equally, it is not necessary to decide if one or more of these problems is due to the child's epilepsy or institutional upbringing: these are coded whether or not they seem to be causes (thereby capturing data that can eventually be used to explore the association statistically). The final axis provides a means for recording how far psychiatric and developmental problems interfere with the individual's everyday life. The five axes of DSM-IV do the same job as the six axes of ICD-10 because DSM-IV allows multiple diagnoses on its axis I, an axis that encompasses both psychiatric disorders and specific developmental disorders.

Subject review

Taylor E, Rutter M. (2008) Classification. *In*: Rutter M *et al*. (eds) *Rutter's Child and Adolescent Psychiatry*, 5th edn. Wiley-Blackwell, Chichester, pp. 18–31.

Further reading

American Psychiatric Association. (2000) *Diagnostic and Statistical Manual of Mental Disorders*. 4th edn, text revision; DSM-IV-TR. American Psychiatric Association, Washington, DC.

Angold A, Costello EJ. (2009) Nosology and measurement in child and adolescent psychiatry. *Journal of Child Psychology and Psychiatry* **50**, 9–15.

Coghill D, Sonuga-Barke EJS. (2012) Categories versus dimensions in the classification and conceptualisation of child and adolescent mental disorders – implications of recent empirical studies. *Journal of Child Psychology and Psychiatry* **53**, 469–489.

Taylor E *et al.* (1986) Conduct disorder and hyperactivity: I and II. *British Journal of Psychiatry* **149**, 760–777. (This elegant study used factor and cluster analyses to identify dimensions and categories respectively, and then validated the findings by examining associated features, developmental history and treatment response.)

World Health Organization. (1993) *The ICD-10 Classification of Mental and Behavioural Disorders: Diagnostic Criteria for Research*. World Health Organization, Geneva.

CHAPTER 3
Epidemiology

Epidemiology can be defined as the study of the distribution of disorders and associated factors in defined populations. The defined population may be a representative community sample, but it might also be a high-risk or particularly informative sample, for example, all children with hemiplegic cerebral palsy in London, or all children living in an area with high lead pollution.

Advantages of an epidemiological approach

1 Essential to estimate incidence and prevalence – relevant for planning service provision for the whole population.
2 Being free (or freer) of referral bias, epidemiological studies are better than clinic-based studies as sources of accurate information about demographic characteristics, associated problems, and natural history. All these benefits are important for studies aiming to improve classification. They are also relevant to aetiology, with causal relationships being suggested, but not proven, by epidemiological associations that are strong, dose-related, and persistent despite controlling for 'confounders' such as socio-economic status. The power of epidemiological studies to distinguish between causal and non-causal associations is increased when the study is longitudinal or capitalises on a 'natural experiment' such as adoption, twin birth or migration.
3 Useful for examining protective factors. For example, why do some children remain well adjusted despite exposure to acrimonious marital conflict? Clinic-based studies are almost bound to miss the children who have benefited most from exposure to protective factors.

Epidemiological studies are not always the best approach

1 A detailed study of a few (unrepresentative) cases may be more instructive than a superficial study of a large and representative population. Understanding phenylketonuria or general paresis of the insane did not require an epidemiological approach.

Child and Adolescent Psychiatry, Third Edition. Robert Goodman and Stephen Scott.
© 2012 Robert Goodman and Stephen Scott. Published 2012 by John Wiley & Sons, Ltd.

2 Epidemiological studies rarely address pathogenesis – different approaches are needed to clarify the processes involved.
3 Sometimes an epidemiological approach gets it wrong. For example, a number of observational surveys showed that women taking Hormone Replacement Therapy (HRT) subsequently had fewer cancers, However, Randomised Controlled Trials then showed that HRT led to *more* cancers – it seems likely that the observational studies underestimated (and therefore made insufficient allowance for) the extent to which the women who chose to take HRT also tended to make healthier lifestyle choices that reduced their chance of developing cancer. If so, this was an example of observational results being misleading because of inadequate adjustment for confounders.
4 In practice, epidemiological studies rarely include the evaluation of an intervention.

Stages in an epidemiological study

1 *Define* the population to be studied: catchment area; inclusion criteria; everyone v. random sample v. stratified random sample. Examples include a random 25% sample of 3-year-olds living in a London borough, and all 5–14-year-olds with new-onset severe head injuries in southeast England.
2 *Identify* individuals who meet the criteria. For community samples, identification is often via some sort of population register (for example, for schools or immunisations). For rare disorders or risks, identification is often via agencies that are particularly likely to be in contact with relevant individuals, for example, doctors, special schools, voluntary organisations. Use of multiple sources (known as 'multiple ascertainment') is likely to identify more relevant individuals than use of any one source. Even with multiple ascertainment, there is still the risk of missing some affected individuals who have never been diagnosed or sent to a special school. There is no straightforward way of estimating the size of this problem.
3 *Recruit* identified individuals. It is far easier to spot problems with recruitment than problems with identification – problems with recruitment show up as low participation rates. Ideally, all studies should compare participants and non-participants on any available information.
4 *Assess* subjects. There are two main possibilities: full assessment of all subjects (known as a 'one-phase' procedure), or use of a two-phase procedure:
   Phase 1: use one or more screening tests (for example, parent, teacher, or self-report questionnaires) to divide the sample up into 'screen positive' and 'screen negative' subjects.
   Phase 2: fully assess a mixture of 'screen positive' and 'screen negative' subjects, sampling disproportionately more of the former (for example, 100% of 'screen positive' and a randomly chosen 20% of 'screen negative' subjects). Inclusion of a random sample of 'screen

negative' subjects makes it possible to determine how often the screening procedure generates false negatives.

Epidemiological findings in child and adolescent psychiatry

The first major epidemiological study of psychiatric disorders in childhood was carried out by Michael Rutter and his colleagues on the Isle of Wight in the late 1960s. It is hardly an exaggeration to say that this study was the beginning of scientific child and adolescent psychiatry; its findings have withstood the test of time remarkably well, with subsequent epidemiological studies from many countries confirming the main findings and extending them in various directions. Box 3.1 illustrates the sorts of findings to have emerged from epidemiological surveys over the past 50 years, drawing on some recent British nationwide surveys.

Box 3.1 British nationwide surveys of child and adolescent mental health

Since 1999, the British Office for National Statistics has been carrying out an extensive ongoing programme of cross-sectional and longitudinal studies of child and adolescent mental health. This box summarises some key aspects of the methods and findings.

Design

The main measures of psychopathology were the Strengths and Difficulties Questionnaire (www.sdqinfo.org) generating scores, and the Development and Well-Being Assessment (www.dawba.info) generating diagnoses. There were additional measures of individual risk factors, family adversities, school factors, and neighbourhood disadvantage. Measures were obtained from multiple informants (parent, teacher and self-report) in a one-phase design, that is, applying all relevant measures on all participants.

Survey of 5–16-year-olds

The sampling frame was a government register of children and adolescents living in private households. Information was collected on around 10,000 5–15-year-olds in 1999 and a separate sample of around 8,000 5–16-year-olds in 2004 (representing a 69% participation rate).

Prevalence of disorders

Disorder (DSM-IV or ICD-10)	(%)
Behavioural disorders (DSM-IV or ICD-10)	5.3
Anxiety disorders (DSM-IV or ICD-10)	3.8
Hyperkinesis (ICD-10)	1.4
ADHD (DSM-IV)	2.2
Depression (DSM-IV or ICD-10)	0.9
Autistic spectrum disorder (DSM-IV or ICD-10)	0.9
*Any DSM-IV disorder**	9.8
*Any ICD-10 disorder**	9.5

Note: *Less than the sum of the individual diagnoses because of comorbidity.

Comorbidity

Many individuals have multiple diagnoses. These are the common overlaps:

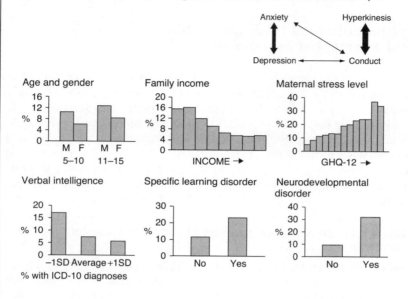

Three-year follow-up

Over 2,500 individuals from the 1999 survey were reassessed three years on – stratified sampling ensured that this follow-up sample included two-thirds of the individuals who had a disorder in 1999, and a fifth of those without.

Persistence

- A quarter of those with emotional disorders initially still had an emotional disorder at follow-up with high persistence associated with high parental stress levels.
- Almost half of those with conduct disorders initially still had a conduct disorder at follow-up. Greater persistence was associated with special educational needs and high parental stress levels.

New onset of disorders

- Onset of new emotional disorders was commoner in adolescents, and was linked to physical illness and stressful life events.
- Onset of new conduct disorders was commoner in boys, and was linked to special educational needs, living with a step-parent and high parental stress levels.

Use of services

Among the children and adolescents who had a disorder in 1999, just under half were seen by specialist services for mental health problems over the next three years, with some using multiple services; 25% had been seen by mental health services, 25% by special educational services, 14% by social services, and 14% by paediatrics.

Looked-after children and adolescents
Roughly 0.5% of British children and adolescents are looked after by local authorities, either living with foster parents or in special institutions. In 2002–3, a national sample of over a thousand looked-after children and adolescents in Britain were assessed using the same measures employed in the previous surveys of children and adolescents living in private households.

Prevalence of disorder

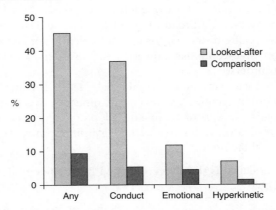

Overall, rates of psychiatric disorder were five times higher than in population controls. Rates were particularly high when children and adolescents were living in institutions rather than with foster families, and when they had experienced repeated changes in placement. It is not clear what is cause and what is effect.

Box 3.2 compares rates of disorders in several countries, all based on surveys using the same measures of psychopathology employed in the British surveys. Such comparisons of findings across countries that differ in language, culture and economic development are obviously are not straightforward to interpret, but using equivalent measures in each country does at least reduce one source of confusion. The findings suggest that there are clinically significant differences in prevalence between countries, but that these differences are moderate rather than large in magnitude.

Box 3.2 Prevalence of psychiatric disorders in five contrasting countries

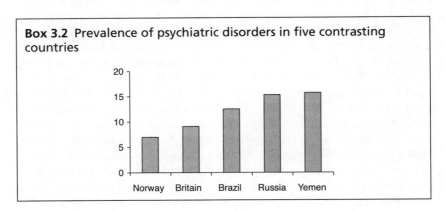

Epidemiological surveys vary not just by geographical location but also by focus:

- A survey may cover a wide age range (for example, the British studies included in Box 3.1) or be focused on a narrower age band, for example 10 and 11-year-olds in the first Isle of Wight survey; very young children in the Preschool to School Study (see Box 22.1); and 14 and 15-year-olds in the Isle of Wight study of adolescence (see Box 23.1).
- The focus may be on a broad range of psychiatric disorders or on just one or two specific disorders, for example, depression, anxiety, hyperactivity, obsessive-compulsive disorder, tic disorders, autistic disorders, or eating disorders.
- The primary focus may be on specific risk factors such as head injury, marital discord or divorce, low-level lead, disasters, or school influences.
- Epidemiological studies of twins and adoptees have increasingly been used to investigate the relative aetiological importance of genetic and environmental factors.

The main conclusions that have emerged from epidemiological studies are discussed below.

Overall prevalence

Recent surveys have generally reported that psychiatric disorders are present in roughly 10–25% of children and adolescents, though some older surveys estimated that up to 50% of children were affected, probably reflecting the inadequacy of DSM-III and DSM-III-R diagnostic criteria. Until DSM-IV, the criteria for a disorder were met when individuals had a particular set of symptoms even if those symptoms had no significant impact on the child's life (in terms of distress or social impairment). As a result, many of the individuals who met DSM-III and DSM-III-R symptom checklists were not in need of treatment and did not correspond to what clinicians recognised as 'cases'. Thus, many of the individuals identified as psychiatrically disordered in epidemiological studies using unmodified DSM-III or DSM-III-R criteria were probably not 'real' cases in any meaningful sense. With DSM-IV and ICD-10 now using impact as well as symptom criteria, prevalence estimates are more conservative (see Box 3.1). At the same time, there is increasing recognition that some children and adolescents have serious mental health problems that warrant treatment but that do not fit neatly into the current diagnostic systems. These are typically individuals who do not have the right number or pattern of psychiatric symptoms to meet operationalised diagnostic criteria, but whose symptoms nevertheless cause substantial distress or social impairment. For every three individuals in an epidemiological survey who meet operationalised diagnostic criteria, there is roughly one other individual whose problems are equally relevant to mental health services, but who does not meet current operationalised criteria. Epidemiological surveys need an element of clinical judgement to detect those individuals who would otherwise slip through the cracks between operationalised diagnoses.

What is common?

Most epidemiological studies show that disruptive behavioural disorders (oppositional-defiant disorder and conduct disorder) are the commonest group of disorders, affecting roughly 5–10% of the population, closely followed by anxiety disorders, affecting roughly 4–6% of the population. Depression is also common in adolescence, when it affects about 2% of the population. The ICD-10 criteria for hyperkinesis are stricter than the DSM-IV criteria for ADHD, and typical prevalence estimates are in the region of 1–2% for the former and 3–6% for the latter.

Comorbidity

Many children and adolescents with psychiatric disorders meet the criteria for more than one psychiatric diagnosis. For example, a child who meets the criteria for generalised anxiety disorder commonly also meets the criteria for other anxiety disorders too, including specific phobias, social phobia and separation anxiety disorder. Similarly, a child who meets the criteria for ADHD commonly also meets the criteria for oppositional-defiant or conduct disorder. For some disorders, comorbidity is the rule rather than the exception. Depression, for instance, is usually accompanied by an anxiety or behavioural disorder. There are several possible explanations for comorbidity. First, the current psychiatric classification may have erred too far in the direction of splitting rather than lumping. If we labelled 'sore throat' and 'runny nose' as separate disorders, many individuals would be comorbid for the two. Second, one disorder may be a risk factor for another. Consider the association of depression and behavioural problems. Perhaps the severe irritability that sometimes accompanies depression leads to aggressive outbursts. Or maybe conduct disorder leads to isolation and criticism, and this, in turn, results in depression. Another possibility is that the same risk factor might simultaneously predispose an individual to several disorders. For instance, a genetic problem with mood regulation could manifest both as behavioural and affective disorders (via irritability and depression respectively).

Most disorders go untreated

Even when children and adolescents do have psychiatric symptoms that result in significant social impairment or distress, only a minority of them are in contact with specialist mental health services. Referral for specialist help is most likely when the problems are a substantial burden to their parents. Conversely, if parents do not feel burdened, their children are unlikely to receive specialist mental health care for their disorders. Some of the children and adolescents with psychiatric problems who are not being seen by specialist mental health services do get help from elsewhere in the health sector, or from education or social services. However, around half of affected individuals get no professional help at all in high-income countries – with even lower rates of getting appropriate help in low- and middle-income countries.

Persistence

When an individual has a disorder at two different ages, the continuity is said to be *homotypic* if the disorders are similar at both ages, and *heterotypic* when the type of disorder has changed with age. For example, when children with conduct disorders are followed up into adult life, some continue to have disruptive and antisocial problems (homotypic continuity) while others become depressed as adults (heterotypic continuity). In this instance, homotypic continuity is more likely in males, and heterotypic continuity in females.

Many studies have shown that conduct problems are somewhat more persistent than emotional problems (see Box 3.1). The continuity from childhood and adolescence into adulthood can be substantial. In the Dunedin longitudinal study, for example, three-quarters of all 21-year-olds with psychiatric diagnoses had previously had a mental disorder when studied between the ages of 11 and 18.

Sex ratio and age of onset

While child and adolescent mental health services tend to see more boys than girls, epidemiological studies do not show marked gender differences in the overall rate of psychiatric disorder: males are more likely than females to have a disorder before puberty, but the reverse is true after puberty. The sex ratio varies markedly with the type of problem (see Table 3.1). The usual age of onset also varies markedly from problem to problem. Some problems characteristically beginning early in childhood, while other adult-type problems are much commoner in adolescence than in earlier childhood (see Table 3.2). It is tempting to suppose that these striking differences in sex ratio and age of onset are important clues to the underlying aetiology or pathogenesis, but sadly the clues remain largely undeciphered.

Table 3.1 Sex ratio of disorders

Marked male excess	Male = female	Marked female excess
Autistic spectrum disorder	Depression (pre-pubertal)	Specific phobias, for example, insects
ADHD	Selective mutism	Diurnal enuresis
Disruptive behavioural disorders	School refusal	Deliberate self harm (post-pubertal)
Juvenile delinquency		Depression (post-pubertal)
Completed suicide		Anorexia nervosa
Tic disorders, for example, Tourette		Bulimia nervosa
Nocturnal enuresis in older children and adolescents		
Specific developmental disorders, for example, language and reading disorders		

Table 3.2 Age at onset of disorders

Characteristic early onset	Mostly teenage onset
Autistic disorders	Depression
Hyperactivity disorders	Mania
Attachment disorders	Generalised anxiety
Selective mutism	Psychosis
Oppositional-defiant disorder	Suicide and deliberate self-harm
Separation anxiety	Anorexia and bulimia nervosa
Specific phobias, for example, insects	Panic attacks and agoraphobia
Enuresis	Substance abuse
Intellectual disability	Juvenile delinquency
Specific developmental disorders, for example, language and reading disorders	

Aetiology

Epidemiological studies have provided evidence for the aetiological importance of psychosocial, genetic and neurological factors. A particularly influential study of psychosocial factors involved a direct comparison of children from a run-down area of inner London with children from the small towns and countryside of the Isle of Wight. The same two-phase measures of psychopathology were applied to representative samples of 10-year-olds from both areas. By comparison with the Isle of Wight children, the inner city children had roughly double the rate of conduct, emotional and reading disorders. These differences seemed to be attributable primarily to higher rates of the following psychosocial problems in the inner city: marital breakdown, parental illness and criminality, social disadvantage, and schools with high turnovers of pupils and teachers.

Epidemiological twin and adoption studies have pointed to substantial genetic contributions to many psychiatric disorders in childhood and adolescence. In the case of autism, for example, epidemiological twin studies have demonstrated a very high heritability for a 'broad phenotype' that includes autism and lesser variants. Genetic factors also seem to play a prominent role in bipolar affective disorders, schizophrenia, tic disorders, and pervasive hyperactivity, and somewhat lesser roles in the common behavioural and emotional disorders.

Child and adolescent psychiatric disorders are often associated with intellectual disability or specific learning disorders. Though these links are well established, the underlying causal mechanisms are still in doubt. In some instances, psychiatric problems such as ADHD may interfere with learning. In other instances, the frustration and stress caused by learning difficulties may lead to psychiatric problems. In yet other instances, both learning and behavioural problems may reflect the operation of some 'third factor', whether psychosocial, genetic or neurological.

Epidemiological studies of children and adolescents with congenital and acquired brain disorders have found particularly high rates of associated psychiatric disorders – much higher rates than those found among children and adolescents with chronic non-cerebral disorders that result in comparable disability and stigmatisation. This persuasive evidence for direct brain–behaviour links is perhaps not surprising given the key role of the brain as the seat of the mind.

Cross-cultural differences

In a multicultural society there is obvious interest and importance in epidemiological studies examining whether children and adolescents from different communities have different psychiatric profiles. How else could one determine whether minority groups were being appropriately served? In addition, our current knowledge of child and adolescent psychiatry is largely based on studies of white samples, so cross-cultural studies are needed to show whether our current ideas on classification, aetiology, prognosis, treatment and prevention apply equally to children and adolescents from all backgrounds. It is important to remember that cross-cultural differences in mental health could arise from many factors, including cultural differences in child-rearing practices; physical and social consequences of migration; different experiences of racism or poverty; or biological differences. Here are a few interesting findings from epidemiological studies in this field:

1 In Britain, a comparison of 5–16-year-olds with 'British Indian' and 'White' ethnicities showed that the British Indians had less than half the rate of psychiatric disorders of British Whites. This British Indian advantage was primarily for behavioural and hyperactivity disorders; was as evident from teacher and clinician ratings as from parent or self-ratings; and was not removed by adjusting for likely confounders such as family composition or functioning. Among the British White sample, there was a strong socio-economic gradient, with middle-class children and adolescents having fewer problems. Among the British Indian sample, there was no such gradient. In effect, the British Indians from all socio-economic groups did as well as the middle-class British Whites – and much the same has been shown for reading ability. Why? This is not yet known, though it is tempting to suppose that a strong cultural commitment to education could be relevant.

2 A London study showed that by comparison with British White children, British African-Caribbean children were more likely to have conduct disorders at school, but were no more likely to have conduct disorders at home. One possible explanation is that the disruptive behaviour of the African-Caribbean children at school was commonly a response to their experience of racism in the school environment. However, the fact that African-Caribbean adolescents self-report more delinquent acts outside the home or school suggests the causes are complex.

3 Several studies from different countries have reported higher rates of autism in the children of immigrants. One possible but unproven

explanation is that this excess of autism is due to prenatal infections with viruses that immigrant mothers had not previously been exposed to in their countries of origin.

Even from these few examples, it is evident that many possible explanations need to be considered when cross-cultural differences are found.

Time trends

A growing body of empirical evidence supports the pessimists' view that things are getting worse as the years go by. Since diagnostic criteria and research tools have changed over time, it is obviously hard to establish whether some particular problem has really become more common, or whether clinicians are setting their threshold lower nowadays, or getting better at recognising particular types of problem. Taking account of these methodological issues, it still seems likely that young people over the past 50 years have become increasingly prone to behavioural problems, crime, substance abuse, depression and suicide – problems which are known to be sensitive to psychosocial circumstances. For eating disorders, the evidence for a real rise in prevalence is suggestive but not conclusive. For autism, it is more likely but not proven that the substantial increase in accepted prevalence in the past 30 years (from less than 1 in 1,000 to around 1%) is due to better recognition and ascertainment rather than a large rise in the number of individuals with the disorder.

Subject review

Costello EJ *et al.* (2005) 10-Year Research Update Review: The Epidemiology of Child and Adolescent Psychiatric Disorders: I. Methods and Public Health Burden. *Journal of the American Academy of Child and Adolescent Psychiatry* **44**, 972–986.

Costello EJ *et al.* (2006) 10-Year Research Update Review: The Epidemiology of Child and Adolescent Psychiatric Disorders: II. Developmental Epidemiology. *Journal of the American Academy of Child and Adolescent Psychiatry* **45**, 8–25.

Further reading

Collishaw S *et al.* (2004) Time trends in adolescent mental health. *Journal of Child Psychology and Psychiatry* **45**, 1350–1362. (Evidence that mental health has worsened over the last quarter of the twentieth century, and that this was not simply a methodological artefact.)

Fleitlich-Bilyk B, Goodman R. (2004) The prevalence of child psychiatric disorders in south east Brazil. *Journal of the American Academy of Child and Adolescent Psychiatry* **43**, 727–734.

Goodman A *et al.* (2010) Why do British Indian children have an apparent mental health advantage? *Journal of Child Psychology and Psychiatry* **51**, 1171–1183.

Green H *et al.* (2005) *Mental Health of Children and Young People in Great Britain, 2004*. Basingstoke: Palgrave Macmillan.

Kieling C *et al.* (2011) Child and adolescent mental health worldwide: evidence for action. *Lancet* **378**, 1515–1525. (A review focused on what is known and what needs to be done in low- and middle-income countries.)

Prince M *et al.* (2003) *Practical Psychiatric Epidemiology*. Oxford University Press, Oxford.

Rutter M. (1976) Isle of Wight studies, 1964–1974. *Psychological Medicine* **6**, 313–332.

PART 2

Specific Disorders and Presentations

CHAPTER 4

Autistic Spectrum Disorders

Childhood autism, also known as 'infantile autism' or simply 'autism' is the best known and best researched of a group of disorders that are variously referred to as *autistic spectrum disorders (ASDs)* or *pervasive developmental disorders (PDDs)*. The other disorders in the group can be thought of as milder variations on the same theme – meeting some but not all of the diagnostic criteria for childhood autism. When people talk of an autistic spectrum, they can mean a variety of things. In a narrow sense, they can be referring simply to autism and related disorders, that is, a set of conditions, all of which are significantly distressing or disabling for the affected individual. In a broader sense, however, the spectrum can refer to a dimension ranging from 'classical' autism at one extreme to 'typically developing children' at the other end – or perhaps extending in the opposite direction to a group of children who have unusually well-developed empathy, mind-reading skills and flexibility. In this broad sense, everyone is somewhere on the autistic spectrum, just as everyone is somewhere on the height spectrum. Having some of the features of autism is not necessarily a disadvantage (unless society makes it so) and may have advantages.

Epidemiology

As the recognition of ASDs has improved, the reported prevalence has increased, with several recent good quality studies suggesting a rate of around 1%. 'Classical' autism accounts for between 25% and 60% of all ASDs. The male:female ratio is approximately 4:1. There is no clear relation to socio-economic status; the links with high socio-economic status reported by early studies were probably due to ascertainment bias. Whereas autism was formerly viewed as an extremely rare condition with a unique combination of the three characteristic features described below, it is increasingly being realised that each of these features is itself a spectrum, present to a greater or lesser extent. Some individuals have just one or two of these features to a marked degree. Studies are underway to

Child and Adolescent Psychiatry, Third Edition. Robert Goodman and Stephen Scott.
© 2012 Robert Goodman and Stephen Scott. Published 2012 by John Wiley & Sons, Ltd.

determine whether autism reflects the co-occurrence of the three features by chance, or whether the combination is more common than would occur by coincidence.

Characteristic features

Childhood autism is defined by the *early onset* of symptoms in three domains:

1 Social impairment
2 Communication impairment
3 Restricted and repetitive activities and interests.

Social impairment

These concern the quality of reciprocal interactions with others. The archetypal young child with autism is aloof, with poor eye contact, shows a lack of interest in people as people (though they may be interested in people as tickling machines, biscuit dispensers, etc.), and fails to seek comfort when hurt. If social interest subsequently develops, as it does in the majority of children with autism, problems persist in social responsiveness, reciprocity and the capacity for empathy. There are difficulties adjusting behaviour according to the social context, and problems recognising other people's emotions and responding appropriately. Attachment to parents is not unusual, and the child may be affectionate (or even over-affectionate), although he or she is more likely to initiate cuddles than to accept cuddles initiated by his or her parents. Nonetheless, a substantial proportion of individuals with autism make secure attachments to their parents. Social interactions are on the child's terms – adults and much younger children typically adjust better to this than children of the same age. Interactions with peers are generally very restricted. Even among older high-functioning individuals with autism, a limited ability to form close friendships (involving mutual sharing of interests, activities, and emotions) is probably the most sensitive index of residual social impairments.

Communication impairment

This affects comprehension as well as expression, and gesture as well as spoken language. Babble may be reduced. Good studies carried out at a time when autism was less commonly recognised suggested that roughly 30% of individuals with classical autism never acquired useful speech. The proportion may be lower nowadays since the concept of autism has broadened and milder cases are now more widely recognised, thereby diluting individuals with a poor prognosis in a much larger pool of individuals with a better prognosis. Among those who do acquire speech, the milestones are typically markedly delayed. A minority of individuals with autism acquire single words and even phrases at the normal time but then lose these skills again. Speech, if it emerges, is typically deviant as well as delayed. Possible abnormalities include: immediate or delayed parroting of words or phrases (echolalia); pronominal reversal (for example, 'you' for 'I'); idiosyncratic use of words or phrases; invented words (neologisms); and reliance on stock phrases or repetitive questioning. Instead of chatting in a to-and-fro way *with* other people, the individual with autism primarily talks *at* other people. For example, some individuals with autism use speech mainly for demanding things. Others talk at length about one of their current pre-occupations, oblivious of the social cues indicating that their listener has long since lost interest in the topic. Speech is often abnormal in intonation or pitch, for example, sing-song or a monotonous drone. Gestures are similarly reduced and poorly integrated (for example, abnormal pointing).

Restricted and repetitive activities and interests

These include: resistance to change so that, for example, a small rearrange-ment of furniture provokes major tantrums; insistence on routines and rituals; hand-flapping, twirling, or other stereotypies; ordering play (for example, lining things up); attachment to unusual objects (for example, a dustbin); fascination with unusual aspects of the world (for example, the feel of zips or people's hair); and intense preoccupations with restricted subjects (for example, train timetables, car prices). Pretend play is typically lacking, except in older higher-functioning individuals; when present, pretend play is often limited to simple repetitive enactments, for example, of just one or two incidents from a favourite story or TV programme.

Early onset

Though the disorder is rarely recognised in the first year of life, it is clear retrospectively in around 70% of cases that development was never entirely normal. For example, the child may never have liked being cud-dled, even as a baby; or speech development may have been significantly delayed. In around 30% of cases, however, there was a clear 'setback': after a period of normal or near normal development, these children went through a phase of regression (most often between 18 and 24 months) when they lost previously acquired skills in social interaction, communication and play. Both ICD-10 and DSM-IV stipulate that at least some symptoms must have been present by 36 months, but this is an arbitrary cut-off and it is sometimes hard to date the onset precisely from retrospective accounts, particularly when the disorder is relatively mild.

While some children meet all four of these criteria and warrant a diagnosis of childhood autism, others meet only some of the criteria and so may warrant a diagnosis of atypical autism (ICD-10) or pervasive developmental disorder, not otherwise specified (DSM-IV).

Asperger syndrome

This differs from classical autism in several respects:

- There is little or no delay in the development of vocabulary and gram-mar, though other aspects of language are abnormal, as in autism. Thus, speech is often stilted and pedantic, with abnormal intonation; gesturing may be restricted or exaggerated; and monologues on favourite topics are easily triggered and hard to stop.

- Early aloofness is less likely than in autism. The child with Asperger syndrome is often interested in other people, although his or her social interactions are gauche, reflecting impaired empathy and social responsiveness. In these respects, the individual with Asperger syndrome resembles higher-functioning individuals with autism who have grown out of their aloofness.
- Restricted and repetitive behaviours are mostly evident in preoccupations or circumscribed interests (such as plane spotting or bar codes) rather than in motor stereotypies such as flapping.
- Marked clumsiness may be commoner in Asperger syndrome than in autism.

While Asperger syndrome is currently distinguished from autism and 'other' ASDs, it is unclear whether this distinction really is useful and whether it should be retained in future.

Associated features of ASDs

Intellectual disability

Many children and adolescents with ASDs also have an intellectual disability: in about 40% this is severe (IQ under 50), and in a further 30% this is mild (IQ 50–69); the remaining 30% have an IQ in the normal range. In autism, the IQ is generally best measured by non-verbal tests. In severe autism, verbal IQ is almost always lower than non-verbal IQ because of the associated language problems. The reverse pattern, with lower non-verbal than verbal IQ, is common in Asperger syndrome and high-functioning autism.

Seizures

These affect about a quarter of individuals with autism and intellectual disability, and about 5% of individuals with autism and normal IQ. Seizures often begin in adolescence. By contrast, when individuals with intellectual disability but without autism develop seizures, the onset is usually in early childhood rather than adolescence.

Other psychiatric problems

In addition to the characteristic features already described, many children with autism have additional problems with ADHD, behaviour and emotions. Parents and teachers commonly complain of over-activity and poor concentration. A careful history often shows that the ADHD-like symptoms are evident for tasks such as schoolwork that are imposed by adults, but not for self-chosen tasks such as lining up toy cars or watching the same video sequence over and over again. In other instances, however, concentration is poor for all activities. Perhaps surprisingly, since individuals with autism can appear indifferent to people, a quarter or more suffer from social anxiety disorder – they get very fearful and avoidant of contact with other people, which is not the same as indifference. Severe and frequent temper tantrums are common and may be triggered by their inability to communicate needs, or by someone interfering with their rituals and routines. Interference by others may also unleash aggressive outbursts. Children and adolescents with autism and intellectual disability are particularly prone to self-injurious behaviours, such as head banging, eye poking or hand biting. Extreme food fads represent one particular form of ritualistic behaviour. Intense fears may lead to phobic avoidance. Some of these phobias are exaggerations of common childhood fears (for example, of large dogs) while others are idiosyncratic (for example, fear of petrol pumps). Hallucinations and delusions are not generally associated with autism. Sleep difficulties are very common and may exacerbate psychiatric problems.

Assessment

A thorough history and examination should be carried out looking for the core features and associated conditions as described above. There are standardised interviews such as the Autism Diagnostic Interview (ADI) that help clarify the diagnosis through algorithms that take into account severity on each of the three featured dimensions. However, a history is not enough and more subtle abnormalities of social interaction and communication may be helpfully assessed using standardised observational tests, such as the Autism Diagnostic Observation Schedule (ADOS). Because such assessments are time-consuming, it can help to use one of a number of screening questionnaires (for example, the Social Communication Questionnaire, SCQ) that have reasonable psychometric properties.

Differential diagnosis

Developmental or acquired language disorders

Unlike individuals with autism, children and adolescents with 'pure' phonological-syntactic language disorders (see Chapter 30) can communicate successfully by gesture and have a good capacity for social interaction. However, there are 'overlap' cases involving a severe phonological-syntactic language problems with a lesser degree of *pragmatic language impairment*, resulting in language difficulties that do affect social interaction, sometimes combined with other mild or patchy features of autism that are too mild to warrant the diagnosis of an ASD (see Chapter 30). In future classifications, such children and adolescents may be classified as having a *Social Communication Disorder*. Acquired aphasia with epilepsy (Landau-Kleffner syndrome, see Chapter 30) may also involve social withdrawal and behavioural disturbance, but is not usually hard to distinguish from an ASD.

Intellectual disability without features of autism

Language and pretend play will be absent if mental age is under 12 months. Simple stereotypies are common. These children are socially responsive in line with their mental age.

Intellectual disability with some features of autism

Many children with intellectual disability have a 'triad' of impairments affecting (1) social interaction; (2) communication; and (3) play, as well as varying degrees of repetitive and restricted behaviours. Only some of these children meet the full diagnostic criteria for autism, but many more can be diagnosed as having atypical autism (though not all clinicians think this is a useful thing to do).

Rett syndrome

This syndrome is usually due to a mutation in the MECP2 gene on the X chromosome, but occasionally results from a mutation in other genes. The mutation is typically new (that is, not present in either parent), but may be inherited from a phenotypically normal mother who has a germline mutation. Male fetuses with the mutation usually die before birth since, unlike females, they lack a second normal X chromosome. As a result, recognised cases of Rett syndrome occur almost exclusively in girls (affecting about one in 10,000 live-born females). The features of the syndrome may be confused with autism. There is global developmental regression with loss of acquired abilities at about 12 months of age, accompanied by: deceleration of head growth; characteristic 'hand washing' stereotypies and restricted hand use; episodic over-breathing and unprovoked laughter; and progressively impaired mobility. Most children with Rett syndrome are appropriately socially responsive once allowance is made for their low mental age and physical disabilities. The disease is progressive and affected individuals are usually in wheelchairs by their late teens and die before 30.

Neurodegenerative disorders with progressive dementia

These need to be considered when a period of normal (or nearly normal) development is followed by the loss of skills and the emergence of features of autism. With time, frank neurological impairments emerge and the affected individual eventually dies. There are many such genetic disorders, all of which are fortunately rare. Examples include adrenoleucodystropy, juvenile Huntington disease and Batten disease. HIV encephalopathy is probably the commonest cause of childhood dementia worldwide.

Disintegrative disorder

Also known as disintegrative psychosis or Heller syndrome, this very rare condition (with a prevalence of roughly 1 in 50,000) involves entirely normal development for two to six years, followed first by a phase of regression (often accompanied by marked anxiety and loss of bladder and bowel control), leading to lifelong severe intellectual disability with pronounced features of autism.

Intense early deprivation

Severe psychosocial deprivation is sometimes followed by persistent features of autism. This has been evident from studies of trans-nationally adopted children who have been deprived in their first year or two of life of adequate nutrition, physical care, cognitive and linguistic stimulation, and ordinary social interaction. Though most such children do remarkably well within a few years of being adopted, a small minority continue to have social and communicative impairments associated with intense circumscribed interests, and preoccupations with specific sensations. In early childhood, the distinction from autism can be difficult. As the children mature, the clinical picture evolves, with loss of autistic-like features in around a quarter, leaving social disinhibition and circumscribed intense interests as the predominant features.

The fragile X syndrome

This is commonly associated with behaviours that bear a superficial resemblance to autism. Social avoidance and poor eye contact are common, but they seem to result from social anxiety rather than social indifference. Setting aside these features that superficially resemble autism, it remains controversial whether the fragile X syndrome is any more likely than other intellectual disability syndromes to result in classical autism.

Deafness

This is often suspected when young children with autism pay no heed to people speaking to them. A careful history usually establishes that they have no difficulty hearing sounds that interest them, for example, the rustle of a crisp packet! Unlike children with autism, deaf children are typically sociable and keen to communicate, for example, by gesture.

Aetiology and pathogenesis

Roughly 10–15% of individuals with autism have identifiable medical conditions. The likelihood of finding an underlying medical cause is probably higher when there is severe or profound intellectual disability. A wide variety of medical disorders have been reported; some may be chance associations and others may reflect a non-specific increase in the rate of autistic disorders in any condition that results in intellectual disability. It is unlikely that the link with intellectual disability is entirely non-specific, however, since autistic disorders are over-represented in some conditions that commonly result in intellectual disability, such as tuberous sclerosis with seizures, but much less commonly seen in others, such as severe cerebral palsy.

For the great majority of children with classical autism who do not have a known medical disorder, genetic factors seem of primary importance, with twin studies demonstrating a heritability of over 90%, almost certainly due to multiple genes of small or moderate effect rather than a single major gene. The heritable phenotype seems to be broad, stretching from classical autism at the one extreme to mild partial variants at the other extreme. The recurrence rate in siblings is roughly 3% for narrowly defined autism, but is about 10–20% for milder variants. Family studies suggest greater genetic overlap for the social/communication features and language features than for the restricted/repetitive activities. Genome-wide association studies and candidate gene studies have identified various loci, some of which have been independently replicated. Perhaps such findings may one day illuminate the pathogenesis of autism or contribute to screening. Genetic factors may be less important in the aetiology of the autistic features associated with severe and profound intellectual disability; these may be primarily determined by widespread brain damage (phenocopies). Obstetric adversity is of dubious aetiological significance.

Though extreme and prolonged early deprivation in grossly inadequate institutions may result in features of autism, there is no evidence that 'ordinary' psychosocial adversities play any part in the aetiology of autism. There is no evidence for theories that autism is caused by an early traumatic event, or by parents' insensitivity or lack of responsiveness to their child. Nevertheless, these views are still held in some quarters, and cause parents unnecessary distress.

Many researchers have hypothesised that autism results from a primary fault in just one neurological system or just one psychological function. It is equally plausible that autism reflects a distinctive combination of structural or functional abnormalities. Neurobiological studies have not identified a characteristic focal deficit: almost every portion of the brain has been implicated by some neuroimaging or neuropathology study and no localisation has been consistently replicated. However, the structural and functional relationships between different brain regions may be abnormal. Since individuals with autism have, on average, larger head circumferences and bigger brains, widespread neurodevelopmental abnormalities may turn out to be more important than focal abnormalities.

Attempts to identify a primary psychological deficit in autism have fared slightly better. Though no one theory has won universal acceptance, two theories have been particularly influential. One theory suggests that the primary deficit in autism is in 'Theory of Mind', that is, the capacity to attribute independent mental states to self and others in order to predict and explain actions (see Box 4.1). This sort of 'mentalising' deficit would disrupt abilities that depended on the capacity to see another person's point of view, but would not interfere with abilities that simply required a mechanical or behavioural understanding of objects and people. Another influential theory is that the primary deficit in autism is in executive function, with the sorts of problems in planning and organisational skills that result in poor performance on 'frontal lobe' tests. Other suggestions for the

> **Box 4.1** The Sally-Anne story: a test of first-order 'Theory of Mind'
>
> The following story is enacted with puppets and props.
>
> Sally has a marble. She puts it in a basket and then goes out. While Sally is out, Anne decides to play a trick on Sally. Anne takes the marble out from the basket and puts it in a box instead. Then Anne leaves. When Sally comes home, she wants her marble. Where will Sally look for the marble?
>
> - *Normal 3-year-olds* fail the test, saying that Sally will look in the box; they know the marble is there and they find it hard to see that Sally does not.
> - *Normal 4-year-olds* pass the test, predicting that Sally will act on her false belief and look in the basket.
> - Children with *Down syndrome* usually pass the Sally-Anne test if they have a mental age of 4 or more (on verbal tests).
> - *Autistic children*, by contrast, usually fail the Sally-Anne test even when they do have a verbal mental age of 4 or more. The minority of high-functioning autistic individuals who do pass the Sally-Anne test nearly always fail more complex tests of mentalising ability.

primary psychological deficit in autism include an innate impairment in the ability to become emotionally engaged with others and an impaired ability to extract high-level meaning by synthesising diverse sorts of information. However, none of these theories accounts satisfactorily for the repetitive and stereotyped behaviours seen in autism, or for the low IQ seen in the majority.

Treatment

The mainstays of treatment are appropriate educational placement and the provision of adequate support for parents. Children with autism generally do best in a well-structured educational setting where the teachers have special experience of the condition. Early placement in specialised nursery schools from the age of 2 or 3 years may be particularly beneficial. Home- and school-based behavioural programmes can reduce tantrums, aggressive outbursts, fears and rituals, as well as fostering more normal development. However, extreme behavioural regimes involving expensive one-to-one tutoring have not been shown to improve symptoms or development any more than good quality moderately intense special educational care. Many families welcome respite care. Membership of a parents' organisation may be helpful, providing access to newsletters, conferences, telephone helplines and contact with other similarly affected families. Structured social skills groups have been shown in trials to help; speech and language therapy has not been rigorously evaluated but is often reported by parents to be useful.

Standard antiepileptic medication is used to manage any associated epilepsy. Psychotropic medication does not cure the core symptoms of autism but may sometimes improve associated symptoms when used for specific indications and as part of an integrated package of psychological and educational interventions. Selective serotonin reuptake inhibitors (SSRIs) are sometimes effective treatments for severe anxiety, depression, self-injury, and obsessional or repetitive behaviour. Stimulants may reduce associated ADHD, though this may be at the cost of an unacceptable increase in irritability or repetitive behaviours. Neuroleptics such as haloperidol, risperidone and aripiprazole have been shown to reduce irritability, hyperactivity, aggression and self-injurious behaviour, though these potential advantages have to be set against the hazards of neuroleptic medication (see Chapter 38).

Prognosis

As described earlier, classical studies showed that roughly 70% of children with the full autistic syndrome acquired useful speech – which may be an underestimate nowadays since autism is more broadly defined and mild cases are more likely to be recognised. Children who have not acquired useful speech by the age of 5 years are unlikely to do so subsequently. Autistic aloofness improves in the majority of cases, being replaced by an 'active but odd' social interest.

Adolescence is associated with several changes:

- The peak age for onset of seizures is 11–14 years.
- Earlier over-activity may be replaced by marked under-activity and inertia.
- About 10% of individuals with autism go through a phase in adolescence when they lose language skills, sometimes with intellectual deterioration as well; this decline is not progressive, but the lost skills are not generally regained.
- Agitation seems more common, sometimes leading to serious aggressive outbursts.
- Inappropriate sexual behaviour can become troublesome.

By adult life, roughly 10% of individuals who initially had the full autistic syndrome are working and able to look after themselves. Fewer have good friends, marry, or become parents. The best predictors of long-term social independence are IQ and whether speech was present by 5 years of age. Individuals with a non-verbal IQ of under 60 are very likely to be severely socially impaired in adult life and unable to live independently. Individuals with higher IQs are more likely to become independent, particularly if they have acquired useful speech by the age of 5. Even with IQ and speech on their side, however, people with classical autism only have around a 50% chance of a good social outcome in adult life. The prognosis is generally better for those milder variants of autism that are now increasingly recognised. Though some individuals with ASDs subsequently develop psychotic symptoms, this is a distinctly unusual outcome.

Subject review

National Institute for Health and Clinical Excellence. (2011) *Autism: Recognition, Referral and Diagnosis of Children and Young People on the Autism Spectrum*. NICE: London. Available at: http://guidance.nice.org.uk/CG128.

Van Engeland H, Buitelaar JK. (2008) Autism spectrum disorders. *In*: Rutter M *et al*. (eds) *Rutter's Child and Adolescent Psychiatry*, 5th edn. Wiley-Blackwell, Chichester, pp. 759–840.

Volkmar FR *et al*. (2004) Autism and pervasive developmental disorders. *Journal of Child Psychology and Psychiatry* **45**, 135–170.

Woodbury-Smith MR, Volkmar FR. (2009) Asperger syndrome. *European Child and Adolescent Psychiatry* **18**, 2–11.

Further reading

Attwood T. (1997) *Asperger's Syndrome: A Guide for Parents and Professionals*. Jessica Kingsley, London.

Frith U. (2003) *Autism: Explaining the Enigma*. Blackwell, Oxford.

Rutter M *et al*. (2007) Early adolescent outcomes of institutionally deprived and non-deprived adoptees. III. Quasi-autism. *Journal of Child Psychology and Psychiatry* **48**, 1200–1207.

Simonoff E *et al*. (2008) Psychiatric disorders in children with autism spectrum disorders: Prevalence, comorbidity, and associated factors in a population-derived sample. *Journal of the American Academy of Child and Adolescent Psychiatry* **47**, 921–929.

Smith T. (2010) Early and intensive behavioural intervention in autism. *In*: Weisz JR, Kazdin AE (eds) *Evidence-Based Psychotherapies for Children and Adolescents*, 2nd edn. Guilford Press, New York, pp. 312–326.

Volkmar FR *et al*. (1999) Practice parameters for the assessment and treatment of children, adolescents, and adults with autism and other pervasive developmental disorders. *Journal of the American Academy of Child and Adolescent Psychiatry* **38 (Suppl. 12)**, 32–54.

Wing L, Gould J. (1979) Severe impairments of social interaction and associated abnormalities in children: Epidemiology and classification. *Journal of Autism and Developmental Disorders* **9**, 11–30. (This is the classic account of the high rate of the 'autistic triad' in children with intellectual disability.)

CHAPTER 5

Disorders of Attention and Activity

Whereas DSM and ICD criteria are identical or almost identical for most disorders, they do differ significantly for disorders of attention and activity. The disorder in DSM-IV is called *attention-deficit/hyperactivity disorder* (*ADHD*), while the disorder in ICD-10 is called *hyperkinesis*. What is the difference between the two? To simplify slightly, hyperkinesis is a severe subtype of ADHD – less common and more likely to respond to medication. As regards brand recognition, there is no doubt that 'ADHD' is the label that is more widely used and recognised. Even fans of the ICD-10 definition often use 'ADHD' in preference to 'hyperkinesis' – and so will we in general.

Epidemiology

Prevalence is around 2–5% for DSM-IV ADHD but only 1–3% for ICD-10 hyperkinesis. The male:female ratio is around 3:1. It is commoner in younger children than in adolescents. ADHD is linked with various markers of deprivation, being commoner in inner cities, very poor rural areas, in families of low socio-economic status and among children reared in institutions.

Defining characteristics

Marked restlessness, inattentiveness and impulsiveness

Children and adolescents with ADHD wriggle and squirm in their seats, fiddle with objects or clothing, repeatedly get up and wander about when they should be seated, have difficulty persisting with any one task, change activity frequently, and are easily distracted. The most obvious abnormality is not in the amount but in the control of activity. In the playground, a child with ADHD is not necessarily more active than anyone

Child and Adolescent Psychiatry, Third Edition. Robert Goodman and Stephen Scott.
© 2012 Robert Goodman and Stephen Scott. Published 2012 by John Wiley & Sons, Ltd.

else. What particularly distinguishes an individual with ADHD is his or her inability to suppress activity when stillness is required, for example, in the classroom or at the meal table. Children and adolescents with ADHD are also likely to be impulsive: acting without due reflection, engaging in rash and sometimes dangerous behaviours, blurting out answers in class, interrupting others, and not waiting their turn in games. However, impulsiveness is also a common feature of most disruptive behavioural disorders (see Box 6.3 on p. 71), so it is not as useful as over-activity and inattention when trying to distinguish ADHD from disruptive behavioural disorders.

Pervasiveness

If symptoms and impact only occur in a single setting, this is not enough for an ADHD diagnosis. Thus DSM-IV stipulates that the symptoms must have an impact in different settings, for example, both at home and at school. ICD-10 has a similar requirement for pervasive symptoms. It is important to note, however, that ADHD symptoms may not be evident during a brief clinic visit since the child or adolescent may be intimidated by unfamiliar professionals, or may be happy to settle to interesting tasks when given plenty of adult attention.

Chronicity and early onset

Both ICD-10 and DSM-IV require chronicity (at least six months of symptoms) and early onset (by or before 7 years of age). Though ADHD generally dates back to the preschool years, referral is often delayed until the early school years. This is the period when the child's inattentiveness, learning problems and disruptiveness become increasingly troublesome.

Exclusion criteria

According to the rules, autistic spectrum disorders (ASDs) are meant to take precedence over ADHD. Though individuals with ASDs can also be restless and inattentive, they should never officially be given an additional ADHD diagnosis. Sometimes this rule makes sense. For instance, a boy with an ASD may be extremely restless and inattentive both at home and at school because he is not interested in doing what his parents or teachers want him to do – so he will have a lot of ADHD symptoms reported by both parents and teachers. However, if careful enquiry establishes that he has excellent attention when lining up toys or memorizing timetables, he should not be diagnosed as having ADHD as well as an ASD.

In other instances, though, the exclusion rule makes much less sense and may be dropped in future revisions of DSM and ICD. This is because some individuals do seem to have mixed features of ASDs and ADHD (perhaps because of shared genes), and both conditions need treating.

Additional exclusion rules specify that ADHD should not be diagnosed when restlessness and poor concentration are due to a mood disorder, an anxiety disorder, or schizophrenia.

Assessment of symptoms

1 Attention is primarily assessed from how long the child or adolescent persists when engaged in a range of tasks including playing alone, reading, drawing, or playing with a friend. Some parents say their children can persist for fairly long periods when playing alone or with others – but closer enquiry makes it clear that they have a brief attention span, switching frequently from one play activity to another. Since even ADHD individuals are often able to watch TV or play computer games for long periods, persistence with these tasks is not a very discriminating measure of attention.

2 Motor activity is assessed from:
   (a) how long the individual can stay seated during the previously mentioned tasks;
   (b) what proportion of the time they are fidgeting;
   (c) how often they wander off on family outings or at the supermarket.

3 Impulsiveness is assessed using questions such as: Does he often blurt out an answer before he has heard the question properly? Is it hard for her to wait her turn? Does he often butt in on other people's conversations or games?

Additional features commonly associated with ADHD

1 *Defiant, aggressive, and antisocial behaviours* are often sufficiently marked to warrant the diagnosis of a disruptive behavioural disorder as well (see Chapter 6). Child and adolescent psychiatrists using DSM-IV will diagnose ADHD alongside either an oppositional-defiant disorder or a conduct disorder; child and adolescent psychiatrists using ICD-10 will use the combined diagnosis of 'hyperkinetic conduct disorder'.

2 *Problems with social relationships.* Children and adolescents with ADHD are often socially disinhibited with adults, being over-familiar and cheeky. Peer rejection is common, partly in response to their disruptiveness and impulsive disregard for rules and turns. Individuals with ADHD are easily led or dared into all sorts of mischief.

3 *IQ under 100* in many but certainly not all affected individuals.

4 *Specific learning problems* (for example, with reading or spelling), even when IQ is taken into account.

5 *Coordination problems* and neurodevelopmental immaturities ('soft neurological signs').

6 A history of specific *developmental delay*, for example, in language acquisition

7 *Deficient emotional self-regulation* (DESR) in a subgroup, with excessive emotional reactions to everyday occurrences.

Differential diagnosis

1 *Normality*. Parents may complain of minor degrees of restlessness and inattention that are well within the normal range. Simple exuberance can be wearing for parents and teachers; this requires sympathy rather than a diagnostic label!

2 *Situational hyperactivity*. Some children and adolescents seem to be hyperactive and inattentive in just one setting, such as at school but not at home, or vice versa. These individuals cannot be diagnosed with ADHD or hyperkinesis under current rules since cross-situational pervasiveness is required. In some instances, situational symptoms may be a milder variant of pervasive symptoms, simply being more recognisable in one setting rather than the other. In other instances, though, situational symptoms reflect situational stresses. For example, symptoms limited to school can be the result of specific learning difficulties, while symptoms limited to the home can reflect home-based difficulties with relationships or behaviour.

3 *Behavioural disorders*. While it is true that ADHD and disruptive behavioural disorders often occur together, it is also possible for 'pure' disruptive behavioural disorders to mimic ADHD. Impulsiveness is a feature of both disorders (see Box 6.3 on p. 71). In addition, children and adolescents with behavioural problems at school may not want to settle to school-work and may wander about the classroom creating trouble. Similarly, children and adolescents with behavioural problems at home may not settle to their chores or their homework. The key question is whether restlessness and inattentiveness persist during chosen activities, such as drawing, reading comics, building models, or playing with friends. If the answer is 'no', this is unlikely to be ADHD; if 'yes', this may be a mixture of ADHD and a behavioural disorder (depending on pervasiveness, age of onset, etc.).

4 *Emotional disorders*. Severe anxiety, depression or mania can all result in restlessness and inattentiveness (in which case, a diagnosis of ADHD is ruled out). When assessing someone with a mixture of ADHD symptoms and emotional symptoms, it is essential to take a careful history to establish which began first. If the emotional symptoms came first, the right diagnosis is probably just an emotional disorder. However, if the ADHD symptoms came first, this may be an acute emotional disorder on top of a chronic ADHD problem.

5 *Tics, chorea, and other dyskinesias*. These may be mistaken for fidgetiness. Observe the movements carefully. Children with tic disorders may also have ADHD and the ADHD may have been evident long before the first tic.

6 *Autistic spectrum disorders*. ASDs are suggested if the restlessness and inattentiveness are accompanied by autistic types of social impairment, communication deviance, rigid and repetitive behaviours, or lack of spontaneous pretend play.

7 *Intellectual disability.* If an individual's attention and activity control are in line with his or her mental age, you should not diagnose ADHD. This is as true for someone with an intellectual disability as for anyone else. Thus, if a 10-year-old boy has a mental age of 6, then you should not diagnose ADHD if his level of attention and activity control is in line with what you would expect of an average 6-year-old. However, you should consider diagnosing ADHD if his level of attention and activity control is at 3-year-old level, that is, well below what you would expect, given his mental age of 6. While intellectual disability does not necessarily result in ADHD, it does increase its likelihood. Overall, ADHD is some 10–30 times more common among children and adolescents with intellectual disability.

Causation

Several lines of evidence from pharmacology, neuroimaging and genetics suggest that two catecholamine neurotransmitters – dopamine and noradrenaline – play a key role in ADHD. However, this evidence is suggestive rather than conclusive. It is still possible that changes in one or both of these catecholamines are the result of some other more fundamental pathophysiology.

Family, adoption and twin studies suggest that genetic factors make a major contribution, with heritability estimates of around 75%. Evidence is accumulating that the risk of ADHD varies with polymorphisms of some of the genes involved in dopaminergic and noradrenergic transmitter systems, for example, the dopamine D4 receptor gene and the DAT1 dopamine transporter gene. However, these identified genes only account for a small proportion of the heritability of ADHD, and genome-wide searches have been negative. What could account for a high heritability that cannot be explained by currently identified genes? Perhaps there are still many susceptibility genes of small effect that have not yet been discovered, but other possible explanations need to be considered. Firstly, gene–gene interactions may be important, such that several genetic effects that are individually small combine to produce a major effect in combination. Secondly, gene–environment interactions may act similarly, with a gene that has little or no effect by itself producing a major effect when combined with some specific environment, such as exposure to lead or some other neurotoxin. Thirdly, ADHD may be caused by many rare genes with major effects. Although such genes would make ADHD highly heritable within a single family, the effects would be hard to demonstrate when pooling a lot of different families, each with its own rare gene. Finding rare but powerful genes may require studies of particularly informative families that have many affected members.

Though epilepsy and other brain disorders do increase the likelihood of ADHD (and other psychiatric problems), most individuals with ADHD have no neurological symptoms or signs: ADHD is not synonymous with overt brain damage, and terms such as 'minimal brain damage' are un-helpful. If neurobiological explanations are to be useful, they need to be as specific and testable as possible. There is growing support from neuroimaging and neuropsychological studies for the idea that ADHD sometimes results from impaired executive functioning linked to structural and functional abnormalities of the prefrontal cortex and basal ganglia. Other evidence links ADHD to delay aversion, that is, a preference for small immediate rewards rather than larger delayed rewards. Executive dysfunction and delay aversion may be alternative routes into ADHD; difficulties regulating arousal may be a third route. It is important to remember that just as a physical syndrome such as hepatitis can have many possible causes (for example, alcohol, viral infections), so too may a psychiatric syndrome such as ADHD.

Despite popular stereotypes, it is not common for ADHD to result from exposure to environmental toxins such as lead, or to be due to pregnancy and birth complications – with the exception that very premature births are more likely to lead to problems with inattention. However, there is rather more evidence for the widely held view that ADHD can be triggered by adverse reactions to specific foods or drinks.

Psychosocial as well as biological factors influence ADHD symptoms, as indicated by the link with deprivation and institutional rearing. The re-sponses of parents, teachers and peers may influence the prognosis. There is growing evidence that parents and teachers who respond to ADHD with criticism, coldness and lack of involvement thereby increase the chance of the affected individual becoming defiant, aggressive and antisocial.

Treatment

Education
The nature of the disorder needs to be explained to the affected individual, the family and the school. ADHD is neither the parents' fault nor their child's fault. Since children and adolescents with ADHD can be extremely exasperating, they often come in for much criticism and little praise. The balance may improve, however, once adults accept that the problems are not just wilful naughtiness. Rules about unacceptable behaviours should be clear, consistently and calmly enforced, and backed up by immediate (but not harsh) sanctions. A key objective of treatment is to reduce the chances of the child acquiring an additional behavioural disorder. Special learning problems may need remedial help, and all teaching will need to take account of the child's limited attention span.

Psychological treatments
Behavioural management is often useful, and may be the only treatment needed for the mildest cases. The most suitable targets are the sorts of dis-ruptive behaviours described in more detail in Chapter 6. Parent-training programmes can improve parents' child-management skills and thereby

reduce family stress and children's negative behaviours. In the process, they may improve the children's long-term outcome by reducing the likelihood of future substance abuse and antisocial personality disorder. It is less clear how useful behavioural or cognitive-behavioural approaches are when targeted on the core ADHD symptoms. It is possible to reward children when they concentrate for progressively longer periods, just as it is possible to teach them cognitive strategies to increase reflectiveness. However, it is not clear how much real-life benefit this confers.

Medication

Stimulant medication is a well-tested treatment for ADHD that is under-used in some places and over-used in others. Indeed, over-use and under-use can occur side by side, with some children getting medication they don't need, while other children with severe ADHD are never tried on a medication that might have brought considerable benefit. The most commonly used stimulant is methylphenidate, but dexamfetamine has very similar properties. A good response to stimulant medication is predicted by severe and pervasive ADHD symptoms, and by the absence of emotional symptoms. Many parents have reservations about medication, and it is true that medication can have side effects and is a symptomatic rather than a curative treatment. It is also true that the short-term benefits of medication may not translate into any long-term advantage. However, much the same could be said of treating a child's fever or headache with paracetamol: the relief of symptoms can be important. Consequently, it may be worth encouraging parents to consider a brief trial of medication if their child seems likely to respond. After seeing the positive and negative effects, the family can then join with professionals in deciding whether medication should be continued when the trial period is over.

When medication does improve attention and activity level, there are often parallel improvements in compliance, peer relationships, family relationships and learning ability. Methylphenidate and dexamphetamine are not addictive for children, do not make them 'high' and do not cause sedation. Side effects are rarely troublesome. Headache, stomach-ache, low mood and jitteriness often wear off spontaneously or respond to reduction in dose. Appetite suppression or difficulty getting to sleep can usually be overcome by adjusting the timing or dosage. Repetitive activities or stereotypies can be provoked by over-medication but these side effects usually disappear when the dose is reduced. Since stimulants can exacerbate tics, they are not usually the first choice in children with tics or a strong family history of tics. Stimulants can be administered for months or years. Long-term use of stimulants is remarkably safe – the only possible complication of long-term use is a very slight reduction in adult height, and even this is controversial.

Atomoxetine is a more recent alternative to stimulants; it has a smaller effect on average, but it may work when stimulants have failed, or when stimulants have unacceptable side effects. Other drugs that are sometimes used for hyperactivity include clonidine, buproprion and tricyclics such as imipramine. Medication should always be part of an integrated treatment package. A good response to medication is the beginning rather than the end of treatment – increasing the chance of successful work with the family and the school to get the child back on to as normal a developmental trajectory as possible.

Diet

Dietary treatment is popular with parents, and often needs to be explored before the family are willing to try anything else. Removal of food colours from the diet results in a small improvement in some children with ADHD, and this is not just suggestibility since it has been confirmed with 'blind' challenges. In addition, several trials have demonstrated that some children improve when specific foods are excluded from their diets – though it is still uncertain whether diet-responsive children are rare or common. It is not possible to predict on the basis of blood or skin tests which children will respond, or which foods are responsible. Additives are rarely the only culprits; one or more natural foods, such as milk, wheat products or oranges, are usually involved as well. As described in Chapter 38, a proper trial of dietary treatment is very hard work for all concerned.

Prognosis

Over-activity typically wanes in adolescence, though many affected individuals have continuing problems with inattentiveness, impulsiveness and an inner sense of restlessness even in adult life. Educational attainments are often poor, which may account for lower occupational status in adult life. Individuals with both ADHD and a behavioural disorder are at high risk of antisocial personality disorder and substance abuse in adult life; individuals with 'pure' ADHD are at less risk of these antisocial outcomes, though they are still vulnerable.

Subject review

Taylor E, Sonuga-Barke E. (2008) Disorders of attention and activity. *In*: Rutter M *et al.* (eds) *Rutter's Child and Adolescent Psychiatry*, 5th edn. Wiley-Blackwell, Chichester, pp. 521–542.

Further reading

Faraone SV *et al.* (2008) Effect of stimulants on height and weight: A review of the literature. *Journal of the American Academy of Child and Adolescent Psychiatry* **47**, 994–1008.
Graham J *et al.* (2011) European guidelines on managing adverse effects of medication for ADHD. *European Child and Adolescent Psychiatry* **20**, 17–37.

Lambek R *et al.* (2010) Validating neuropsychological subtypes of ADHD: how do children *with* and *without* an executive function deficit differ? *Journal of Child Psychology and Psychiatry* **51**, 895–904. (Suggests at least two different paths to ADHD, one involving executive dysfunction and the other involving delay aversion.)

Neale BM *et al.* (2010) Meta-analysis of genome-wide association studies of attention-deficit/hyperactivity disorder. *Journal of the American Academy of Child and Adolescent Psychiatry* **49**, 884–897. (Results are negative so far, but it is not yet time to give up.)

Rommelse NNJ *et al.* (2010) Shared heritability of attention-deficit/hyperactivity disorder and autism spectrum disorder. *European Child and Adolescent Psychiatry* **19**, 281–295.

Schachar R *et al.* (1987) Changes in family function and relationships in children who respond to methylphenidate. *Journal of the American Academy of Child and Adolescent Psychiatry* **26**, 728–732.

Stevenson J. (2010) Recent research on food additives: Implications for CAMH. *Child and Adolescent Mental Health* **15**, 130–133.

Surman CBH *et al.* (2011) Deficient emotional self-regulation and adult Attention Deficit Hyperactivity Disorder: A family risk analysis. *American Journal of Psychiatry* **168**, 617–623.

Young S, Amarasinghe JM. (2010) Non-pharmacological treatment for ADHD: A lifespan approach. *Journal of Child Psychology and Psychiatry* **51**, 116–133.

CHAPTER 6
Disruptive Behaviour

According to most epidemiological studies, the commonest sort of child and adolescent psychiatric disorder involves *persistent failure to control behaviour appropriately within socially defined rules*. It is often persistent, costly for society, and not treated successfully. There are three overlapping domains of disruptive behaviour: *defiance* of the will of someone in authority, *aggressiveness* and *antisocial behaviour* that violates other people's rights, property, or person. None of these is in itself abnormal or pathological and indeed there are occasions when one tries to promote some of these behaviours in over-dependent children. Some disobedient and destructive behaviour is a part of normal development that usually diminishes with maturity, and a diagnosis should only be made when the behaviours are both extreme and persistent.

The naming of disruptive behavioural disorders involves a mixture of straightforward and confusing elements. Let's start with the straightforward bits. Both ICD-10 and DSM-IV recognise a category of *oppositional-defiant disorder* (ODD) where, as the name suggests, defiance is a major ingredient. The other major behavioural disorder in DSM-IV is called *conduct disorder* (CD) and has aggression and antisocial behaviour as its major ingredients. In DSM-IV, ODD and conduct disorder are alternatives – you either have one or the other, but you are not officially allowed to have both. So far, so good. Now for the confusing bit. In ICD-10, the term 'conduct disorder' refers to any sort of disruptive behavioural disorder – including ODD and what DSM calls conduct disorder. You can imagine how this muddles clear communication. For the ICD-orientated clinician, ODD is a sub-type of (broadly defined) conduct disorder; for the DSM-orientated clinician, ODD is different from a (narrowly defined) conduct disorder. Beware! Whenever you see the term 'conduct disorder', make sure you know if this is the narrowly defined DSM term or the broadly defined ICD term. In this book, we use the term *disruptive behavioural disorder* to denote the broader term.

Child and Adolescent Psychiatry, Third Edition. Robert Goodman and Stephen Scott.
© 2012 Robert Goodman and Stephen Scott. Published 2012 by John Wiley & Sons, Ltd.

Psychiatric labelling and social control

Should children and adolescents be given a psychiatric label simply because their behaviour is unacceptable to people in authority? Totalitarian regimes have used similar rationales in order to justify the incarceration of dissidents in psychiatric hospitals. Partly for this reason, some psychiatrists will only make a diagnosis of a disruptive behavioural disorder if a further criterion is met, namely that the disruptive behaviour results in impairment in everyday functioning (for example, in interpersonal relations or schoolwork). This impairment criterion is included in DSM-IV, but not in ICD-10.

Dimension or category?

It is, arguably more appropriate to think of disruptive behaviour as a dimension than as an all-or-nothing category. In medicine, cut-offs are often imposed on continuous variables in order to distinguish between normality and abnormality. In psychology, the thinking is much more likely to be in dimensional terms, retaining the continuous variable and investigating the extent to which increasingly abnormal scores have increasingly maladaptive outcomes. In the case of disruptive behaviour, both dimensions and categories have advantages and disadvantages.

Advantages of a dimension
As the variety and severity of disruptive behaviour increase, so the prognosis progressively worsens. There is not a relatively sudden transition from a good prognosis for children and adolescents just below the threshold for a disruptive behavioural disorder to a bad prognosis for those above the threshold (although it does seem to be the case that individuals with disruptive behaviour confined to just one area, such as aggression, do have a relatively good prognosis). An advantage of seeing disruptive behaviour as a dimension and hence an exaggeration of normal behaviour is that the environmental determinants causing or exacerbating the behaviour may be more thoroughly examined, and hopefully put right.

Disadvantages of a dimension
Coexisting difficulties may be missed because they are not part of the same dimension, for example, reading problems, ADHD.

Advantages of a category
It is simpler and focuses on the most severely affected individuals; they are particularly relevant clinically and most studies of causation and treatment have been based on this group. An advantage of giving a diagnosis is that it implies the need to look for known associated features outside the core phenomenology (for example, poor parenting, ADHD, reading delay, poor

social and relationship skills), gives information regarding prognosis, and carries information about which treatments are likely to be effective.

Disadvantages of a category

There is the risk that an all-or-nothing classification that divides individuals into those with and without a disruptive behavioural disorder might create an us-and-them attitude that adds to the marginalisation of troubled families. A diagnosis can also lead to the belief that the individual has an immutable, biologically determined entity, for which little can be done. A further disadvantage is that many professionals (for example, teachers and social workers) and lay people outside medicine are not familiar with the terms 'conduct disorder' or 'oppositional-defiant disorder' so that often it does not help their understanding or management of children with the problem.

In summary, both approaches have their advantages, and the wise practitioner will try to bring the best of both to bear.

Is disruptive behaviour a psychiatric problem?

Whether disruptive behaviour should be assessed or treated by child and adolescent mental health professionals is debatable. Certainly, the difficulty is one of behaviour that is beyond the normal range and is causing impairment or burden to others. However, so is smoking 40 cigarettes a day as a teenager or driving motorcycles at 100 mph, yet these are more likely to be seen as social or moral problems than health problems.

Perhaps those cases of disruptive behaviour that are clearly socially determined and where management is solely a matter of discipline or behaviour management could be seen as the province of social services, education, or voluntary agencies. To be maximally effective, these other agencies would need to acquire a wide range of assessment and management skills, many of which were originally developed within mental health disciplines. They would need to be able to recognise the minority of individuals with problems such as ADHD or depression who could benefit from referral to mental health professionals, and to recognise learning problems that could benefit from referral to specialist educational services. They would also need to be able to offer, or refer families to, evidence-based parenting groups, which are becoming more available. Given the high prevalence of disruptive behaviour, and the relatively small number of child and adolescent mental health professionals, the practicalities of effective service provision demand some such spread of expertise and responsibility, as discussed in Chapter 43 on the organisation of services. The long-term financial cost to the public of disruptive behaviour in children and adolescents is great, at least ten times that of controls, and falls on many agencies, so there is a justification on economic grounds for several government departments to become involved in contributing to treatment and prevention.

Symptoms and signs

The manifestations change with age. Younger children are more likely to show the signs of oppositional-defiant disorder (ODD), which is a subtype of CD in ICD-10 but a separate condition in DSM-IV. The criterion behaviours for ODD (see Box 6.1) should occur much more often than in other children or adolescents of the same developmental age. The DSM-IV criteria for CD (see Box 6.2) are more likely to be met by adolescents, and are closer to those for adult antisocial personality disorder. This definition is less likely to include girls than previous definitions since early sexual experience, early substance abuse and chronic violation of rules have been dropped.

Box 6.1 ICD-10* criteria for oppositional-defiant disorder (ODD)

At least four of the following eight items have been present for at least six months:

Irritable items
1 Unusually frequent or severe temper outbursts.
2 Often touchy or easily annoyed.
3 Often angry or resentful.

Headstrong items
4 Often argues with adults.
5 Often defies adult requests or rules.
6 Often deliberately annoys other people.
7 Often shifts blame to others.

Hurtful items
8 Often spiteful or vindictive.

  Recent studies suggest that when irritable items are particularly prominent, there is a high concurrent and future risk of anxiety or depression. Likewise, headstrong items seem linked to ADHD, and hurtful items to psychopathy.
Note: *DSM-IV criteria for ODD are similar to *The ICD-10 Classification of Mental and Behavioural Disorders: Diagnostic Criteria for Research* (World Health Organization, 1993).

Associated features

Psychiatric symptoms

1 *ADHD features*: restlessness, inattentiveness, impulsiveness and general over-activity often co-exist but are often been under-recognised in the UK. The combination makes the outcome worse.
2 *Low mood*: about a third show significant emotional symptoms, most commonly unhappiness and misery. When present, these symptoms carry an increased risk for depression and deliberate self-harm in the teenage years and adulthood.

Box 6.2 ICD-10* criteria for conduct disorder (CD)‡

At least three of the following items in the previous six months:

- Cons others.
- Often starts fights.
- Has used serious weapons.
- Often out at night without permission (onset before13 years).
- Physically cruel to people.
- Physically cruel to animals.

- Deliberately destroys others' property.
- Fire-setting to cause damage.
- Stealing without force.
- Often truants (onset before 13 years).
- Ran away from home overnight at least twice.
- Stealing with force.
- Has forced someone into sexual acts.
- Often bullies, threatens or intimidates.
- Has broken into car or house.

Notes: * DSM-IV criteria for conduct disorder are generally similar, though the reference period is the past 12 months. *The ICD-10 Classification of Mental and Behavioural Disorders: Diagnostic Criteria for Research* (World Health Organization, 1993).

‡ Narrowly defined, i.e. not including oppositional-defiant disorder.

Educational failure

Many affected individuals have poor achievements in terms of grades and level of work, and often have specific learning deficits. On testing, up to a third of those with a disruptive behavioural disorder have specific reading disorder (SRD), commonly defined as being more than two standard deviations below the reading level expected for their age and intelligence (see Chapter 31). Conversely, up to a third of those with SRD have a disruptive behavioural disorder. The association between disruptive behavioural disorders and SRD could be due to any of three possibilities, and each needs to be considered in individual cases. First, disruptive behaviour may interfere with classroom learning. Second, individuals who do not have the ability to understand and participate in class may become frustrated and disruptive as a result. Third, both disruptiveness and reading problems may stem from a third factor such as ADHD or unsupportive and negative parenting. Independently of poor achievement, lower IQ is associated with disruptive behavioural disorders.

Poor interpersonal relations

Disruptive children and adolescents often become unpopular with their peers and frequently have no enduring friends. They commonly show poor social skills with both peers and adults, for example, they have difficulty sustaining a game or promoting positive social interchanges. Poor peer relationships predict an unfavourable outcome. ICD-10 divides

CD into 'unsocialised' and 'socialised' types according to whether peer relationships are normal or not. DSM-IV has no comparable categories. In clinical practice, the great majority of children and adolescents with CD do have impaired peer relationships. Nevertheless, there is limited evidence from cluster analytic studies for a relatively small group of conduct-disordered individuals who do make enduring friendships, display altruistic behaviour, feel guilt or remorse, refrain from blaming others and show concern for others. These individuals with socialised CD tend to be older and to engage in less aggressive antisocial acts such as stealing, truanting and drinking alcohol. They could be considered 'well-adjusted criminals' who are not regarded as deviant within their own subculture. In contrast, there is increasing interest in a subgroup who display *psychopathic tendencies*, most notably callous-unemotional traits (lack of feeling for the distress of others despite being aware of it, typically associated with insensitivity to punishment). Such individuals are more often bullies and are prone to be cruel to animals.

Differential diagnosis

There is usually not much doubt about the diagnosis if detailed information is obtained from more than one source. Multiple informants are vital, since disruptive behaviour may only occur in one setting, for example, just at home or just at school. Epidemiological studies have shown that there is a fairly low correlation between teacher and parent ratings of disruptive behaviour, often around 0.3.

Differential diagnoses include:

1 *Adjustment disorder*: this can be diagnosed when onset occurs soon after exposure to an identifiable psychosocial stressor such as divorce, bereavement, adoption, trauma, and abuse (within one month according to ICD-10 and within three months according to DSM-IV) and when symptoms do not persist for more than six months after the cessation of the stress or its consequences.

2 *ADHD*: disruptive behavioural disorders can be mistaken for ADHD and vice versa. This is partly due to overlap in symptoms, as shown in Box 6.3. Defiance, aggression and intentionally antisocial behaviour are not part of pure ADHD. In clinically referred populations, disruptive behavioural disorders and ADHD often co-exist, when there is a danger of missing the ADHD.

3 *Normality*: the child or adolescent's behaviour is within the normal range, but parents or teachers have unrealistically high expectations.

4 *Subcultural deviance*: some children and adolescents are antisocial but not particularly aggressive or defiant, and they are well adjusted within a deviant peer culture that approves of drug use, shoplifting, etc. It might be accurate to apply an ICD-10 diagnosis of socialised CD, but it is arguably a mistake to pathologise what can be seen as a cultural variant.

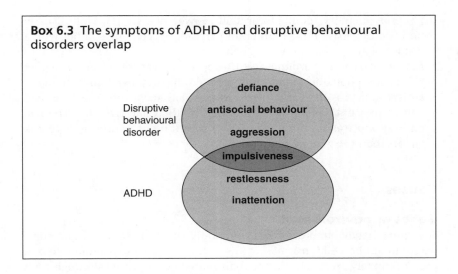

Box 6.3 The symptoms of ADHD and disruptive behavioural disorders overlap

Disruptive behavioural disorder

defiance
antisocial behaviour
aggression

impulsiveness

ADHD

restlessness
inattention

5 *Autistic spectrum disorders*: these are often accompanied by marked tantrums or destructiveness, and the disruptive behaviour is occasionally the principal cause for referral. A number of children and adolescents meet the criteria for a disruptive behavioural disorder while also having some traits on the autistic spectrum (but not enough for a diagnosis).

Epidemiology

A disruptive behavioural disorder was diagnosed in 4% of children in the classic Isle of Wight study, and more recent Office of National Statistics surveys of children and adolescents confirm an overall rate of 5%; many other studies have reported even higher rates. The prevalence is particularly high in deprived inner-city areas. Boys display disruptive behavioural disorders around three times more commonly than girls. Disruptive behavioural disorders are associated with lower socio-economic status (this covers a multitude of variables), and large family size. The age of onset can vary considerably. The Dunedin study found a clear distinction between early and late onset conduct symptoms:

- *Early onset* (typically around age 3–7 years) was found in 7% of the population and led to a pattern of persistent antisocial and offending behaviour that in over half carried on into adulthood, so that there was no diminution when the participants were last studied in their thirties. This *early onset, lifetime persistent* pattern is characterised by increased levels of many parenting risk factors (teenage parent, harsh and inconsistent discipline, family conflict, maternal mental health problems, changes of primary caregiver) and neurocognitive risk factors (hyperactivity, lower

IQ, poor memory, poor motor skills, lower heart rate). Not all early onset cases persist, but a marker for persistence is having a father with a history of antisocial or criminal behaviour.

- *Late onset* (typically around age 13–15 years) was found in a separate 7% of the population, and while as a group they performed as many antisocial acts as the early onset group as late teenagers, this level had halved (but not gone down to normal) by their late twenties. The late onset group was no more exposed to parenting or neurocognitive risk factors than the general population.

Causes

Genes or environment?

Disruptive behavioural disorders commonly cluster in families, and compared to other child psychiatric disorders, shared environment has a proportionately greater influence than shared genes. Thus, although twin studies have shown a high concordance for monozygotic pairs, the concordance for dizygotic pairs is also high. Adoption studies have shown the influence of the biological parents to be less than that of the adoptive ones. However, they show a strong interaction effect, whereby the combination of high congenital risk, as indexed by having criminal or alcoholic biological parents, plus an unfavourable rearing environment, as indexed by having alcoholic or criminal adoptive parents, leads to a far higher rate of antisocial behaviour and criminality than would be expected by addition (see Box 33.2). This gives grounds for some therapeutic optimism, since even if a child is born with considerable congenital risk factors, if the parenting and general rearing environment are favourable, they can do relatively well. However, genetic influences seem to play a stronger role in the development of adult antisocial personality and criminality. Cytogenetic studies have added little so far, and the case studies reporting that individuals with the XYY karyotype are particularly prone to severe aggression have not been supported by population-based surveys. Molecular genetic studies are beginning to emerge. For example, the Dunedin study was the first to show an interesting gene–environment interaction, whereby children with one particular variant of the monoamine oxidase A gene are at an increased risk of developing antisocial behaviour, but only if they receive relatively poor parenting (in the worst third of the population); otherwise they are not at increased risk of antisocial behaviour. Subsequent studies have confirmed this finding, albeit with a relatively small effect. Within subtypes of antisocial behaviour, those with callous-unemotional traits have greater heritability – 80% in one study – than those without, where environmental influences predominate.

Child-based mechanisms

1 *Constitutional characteristics* proposed include neurotransmitter imbalance, hormonal excess (notably testosterone) and metabolic variations

such as low cholesterol. There are also abnormal arousal patterns with failure to calm down after frustration. However, the only reliably replicable findings are that some children and adolescents with disruptive behavioural disorders have lower heart rates, and are more generally under-aroused. Infants with temperaments classified as 'difficult' are more likely to be referred for aggressive problems later on. MRI scans are beginning to show differences in brain activation patterns in individuals with disruptive behavioural disorders during a range of neurocognitive tests but no consistent pattern is yet apparent. Children and adolescents with neurodevelopmental disorders such as cerebral palsy and epilepsy are more likely to have problems with irritability and defiance, but are no more likely than other children to engage in severe antisocial behaviour.

2 *Psychological processes.* Significant cognitive attributional bias has been shown in aggressive children and adolescents, whereby they are more likely to perceive neutral acts by others as hostile. As the individual gets more disliked and rejected by his or her peers, the opportunity for seeing things this way increases. Social skills are lacking. Emotional processes in individuals with disruptive behavioural disorders have been little studied, although self-esteem is often low and co-existent misery common. The role of academic achievement is discussed above.

Immediate environment

1 *Parental psychiatric disorder.* This is an important influence but is mainly mediated through marital discord and child-rearing practices and is not specific to any particular psychiatric condition in the parents.

2 *Parental criminality.* Similar environmental considerations apply, although an irritable or callous temperament may be passed on genetically.

3 *Child-rearing practices.* Disruptive behavioural disorders are strongly associated with discord between parents, hostility directed at the child, lack of warmth, and lack of involvement with their child. While these factors may partly be a reaction to the individual's disruptive behaviour, follow-up and intervention studies show they have a causal role in initiating and maintaining that behaviour. Lack of supervision and inconsistent discipline are also clearly associated with disruptive behavioural disorders, perhaps because the individual is not given the opportunity to experience and learn predictable social rules. Harsh discipline is also associated with disruptive behavioural disorders.

4 *Parent–child interaction patterns.* Fine-grained analysis has shown that disruptive behaviour escalates if this enables children and adolescents to get more attention, avoid unpleasant demands or get their own way more often. By responding in ways that reward disruptive behaviour, and by failing to encourage socially acceptable behaviour, parents are inadvertently training their children to behave antisocially. Interventions to break this cycle have been shown to be effective.

5 *Sexual abuse* can lead to the emergence of disruptive behaviour in girls or boys who were previously free of such problems.

Wider environment

1 *School factors* have been shown to affect the rate of disruptive behavioural disorders independently of home background: poorly organised, unfriendly schools with low staff morale, high staff turnover and poor contact with parents have higher rates of disruptive behavioural disorders even when catchment area characteristics have been allowed for.

2 *Wider social influences.* Though disruptive behaviour is associated with overcrowding, poor housing, and poor neighbourhoods, it is still unclear if these factors are causal or simply markers for other family or socio-economic variables. A prevailing set of values in a neighbourhood that gives youths kudos for stealing, carrying knives, truanting and gaining 'respect' from others through frightening violence and joining a gang is associated with more conduct disordered behaviour by residents.

Assessment

The severity and frequency of defiant, aggressive and antisocial acts in the last month or so should be established in detail. Some parents are prone to catalogue all 'bad' things done over the last year or even since birth. Attention and activity should be enquired about in the same detailed way (see Chapter 5) since ADHD is a common and easily overlooked accompaniment (or differential diagnosis) of disruptive behavioural disorders. Though it is worth enquiring about impulsiveness, this could be part of either ADHD or a disruptive behavioural disorder. Do not forget to enquire about emotional symptoms, particularly unhappiness and misery. Part of the problem may derive from things that are upsetting the child or adolescent, for example, a father who often fails to turn up for his access visits, or a mother who never seems to appreciate her child's efforts, however hard he or she tries. The strength of these concerns may only come out in an individual interview, and could easily be missed if the family is only ever seen together. Remember to ask about autistic traits (see Chapter 4) and also callous-unemotional characteristics.

Parenting practices should be enquired about in detail, with a blow-by-blow account of what happens before, during and after a recent episode of troublesome behaviour. Who 'won' the encounter? What was said? What punishments or consequences were used and did they work? How long did it take for relations to return to normal? More generally, ask how much praise and encouragement is given for constructive behaviour, and how much time is spent in joint activities. Get detailed recent examples. Try to gauge the parents' sensitivity to their child's moods and needs, and how much they take these into account when negotiating how to settle disagreements and planning their child's life.

Consider the parents' emotional tone and attitude towards their child. Asking about the child's good qualities can be helpful. Is there some warmth and approval despite the child's difficulties, or is the tone entirely negative? Powerful beliefs may be discovered, which will need to be addressed if treatment is to progress, for example, 'There's something wrong in his head,' or, 'He's just like his father. He was rotten too.'

Find out about the family history, especially 'the four Ds':

- *Deviance* and criminality in the father (who may use abusive discipline, or transmit antisocial values).
- *Depression* in the mother (she may be able to be reasonably bright and responsive during the assessment, but spend half the day in bed and not be able to respond to her child's needs).
- *Drug* misuse by either parent.
- *Domestic* violence between the two.

Direct observation of parents with their children is invaluable in getting a picture of their interactions, albeit in atypical circumstances. Are clear boundaries set, or is the child allowed to get away with almost anything? For example, how do the parents react when the child tries to leave the room? Is good behaviour praised or ignored? Is the child handled sensitively?

A school report is essential, covering antisocial behaviour, ability to concentrate and sit still, peer relations, and scholastic attainments, including test results. There are occasions when troublesome behaviour in class can take up so much of the teacher's time that significant intellectual disability or reading difficulty can be overlooked or simply regarded as a consequence of the bad behaviour. Poor school attainment should lead to serious consideration of psychometric tests being carried out.

Treatment

Family- and school-focused

1 *Family work* is essential to engage with the parents and come to a shared formulation about the causal factors. Parents of children and adolescents with conduct disorder are likely to feel ashamed and may be suspicious of authority – so considerable skill is required to form a working alliance with them and their child, thereby setting the scene for more specific therapeutic work.
2 *School.* Often class teachers appreciate advice on management strategies and are glad the problem is being tackled. Feedback about significant results of psychometric testing should lead to a different teaching approach. If there are significant comorbid problems such as ADHD and autistic traits, the school needs to know this.
3 *Parent management training* is the best established approach, with scores of randomised controlled trials attesting to its effectiveness. It makes parents pay attention to desired behaviour rather than get caught up in lengthy slanging matches; positive aspects of parent–child relationships are promoted, and parents are also taught effective techniques for handling undesired behaviour. It can be given more economically in groups while maintaining effectiveness. It is based on behavioural methods, see Chapter 39.

4 *Family therapy* is fairly frequently used but has hardly been evaluated. Judging from clinical experience, it is often useful in fairly
well-functioning families where after only a few sessions parents may
collaborate in setting clear boundaries for their child and improve the
emotional atmosphere; it is less useful for chaotic, disorganised families
who lack coping skills; see Chapter 41.

5 *Social work referral*. This should be considered if the child or adolescent is
at risk of significant harm, either from abusive or neglectful parenting,
or is so out of control that he/she is a risk to others.

Child- or adolescent-focused

1 *Behaviour modification* can be very effective in modifying one or two
specific antisocial behaviours, but does not usually generalise; see
Chapter 39.

2 *Problem-solving skills training and social skills training* have been shown to
have definite effects but are best combined with parent training.

3 *Individual psychotherapy* is usually unfruitful as these individuals have
little insight into why they behave the way they do, and there is no trial
evidence to support its use. Furthermore, when they can identify what
is upsetting them, they are not usually in a position to modify it or find
another way of coping. Further, there is risk that outside agencies may
believe that 'something is being done' and avoid addressing parenting
and other issues.

4 *Medication*:

   (a) When a child or adolescent has ADHD as well as a disruptive behavioural disorder, it may be appropriate to treat their restlessness
   and inattention with medication (see Chapter 5). When stimulant
   medication reduces restlessness and inattention, it may well reduce
   defiance, aggression and anti-social behaviour too. There is no
   evidence that stimulants reduce disruptive behaviour in individuals
   who do not also have ADHD.

   (b) There is some very limited evidence that neuroleptics ('antipsychotics') such as aripiprazole and risperidone, and also lithium
   may be of value for children and adolescents who have explosive
   outbursts in response to minimal provocation, and who have not
   responded to appropriate psychological management, but it is very
   rarely prescribed for this purpose, and has a wide range of potentially serious side effects.

5 *Diet*. When diet helps ADHD symptoms, it often reduces irritability too.
In the absence of ADHD, there is no reliable evidence that diet helps
conduct symptoms, although there have been one or two trials, for
example, of oils containing omega fatty acids.

Community-focused

• *Prevention programmes* are currently under evaluation. Effect sizes are
typically modest, although this may be useful for a total population.
They include selective approaches that screen whole populations at

school and offer, for example, parent training and social skills to those at risk. To date, there have been few follow-up studies of long-term effectiveness.

Continuity and outcome

1 *Forwards continuity*: 40% of children and adolescents with disruptive behavioural disorders become delinquent young adults with ongoing behaviour problems and disrupted relationships.
2 *Backwards continuity*: 90% of young adult delinquents had disruptive behavioural disorders as children.

Factors predicting outcome

1 *In the child or adolescent*: A poor outcome is predicted by early onset, a wide range and high total number of symptoms, greater severity and frequency of individual symptoms, pervasiveness across situations (home, school and other), associated hyperactivity, and callous-unemotional traits. Conversely, having only one area of problem behaviour, such as aggressiveness alone, has a good prognosis provided there are no problems in other areas, including peer relationships and educational achievements. The presence or absence of a constellation of problems is what is important.
2 *In family*: A poor outcome is predicted by parental psychiatric disorder, parental criminality, high hostility and high discord focused on the child.

Type of adult outcome

1 *Homotypic* continuity – with the symptoms remaining much the same – occurs more often in males, with continuing aggressiveness and violence, antisocial personality, alcohol and drug misuse, crime.
2 *Heterotypic* continuity – with different types of symptoms coming to predominate – occurs more often in females, with a switch to a wide range of emotional and personality disorders, with less aggressiveness and criminality.

In addition to being at greater psychiatric and forensic risk, individuals with a history of CD are also more likely to be socially impaired in adulthood, being more likely to have few, if any, educational qualifications, a poor job history and impaired social relations, for example, more marital breakdown.

Subject review

Bloomquist ML, Schnell SV. (2005) *Helping Children with Aggression and Conduct Problems*. Guilford Press, New York.

Moffitt TE, Scott S. (2008) Conduct disorders of childhood and adolescence. *In*: Rutter M *et al.* (eds) *Rutter's Child and Adolescent Psychiatry*, 5th edn. Wiley-Blackwell, Chichester, pp. 543–564.

Scott S. (2008) Parenting programs. *In*: Rutter M *et al.* (eds) *Rutter's Child and Adolescent Psychiatry*, 5th edn. Wiley-Blackwell, Chichester, pp. 1046–1061.

Further reading

Kazdin AE. (2005) *Parent Management Training*. Oxford University Press, New York.

National Institute for Health and Clinical Excellence (NICE) (2012) *Conduct Disorders and Antisocial Behaviour in Children and Young People: Recognition, Intervention and Management (Guideline)*. NICE, London.

Scott S, Dadds M. (2009) When parent training doesn't work: Theory-driven clinical strategies. *Journal of Child Psychology and Psychiatry* **50**, 1441–1450.

Scott S *et al.* (2010) Randomized controlled trial of parent groups for child antisocial behaviour targeting multiple risk factors: The SPOKES project. *Journal of Child Psychology and Psychiatry* **51**, 48–57.

Stringaris A, Goodman R. (2009) Longitudinal outcome of youth oppositionality: irritable, headstrong, and hurtful behaviors have distinctive predictions. *Journal of the American Academy of Child and Adolescent Psychiatry* **48**, 404–412.

World Health Organization. (1993) *The ICD-10 Classification of Mental and Behavioural Disorders: Diagnostic Criteria for Research*. World Health Organization, Geneva.

CHAPTER 7
Juvenile Delinquency

The definition of juvenile delinquency is legal and is not directly related to mental health. In the UK, it refers to a person between the ages of 10 and 17 who has been found guilty of an offence that would be criminal in an adult. Contrary to popular belief, more than 90% of the offences are against property rather than persons: thieving, driving away cars, breaking in, and destructive vandalism. Personal violence, drug offences and sex offences comprise less than 10%. Comparisons between official records and delinquents' self-reports and the results of victim surveys suggest that official records only cover about one-tenth of all offences committed. This discrepancy between actual and reported offences applies mainly to smaller crimes; more serious ones are reported in the majority of cases. For relatively minor offences, the chance of being caught decreases if the perpetrator is white, attends a high-achieving school, is from an orderly home and is of normal intelligence. This is not true for more serious offences – personal and demographic characteristics are closely similar whether judged from self-reports or from official records. Once caught, the chances of being charged are increased if there is a previous criminal record, if the type of offence is considered serious and if the individual is older or black. Characteristics of Young Offenders in Britain from a large survey are given in Box 7.1.

Epidemiology

Age

There is an overall peak in law-breaking in the late teens, when theft and property offences are at a maximum; violence peaks in the early twenties and there is a rapid decrease overall by the mid-twenties. One half to three-quarters of people convicted will never be convicted again, leaving a 'hard core' of around a quarter who repeat offences. The characteristics which predict repeaters are similar in kind to those which predict delinquency overall, but are more marked. Starting young is a major predictor of persistence. Thus, in the influential 'Cambridge' Longitudinal Study

Child and Adolescent Psychiatry, Third Edition. Robert Goodman and Stephen Scott.
© 2012 Robert Goodman and Stephen Scott. Published 2012 by John Wiley & Sons, Ltd.

Box 7.1 Findings from the ASSET survey of 3,395 young offender in Britain

Personal characteristics
- 82% were male and 18% were female.
- 90% were White and 10% were from minority ethnic groups.
- 31% were aged 10–14 and 69% were aged 15 and over.

Family and friends
- Only 30% of the young people were living with both their mother and their father.
- Only 55% had contact with both their mother and their father.
- Of those young people who did not live with their father, only 36% had contact with him outside of the home environment.
- 40% of the young people were assessed as associating with pro-criminal peers.
- Nearly 25% had friends who were all offenders.

Education
- 5% were currently excluded from school.
- 27% had previous permanent exclusions.
- 32% had experienced fixed-term exclusions in the last year.
- 41% were regularly truanting.
- 42% were rated as under-achieving at school.
- 25% of cases had special needs identified, of which just over 60% had a statement of SEN.

Behaviour
- 74% were considered to be impulsive and to act without thinking.
- 44% were assessed as being easily bored/having a need for excitement.
- 43% were assessed as giving in easily to pressure from others.
- 20% were considered vulnerable to harm because of the behaviour of other people, specific events or circumstances.
- 25% were vulnerable because of their own behaviour.
- 9% were considered to be at risk of self-harm or suicide (15% in the case of females).

---

carried out in inner London by West and Farrington, three-quarters of those with more than three convictions as a juvenile went on to repeated offending as a young adult.

Sex

Both in Europe and North America, male delinquents are three to ten times commoner than female delinquents, irrespective of whether this is judged from official records or self-reports. The male preponderance is most marked for aggressive offences. Some offences, most notably shoplifting, are commoner in females. There are many possible explanations for the gender differences, ranging from the biological, supported by the cross-cultural invariance and parallel gender differences in non-human primates, to the cultural, looking at which behaviours are differentially encouraged and sanctioned in boys and girls. Current evidence suggests that both biological predisposition and psychosocial factors are relevant. Thus, boys are more liable to biologically based syndromes, such as ADHD, that increase the risk of delinquency; and boys are also more likely to be accepted and praised when they display aggression, as part of a wider subculture that gives kudos for offending and violence.

Socio-economic status (SES)

There are substantial effects of SES, although many authors like to play this down as it co-varies with many other factors. The magnitude of the SES gradient is evident from UK surveys showing that the rates of juvenile delinquency were around 5% for professional and managerial families, as opposed to around 25% for unskilled manual workers' families. Self-reports confirm this trend for the more serious offences, but the ratio comes down to 2:1 for less serious ones.

Race

In the UK, both official records and victim reports suggest that African-Caribbean youths are between five and ten times more likely than their White counterparts to be involved in assault, robbery, violence and theft. This was not true for first-generation African-Caribbean immigrants 50 years ago. For other juvenile offences, the current African-Caribbean rates are around double the White rates. These Black–White differences are partly, but not totally, explained by socio-economic factors and family characteristics; decades of prejudice and harassment may also have much to answer for. At present, delinquency rates for 'Asian' youths are lower than, or equal to, White rates.

Epoch

Historical accounts seem to indicate that violent crime was very prevalent in the middle of the eighteenth century, but then declined, reaching a trough in the late nineteenth and early twentieth century, before rising again. The past 50 years have probably seen a fairly steady rise in juvenile offending. Internationally, officially reported crime rates have mostly increased by a factor of between two and six in most countries over this period, though this is partly attributable to better recording. Changes in officially recorded juvenile delinquency rates are more inconsistent, at least partly because these official rates are very sensitive to changes in policy. For example, the official delinquency rates can dramatically increase or decrease if the police switch from unrecorded warnings to recorded cautions, or vice versa. Over recent decades, the proportion of offences involving violence has stayed fairly constant at well under 10%, but the proportion of women perpetrators involved has increased from around one-tenth to around one-fifth. In the UK, use of knives and guns in violent crimes by youths has increased considerably in the last decade, although overall the rate of violent crime has been static.

Locality

There are clear neighbourhood differences in delinquency rates that cannot be entirely explained by social class or other socio-economic factors. The architectural design of buildings on estates has been shown to have some effect; the ability to keep an eye on people and the feeling of responsibility for what has been termed 'defensible space' seem important. At a broader level, the Isle of Wight/Inner London comparison found more than double the rate of conduct disorders in the inner-city area compared with a rural area, and this was mostly accounted for by psychosocial family factors, such as parental psychiatric disorder, parental criminality and family discord, with neighbourhood factors, such as poor schools, also contributing. It has been suggested that where there are stable cohesive neighbourhoods without too much change in those living there, the social network inhibits crime. The Cambridge study found that convicted juveniles who then moved out of a deprived area of inner London had a lower reconviction rate than those who stayed, even when other risk factors were controlled for.

Associated factors

Family

- *Size*. Particularly in lower socio-economic groups, there is a strong association with large family size, with the number of brothers being more influential than the number of sisters. Conversely, the delinquency rate is considerably lower among only children.
- *Income*. Low income is strongly associated with greater delinquency.
- *Criminality*. Serious juvenile offences are particularly strongly associated with a history of criminality in parents or siblings. Is this due to shared genes, shared deprivation, or social learning? Twin and adoption studies of adult recidivist criminals do suggest a substantial genetic influence. Studies of juvenile delinquency also suggest a genetic influence, but shared environmental effects generally seem equally important. There are interactional effects at play. Thus, observational studies of early adopted children show that the adoptive parents of children who had criminal birth parents use twice as much harsh and physical punishment as those of children who did not have this heritage, suggesting that child temperamental differences elicited more harmful parenting.
- *Child-rearing experiences*. Juvenile delinquency, like conduct disorder, is strongly associated with lack of caring supervision and broken homes. The emotional tone is frequently one of hostility and discord. There is often a lack of house rules, and a low level of monitoring of the child's behaviour and feelings; parents respond infrequently to either desired or deviant behaviour, so that any punishments are inconsistent and such

praising as there is, can be irregular. A lack of techniques for dealing with family crises and problems means that conflict leads to ongoing tension and disputes. Physical, emotional and sexual child abuse are not uncommon.

Individual factors

- *Behaviour*. Around 90% of recidivist delinquents were antisocial enough to meet criteria for conduct disorder in middle childhood. Thus, the notion that the majority of this persistently delinquent group were fine initially but then 'fell in with a bad crowd' in adolescence is a myth. On the other hand, the majority of one-time offenders have unremarkable earlier histories – it is indeed often part of 'a phase teenagers commonly go through'. However, repeaters who only start in adolescence do not necessarily stop in early adulthood – half continue low-level offending.
- *Intelligence*. There is a fairly strong association between lower IQ and greater delinquency. Thus, in one study, 20% of youths with an IQ of less than 90 were recidivist, as opposed to 2% of youths with an IQ of 110 or more. Self-report figures show the association between delinquency and low IQ is not simply due to brighter delinquents escaping detection. Perhaps the link between low IQ and delinquency is mediated by educational failure, poor self-esteem and frustration. Alternatively, low IQ may simply be a marker for other biological or social disadvantages. It is interesting that the link between low IQ and conduct problems has been found at as young an age as 3 years old.
- *Biology*. The general genetic contribution to adult criminality has already been mentioned. By comparison with controls, adult criminals have been shown to have less autonomic reactivity to stress, impaired passive avoidance learning, greater aggression, poorer attention skills and a greater tendency to seek thrills. Whether these characteristics are acquired or inherited is unclear. Offending is only rarely attributable to specific organic syndromes. Though EEG studies of delinquents do not show any consistent abnormalities, seriously aggressive outbursts are sometimes attributed to an 'episodic dyscontrol syndrome', perhaps linked to temporal lobe pathology and complex partial seizures. The XYY chromosome anomaly is not associated with an increase in violent crime, but does seem to be associated with an excess of petty criminality, perhaps mediated by the link with low intelligence.
- *Relationships*. Juvenile delinquents are more likely than non-delinquents to have impaired and disharmonious relationships with same-sex peers and with members of the opposite sex. The greater part of juvenile delinquency is committed with other antisocial peers, and there is abundant evidence that associating with them increases the likelihood of persistence of criminal behaviour. As discussed below, this means that intervention programmes and prisons that put antisocial youths together without very close control of what they say and do may well be actively harmful. Lifetime studies of delinquents in 1950s America showed that

marrying a non-antisocial wife led to reductions in criminal behaviour, as did service in the army.

• *Attitudes*. Do delinquents have a consistently anti-establishment set of values? Early studies suggested not, since when asked why they commit offences, young delinquents commonly mention the thrill, the relief from boredom and the satisfaction of demonstrating their prowess to peers; material gain is often not the main objective. However, studies of young offenders' moral reasoning show more egoism and less altruism; they are less able to take another person's point of view into account or think about the consequences of actions. They are also much more likely to believe that use of violence will resolve a conflict situation, and that fighting and antisocial behaviour (including heavy drug and alcohol use) gain 'respect' among their peers. Affection and respect for school, and identification with its values are less than in non-delinquent controls.

• *Personality*. There have been no consistent differences on personality measures, but recent research has indicated a subgroup with increased callousness and lack of emotional responsiveness to the plight of others. The use of the term 'personality disorder' is controversial in childhood and adolescence. Yet for all types seen in adulthood, the pattern is evident by late adolescence in the vast majority of cases. DSM-IV antisocial personality disorder (ASPD) is predominantly a behavioural description of acts carried out, such as persistent aggression and ir-responsibility; it has as a requirement that the person had conduct disorder as a youth. Between 50–80% of repeat offenders meet DSM criteria for ASPD, but only 15–30% meet criteria for psychopathy (not currently categorised as a personality disorder), who may constitute a subgroup of ASPD. Callousness, deceitfulness, shallow affect and lack of remorse characterise psychopathy, where the core deficit may be lack of interpersonal emotional responsiveness. While biological factors may predispose towards this, psychopaths have worse, more abusive childhoods than non-psychopathic offenders with ASPD.

Risk assessment

When assessing a juvenile delinquent, a usual, full psychiatric assessment should be supplemented by an assessment of the risk of dangerousness to others and to the young person themselves. Traditionally, forensic psychiatry has relied on a 'clinical wisdom' approach that has focused more on the person than their environment, more on risk to others rather than to self, and has lacked much scientific validation in terms of reliability and validity. The adage 'the pattern of past violence predicts future violence' remains true, and is indexed by the number and type of offences. Unfortunately it is only a rough guide, or, to put it another way, it predicts only a relatively small proportion of the variability of outcomes: some youths with many previous offences and risk factors do not offend again, others with fewer do. This makes reliable decisions about who needs to be detained in a secure facility difficult. There are now instruments for assessing and weighting various risk factors, for example, the Early Assessment Risk List (EARL) in North America is well validated, as is the ASSET system in the UK. The latter, for example, predicts reconviction within two years with 70% accuracy. Factors assessed are shown in Box 7.2.

Box 7.2 Factors to take into account in a risk assessment of young offenders

Index offence
- Seriousness
- Nature and quality
- Victim characteristics
- Intention and motive
- Role in offence
- Behaviour
- Attitude to offence
- Empathy for victim
- Compassion for others

Past offences
- Juvenile record
- Number of previous arrests
- Convictions for violence
- Cautions
- Self-reported offending

Past behavioural problems
- Violence
- Self-harm
- Fire-setting
- Cruelty to children
- Cruelty to animals

While society is concerned about the safety of others, it is wise to remember the high rate of self-harm in young offenders, especially when locked up, and assess this too (see Chapter 12 on deliberate self-harm and suicide). Attention should also be given to the environment the young person has come from, including protective factors such as non-deviant friends, a supportive relationship from a non-criminal adult, or skills giving self-esteem and the opportunity for constructive activity or employment. Conversely, the risks inherent in the environment, as well as the person, should be assessed, since offending behaviour also requires opportunity and stimuli, which are often less predictable. Does the young person go out at night to notorious drug spots? Do his friends inject narcotics? Are any of them HIV positive? Does he see friends outside nightclubs known for violence? Does his father come home drunk and hit him? There are a number of instruments to help assess risk, as noted above.

Management

Most effort is directed at the 25% of offenders who repeatedly break the law. There is little evidence for the effectiveness of punishments such as prison or other judicial approaches, and beliefs in 'short, sharp shocks' at one extreme and prolonged individual therapy at the other owe more to fashion and political ideology than empirical evidence. Three treatment approaches have been reasonably well evaluated and shown to be effective: (1) Functional Family Therapy; (2) Multisystemic Therapy (MST); and (3) Multidimensional Treatment Foster Care (MTFC).

1 *Functional Family Therapy*, developed by James Alexander, is the least intensive, involving an individual therapist who works with each family in their home over 10–12 weeks. It has three phases: the first is designed to motivate the family to change, the second teaches the family how to change a specific problem, and the final phase helps the family generalise their problem-solving skills. There have been six trials in the world, including two independent ones in Europe. Reoffending was reduced by 20-40%.

2 *Multisystemic Therapy (MST)*, developed by Scott Henggeler, also lasts for about three months. It is based on sound developmental research that shows that multiple factors determine serious antisocial behaviour, and that many of these are in the immediate environment of the young person. It therefore makes no sense temporarily to isolate the young person from these factors, increase the level of one of the most potent aggravating factors, and then return him to the old criminogenic surroundings that have not been changed at all. Yet this is what the current juvenile justice system does by jailing young offenders with other highly antisocial peers. MST takes the opposite tack, and instead of pouring resources into incarceration, puts them into trying to alter the environment around the youth. MST has six elements that are flexibly applied according to the needs of the young person (see Box 7.3). It has been shown in replicated studies in the USA to reduce re-offending rates by a third to a half, and to increase sociable behaviour. However, quality assurance is key, and to address this, there needs to be a team of staff to ensure adequate ongoing support and supervision of the therapists; there is good evidence that in centres where treatment fidelity is not upheld, outcomes worsen. Also the good results in the USA are helped by two factors. First, if the young person and family do not attend, the youth typically has to go straight to jail, whereas in Europe they remain in the community. This helps compliance! Secondly, management as usual, in the control arm, is usually better in countries with more public services, and, for example, a large trial in Canada and a small one in

---

Box 7.3 Elements of Multisystemic Therapy (MST)

1 Family therapy which focuses on effective communication, systematic reward and punishment systems, and taking a problem-solving approach to day-to-day conflicts.

2 Encouragement to spend more time with peers who do not have problems, and to stop seeing other delinquents.

3 Liaison with school to improve learning and homework performance, and restructure after-school hours.

4 Individual development, including assertiveness training against negative peer influences.

5 Empowerment of youths and their parents to cope with family, school, peer and neighbourhood problems. The emphasis is on promoting the family's own problem-solving abilities, not providing ready-made answers.

6 Coordination with other agencies, for example, juvenile justice, social work, mental health, education.

Sweden failed to find any superiority of MST over management as usual, though one in England did.

3 *Multidimensional Treatment Foster Care (MTFC)* was developed by Patricia Chamberlain. It is the most intensive of the three approaches and is also rooted in sound research on the causes of delinquency. Here, the young person is put into a foster home for around six months and taught life skills and kept away from antisocial peers. A tight regime gives immediate rewards for all positive behaviour and sanctions for rule breaking. This is delivered through a points system carefully tailored to the individual's needs and interests. During this time the birth family are taught skills in managing and supervising the young person. Offending rates one year after return home are again reduced by a third to a half. Parent training has also been shown to reduce offending rates, but at considerable emotional cost to staff involved.

Preventative programmes are theoretically attractive as they operate before antisocial behaviour is thoroughly ingrained. These programmes are aimed at early or middle childhood and can be at one of three levels: (1) universal interventions for all children; (2) targeted interventions for children at high risk of becoming offenders; and (3) indicated interventions aiming for the secondary prevention of offending behaviour in referred populations who already have established conduct problems. Few universal programmes have yet been evaluated, but there are promising targeted programmes for primary school-aged children that involve the following three components: (1) parent-management training; (2) reading remediation; and (3) teacher-training in classroom management techniques. Secondary prevention may well be feasible since parent-management training has been shown to reduce conduct problems in middle childhood, though it has yet to be established that this does reduce subsequent delinquency. One problem with all prevention approaches is the difficulty of enrolling those families whose children are most likely to need this help.

Subject review

Bailey S, Scott S. (2008) Juvenile delinquency. *In*: Rutter M *et al*. (eds) *Rutter's Child and Adolescent Psychiatry*, 5th edn. Wiley-Blackwell, Chichester, pp. 1106–1125.

Farrington D, Welsh B. (2009) *Saving Children from a Life of Crime: Early Risk Factors and Effective Interventions*. Oxford University Press, Oxford.

Further reading

Bailey S, Tarbuck P. (2012) *Forensic Child and Adolescent Mental Health*. Cambridge University Press, Cambridge.

Baker K *et al*. (2005) *Further Development of Asset*. Available at: http://www.yjb.gov.uk/publications/Asset.

Chamberlain P. (2003) *Treating Chronic Juvenile Offenders*. American Psychological Association, Washington, DC.

Henggeler SW *et al*. (2009) *Multisystemic Treatment of Antisocial Behaviour in Children and Adolescents*, 2nd edn. Guilford Press, New York.

Independent Commission on Youth Crime. (2010) *Time for a Fresh Start*. Available at: http://www.youthcrimecommission.org.uk.

Lipsey M. (2009) The primary factors that characterize effective interventions with juvenile offenders: A meta-analytic overview. *Victims & Offenders* **4**, 124–147.

CHAPTER 8
School Refusal

Roughly 5% of referrals to child and adolescent mental health services present with refusal to attend school associated with anxiety or misery. This presentation is labelled 'school refusal'. The term 'school phobia' is probably best avoided since refusal to go to school is not a diagnosis: it is a presenting complaint that can reflect a variety of problems in the child or adolescent – or indeed in the family or school system as a whole. It is also worth noting that school refusal is salient because we live in a society that particularly values schooling and makes it compulsory. There is no administrative or psychiatric category for 'shopping refusal' or 'weeding refusal', though there probably would be if children were expected and obliged to spend much of their time shopping or weeding the garden.

Epidemiology

School refusal peaks at three ages: on starting school; after school transfer; and in the early teens. Though many young children are reluctant to go to school, their parents are generally able to get them there anyway. 'Successful' school refusal is commoner among older schoolchildren, partly because it is harder to compel them to attend school against their will. In the Isle of Wight survey, no cases of school refusal were found among over 2,000 children aged 10 and 11 (in their last two years of primary school). When the same children were assessed at 14 and 15 years of age, there were 15 cases of school refusal (representing a prevalence of 0.7%). School refusal is equally common in boys and girls. No one socio-economic group is particularly vulnerable.

Characteristic features

The child or adolescent either refuses to go to school or sets out for school but returns home before or shortly after arriving at school. In some cases, the child or adolescent explicit says that he or she is frightened

---

Child and Adolescent Psychiatry, Third Edition. Robert Goodman and Stephen Scott.
© 2012 Robert Goodman and Stephen Scott. Published 2012 by John Wiley & Sons, Ltd.

to leave home or attend school. In other cases, school refusal assumes a 'somatic disguise' without overtly expressed fears. For example, there may be complaints of headache, stomach-ache, malaise or tachycardia before leaving for school or once at school. The absence of complaints at weekends or during school holidays is a helpful clue.

Attempts to force the school refuser to attend school are met with tears, pleading, tantrums or physical resistance. In contrast to truancy, school refusers do not make a secret of their non-attendance: the parents know where their child is, generally because their child is in or near the home.

The onset of school refusal may be abrupt, or may be gradual, with the individual expressing increasing reluctance to attend school and staying away for more and more days each week. Precipitating factors can often be identified, for example, a change of teacher, a move to a new school, the loss of a friend, or an illness. The onset is more likely to be insidious in adolescence, with a progressive withdrawal from peer group activities that were previously enjoyed. Onset or relapse of school refusal is particularly common after a period off school due to holiday or illness.

School refusal can be a manifestation of a variety of underlying family dynamics and psychiatric disorders. These underlying problems commonly result in symptoms other than the school refusal itself, and these additional symptoms provide useful clues to the nature of the school refusal. For example, a child who refuses to go to school because of separation anxiety may also refuse to go to sleep-overs or birthday parties. By contrast, a child who refuses to go to school because of fear of being bullied may be happy to go to sleep-overs or parties. An underlying depressive disorder is suggested when symptoms of misery and hopelessness persist even when there is no pressure to attend school, for example, at weekends or during school holidays. In contrast, a timid child who will attend on the few occasions when his father drives him to school, but not on most days, when it is his mother's role, may have some underlying fears compounded by having learned that his mother will give in.

Associated features

Family factors

As well as the child or adolescent's unwillingness to attend, there is often a lack of effective pressure from the parents to get their child to school and keep him or her there. In some cases this may seem justified by the marked distress experienced by their child. Often, however, it reflects some combination of three family processes:

1 *Ineffectual home organisation and discipline*. This may be apparent in a general lack of enforced house rules, and is more likely to occur if the father is absent or ineffectual.
2 *Emotional over-involvement*. For example, the mother may fail to be firm because she is anxious not to incur her child's disapproval; or she may

herself feel happier and more secure when she has her child around during the day. The child or adolescent may always have been perceived as particularly precious or vulnerable, for example, having survived a very premature birth, contrary to the doctors' expectations.

3 *Difficulty negotiating with outside agencies*. For example, the family may find it hard to liaise with the school to address bullying or academic stress, or getting help for emotional difficulties.

Intelligence and attainments

As a group, school refusers are of average intelligence and academic ability. Problems with schoolwork may be present but are not usually the main factors leading to school refusal. Objective measures of attainment level (from school tests or psychometric tests) are frequently useful, if only to reassure the individual and the family.

Personality

The school refuser may have been a rather quiet conformist who had relatively few friends and was easily 'thrown' by minor mishaps. On the other hand, the previous personality may have been unremarkable or even outgoing. There is commonly a history of previous separation difficulties when first attending nursery or school.

Family composition

Family size is irrelevant, that is, there is no over-representation of only children or children from large families. Youngest (rather than middle or eldest) children are probably at greatest risk.

Differential diagnosis

1 *Truants* stay away from school to engage in other activities without parental permission. In many schools, this is the commonest cause of non-attendance in the last year or so before adolescents are officially allowed to leave school. In most cases truants spend the day in groups, and their parents are unaware of their whereabouts. Whereas school refusal is often secondary to an emotional disorder, truancy is often linked to disruptive behavioural disorders. Unlike school refusal, therefore, truancy is associated with the predictors of a conduct disorder: male sex, social disadvantage, large family, parental criminality, marital discord, poor school attainment, inconsistent discipline and lax supervision.

2 Some children are deliberately *withheld from school by their parents*, either because the parents think school is useless or because they need their child's help. An ill mother, for example, may choose to keep one of her children at home for company or to do the housework. The distinction between withholding and school refusal is not always clear since the parents of school refusers are often anxious themselves and may collude with their child's decision to stay at home.

3 *Physical illness* is by far the commonest reason for non-attendance at school, except during the last year or so of compulsory education, when truancy rates are often high. It is not always easy to distinguish between physical illness and school refusal in a 'somatic disguise'. Being better at weekends is not an infallible guide: physical illnesses may be aggravated by school-related stresses, and most children are capable of exaggerating genuine symptoms when it suits them.

Underlying psychiatric conditions in the child

- School refusal can be the presenting complaint for children with a variety of underlying disorders, with *separation anxiety* being the commonest diagnosis, particularly among younger children. In many cases, school refusal results from the combination of: a child who does not want to separate and parents who do not insist very forcefully on school attendance, either because they are poor at imposing limits in general or because they share their child's anxieties about separation.
- In a minority of cases, school refusal arises not from anxiety about leaving home but from a *specific phobia* related to school or to the journey to and from school. There may be a specific travel phobia, a fear of bullies, of one particular teacher, or of one particular subject. Complaints about school may be a smokescreen for separation anxiety, but they should not be dismissed without investigation.
- *Depression* is particularly important as a cause of school refusal in adolescents, though different studies have generated very different prevalence estimates.
- *Psychosis* is a rare cause of adolescent school refusal.

Treatment

A behavioural 'back to school' approach is particularly likely to be successful when refusal to attend school began recently and relatively suddenly. A rapid return to full-time school is often possible once parents are persuaded that consistent firmness is in their child's best interests. With motivated parents and supportive teachers, this approach can be very effective. When the anxiety level in the school refuser or parents is particularly high, or when the child or adolescent has been out of school for a long time, a gradual desensitisation approach may be more appropriate, for example, initially visiting the school out of hours and then spending progressively longer periods at school every day.

Parents are usually already well aware of the academic and social disadvantages of their child being out of school – it is not generally necessary to rub this in and risk making the parents feel more like failures than they do already. It is more productive to empower parents to set firm boundaries and exert control over their child, while reducing over-involvement.

Once school refusal has become chronic, there are a variety of additional obstacles that need to be overcome. For example, it is harder to get back to school if you are way behind with schoolwork, if your former friends have made new friends, and if you cannot find a good explanation for why you have been away from school for so long. At the same time, extra parental attention while at home all day may be very rewarding. If the individual is to return to school, the obstacles need to be overcome, for example, by providing coaching on how to explain their absence to classmates. Overall, the balance of rewards and disincentives needs to be altered to favour school attendance rather than non-attendance.

Liaison with the school is essential. Teachers need to be as well prepared as possible to support the return to school. They may need to be backed up by social workers and psychologists working with the school. Providing home tuition during the period when the pupil is out of school is often inappropriate since it reduces the pressure on all concerned to achieve a more definitive solution and legitimises the individual spending all day at home. If return to school is delayed, attending a tutorial unit with other people of their own age is a more satisfactory interim solution. Though families often maintain that a change in school would solve the problem, this is rarely the case. Instead, the slow process of arranging a school transfer delays the implementation of a more appropriate solution. Even when school factors (such as bullying) are important, the school should generally be given a reasonable chance to overcome the problems rather than opting at once for a school transfer.

The evidence does not generally favour the use of medication for school refusal that is due to separation anxiety disorder. One possible indication for medication is the use of tricyclics for adolescents whose school refusal is associated with panic attacks. The value of medication is also uncertain when school refusal is due to depression. As discussed in Chapter 10, tricyclic antidepressants are ineffective in the treatment of childhood or teenage depression. While fluoxetine – a selective serotonin reuptake inhibitor (SSRI) – may be helpful for severe depression, a psychological treatment is generally preferable for mild or moderate depression.

In-patient treatment is sometimes appropriate when problems are so severe or entrenched that there is no response to other forms of treatment, and when the family environment actively maintains the disorder and blocks effective treatment.

Prognosis

Even though many reported studies include a disproportionate number of severe cases, the success rate for return to school is generally 70% or better. This success rate is higher when the individual is younger, when the symptoms are less severe and when intervention occurs soon after the onset. It is therefore very important to try to get the child or adolescent back to school as soon as possible. Even when return to school is successful, emotional symptoms and relationship problems commonly persist. Though most school refusers become normal adults, social relationships may be somewhat limited and around a third have persisting emotional disorders. Only a small minority develop agoraphobia or become unable to face going to work.

Subject review

Heyne D, Rollings S. (2002) *School Refusal*. John Wiley & Sons, Chichester.
Heyne D *et al.* (2004) *School Refusal in Adolescence*. No. 18 in the PACTS Series, edited by Martin Herbert. British Psychological Society, Leicester.
King NJ, Bernstein GA. (2001) School refusal in children and adolescents: A review of the past ten years. *Journal of the American Academy of Child and Adolescent Psychiatry* **40**, 197–205.

Further reading

Bernstein G *et al.* (2000) Imipramine plus cognitive-behavioral therapy in the treatment of school refusal. *Journal of the American Academy of Child and Adolescent Psychiatry* **39**, 276–283.
Egger, H *et al.* (2003) School refusal and psychiatric disorders: A community study. *Journal of the American Academy of Child and Adolescent Psychiatry* **42**, 797–807.
Heyne D *et al.* (2011) School refusal and anxiety in adolescence: Non-randomized trial of a developmentally sensitive cognitive behavioral therapy. *Journal of Anxiety Disorders* **25**, 870–878.
McCune N, Hynes J (2005) Ten year follow-up of children with school refusal. *Irish Journal of Psychological Medicine* **22**, 56–58.
Thambirajah M *et al.* (2008) *Understanding School Refusal: A Handbook for Professionals in Education, Health and Social Care*. Jessica Kingsley, London.

CHAPTER 9
Anxiety Disorders

Worries, fears and misery often cluster together, along with somatic complaints in many cases. Given the considerable overlap, children and adolescents with socially incapacitating fears, worries or misery were traditionally 'lumped' into a relatively broad-band category of emotional disorders of childhood. Over the past 15–20 years, the 'splitters' have been more influential, delineating the large number of specific anxiety and depressive disorders included in ICD-10 and DSM-IV. This attempt to increase diagnostic precision has its drawbacks. Some individuals have difficulties that do not quite match any set of operationalised diagnostic criteria, while others with broad-band symptomatology qualify for several labels simultaneously.

Epidemiology

Around 4–8% of children and adolescents have clinically significant anxiety disorders that cause substantial distress or interfere markedly with everyday life. This makes anxiety disorders the second commonest group of psychiatric disorders among children and adolescents, second only to disruptive behavioural disorders and ahead of ADHD and depressive disorders. For every child or adolescent with an anxiety disorder, there are several others in the community with multiple fears or worries, but who do not get classified as having a disorder because their symptoms do not cause them much distress or social impairment. The effects of gender and age on prevalence vary from one anxiety disorder to another.

Causation

Anxiety disorders run in families: affected parents are more likely to have affected children, and vice versa. Twin studies suggest moderate heritability, but the pattern does not point to   different genes for each anxiety

Child and Adolescent Psychiatry, Third Edition. Robert Goodman and Stephen Scott.
© 2012 Robert Goodman and Stephen Scott. Published 2012 by John Wiley & Sons, Ltd.

disorder. Instead, what is inherited seems to be a broad vulnerability to many anxiety disorders (though post-traumatic stress disorder and obsessive compulsive disorder seem to be special cases). An inherited vulnerability to a broad range of anxiety disorders may extend even further, encompassing depression and irritability as well. Shared genetic liability to depression and generalised anxiety disorder is one indication of particularly close links between these two disorders that are sometimes jointly described as 'distress disorders'. The clustering of anxiety disorders in families may reflect not just genetic effects but also parent-to-child transmission through learning and modelling.

Catastrophic but rare life events are clearly relevant to post-traumatic stress disorder. Other anxiety disorders can also be related to adverse life events, including relatively common experiences such as permanently breaking up with a best friend, going through a period of financial hardship as a result of parental unemployment, or experiencing parental separation and divorce. Children and adolescents may cope with a single such event, but develop an emotional disorder when exposed to several such events in combination or rapid succession – emphasising the importance of thinking about the cumulative impact of life experiences.

Many theories suggest that anxiety is due to experiencing threat (while depression is due to experiencing loss). According to Bowlby's influential formulation based on attachment theory (see Chapter 32), anxiety, and particularly separation anxiety, often arises from threatened or actual separations from key attachment figures (for example, when parents punish their children by threatening to send them away).

Psychodynamic theories formulate the threat in terms of intrapsychic conflicts. Classical conditioning can potentially explain the way in which previously neutral stimuli can, by association with a frightening experience, become fear-evoking in themselves. Operant conditioning theory predicts subsequent avoidance of these stimuli (thereby blocking the opportunity for natural exposure and the extinction of the fear).

Temperament also seems relevant. Prospective studies show that temperamentally shy, inhibited infants and toddlers are at increased risk of developing anxiety disorders later on.

Prognosis

Anxiety disorders are not quite as likely to persist into adult life as disruptive behavioural disorders, but they certainly cannot be dismissed as inevitably transient. Prospective studies show that a substantial minority of children and adolescents with anxiety disorders will still have at least one anxiety disorder in adult life, and others will have developed depressive disorders. Retrospective studies also show that a substantial proportion of adults with anxiety or depressive disorders have previously experienced anxiety disorders as children or adolescents.

Varieties of anxiety disorder

The three most common anxiety disorders are specific phobias, separation anxiety disorder and generalised anxiety disorder. Social anxiety disorder and panic disorder are less common, as is post-traumatic stress disorder (PTSD) (see Chapter 13).

Specific phobias

Characteristic features

Specific fears of circumscribed stimuli are very common in childhood and adolescence, with different fears peaking at different ages, for example, fear of animals peaks at age 2–4 years, fear of the dark or of imaginary creatures peaks at age 4–6, and fear of death or war is particularly common during adolescence. To be classified as a specific phobia, a fear must result either in substantial distress or in a level of avoidance that interferes significantly with the individual's everyday life. For example, a fear of dogs is common in childhood and only warrants a phobia diagnosis if the child often experiences intense and prolonged fear, or if the child's avoidance of dogs leads to marked social restriction, for example, refusal to go to the park to play, or refusal to visit friends' houses when they have dogs. The definition of a phobia in adults includes the criterion that they recognise that their fear is excessive or unreasonable. This criterion need not apply to children since they may lack the cognitive maturity to recognise the irrational nature of their own fears.

Epidemiology

Severe specific phobias affect around 1% of children and adolescents. Girls report more fears than boys at all ages, but severe specific phobias are only slightly commoner in girls. Similarly, although younger children report more fears than adolescents, severe specific phobias are only slightly commoner in children than adolescents.

Treatment

Desensitisation, contingency management and cognitive techniques are all useful. It is extremely valuable when treating younger children to recruit parents as co-therapists. For example, parents can be taught to provide graded exposure as 'homework' between formal treatment sessions, adjusting the pace of exposure to what their child can manage. Adolescents with specific phobias are better able to manage their own 'homework', but active parental involvement is usually helpful at this age too.

Course

Though mild fears are often transient, true phobias (particularly if they are severe) are more likely to be persistent and may continue into adulthood in the absence of treatment. This is a great shame since specific phobias are among the most treatable of all child and adolescent disorders. It often takes only a few hours of skilled treatment to bring about a complete and lasting cure.

Separation anxiety disorder

Anxiety about separation from parents and other major attachment figures usually emerges at around six months and remains prominent during the preschool years, subsequently waning as the child acquires the ability to keep attachment figures, and the security they provide, 'in mind' even when they are not physically present. Separation anxiety disorder is diagnosed when the intensity of separation anxiety is developmentally inappropriate and leads to substantial social incapacity, for example, refusal to go to school. ICD-10 criteria stipulate early onset (before the age of 6) whereas DSM-IV criteria are less restrictive, allowing the diagnosis to be made provided the onset occurs before the age of 18.

Causation

Constitutional factors and family environment may both be important. Styles of parental interaction that may contribute include: modelling avoidant or anxious behaviour through over-protectiveness; evoking anxiety through harsh child-rearing practices that may include threats of abandonment; and failure to soothe children effectively when they do become anxious.

Characteristic features

Affected children (and more rarely adolescents) worry unrealistically that their parents will come to harm or leave and not return. They also worry about themselves, fearing that they will get lost, be kidnapped, be admitted to hospital, or be separated from their parents as the result of some other calamity. These worries may also emerge as themes of recurrent nightmares. Affected individuals are commonly clingy even in their own home, for example, following a parent from room to room. There may be reluctance or refusal to attend school, or to sleep alone, or to sleep away from home. Separations, or the anticipation of separations, may result in pleading, tantrums and tears, or may result in purely physical complaints, for example, headaches, stomach-aches, nausea.

Epidemiology

Separation anxiety disorder affects about 1–2% of children and adolescents, being commoner in prepubertal children than adolescents, and affecting roughly equal numbers of males and females.

Treatment

Operant techniques (for example, star charts or contingency management) may be used to alter the balance of rewards and disincentives that favour clinging rather than separation. Graded exposure to increasingly more demanding separations can be useful. Cognitive therapy may have a place, teaching the child or adolescent to use coping self-statements. If separation anxiety is increased or maintained by the parents' own need to stay close to their child, by the parents' own anxieties, or by the parents' underestimation of their child's capacity for independence, then these issues can be the focus for work with the parents or with the family as a whole. Parents can be encouraged to take practical steps to make their child feel more secure, for example, providing adequate warning and explanation before going out and leaving a baby-sitter in charge. There is no convincing evidence that tricyclic antidepressants or benzodiazepines are helpful. There is limited evidence that selective serotonin reuptake inhibitors (SSRIs) provide symptomatic relief, but no evidence that this benefit persists when medication is discontinued.

Course
Some affected individuals experience a chronic low level of separation anxiety that is punctuated by episodes of exacerbated anxiety, for example, precipitated by a change of school or by illness in a parent. Over the years, anxieties about separations may be replaced by a wider range of anxieties more typical of generalised anxiety disorder. Follow up into adult life suggests a particular vulnerability to panic disorder and depression.

Generalised anxiety disorder
The adult criteria for generalised anxiety disorder in DSM-IV are slightly modified for use with children, requiring fewer somatic symptoms. Similarly, although ICD-10's criteria for generalised anxiety disorder require a relatively large number of somatic symptoms, there is an alternative set of criteria provided for use with children and adolescents, and these criteria require fewer somatic symptoms.

Characteristic features
Children and adolescents with generalised anxiety disorder are marked and persistent worriers whose anxieties are not consistently focused on any one object or situation. Typical worries focus on the future, on past behaviour, and on personal competence and appearance. To meet diagnostic criteria, worries must be present on more days than not, be hard for the individual to control, and have caused clinically significant distress or social impairment. The worries are commonly accompanied by restlessness, fatigue, irritability, poor concentration, tension, inability to relax and sleep problems. Other common symptoms are self-consciousness, need for frequent reassurance, and somatic complaints, such as headaches and stomach-aches.

Epidemiology
Roughly 1–2% of young people are affected, with substantially higher rates in adolescents than prepubertal children, and slightly higher rates in females than males. Many children with generalised anxiety disorder also fulfil the criteria for other DSM-IV and ICD-10 diagnoses, particularly relating to separation anxiety, depression and specific phobias.

Treatment

It is often possible to enlist the help of parents and teachers to reduce avoidable stresses in the young person's life. It may also be helpful to teach the young person (and perhaps the rest of the family) cognitive-behavioural strategies for managing the remaining anxieties. Selective serotonin reuptake inhibitors (SSRIs) may reduce symptoms for as long as medication is taken. For the present, the most promising long-term approach seems to be a combination of stress reduction and cognitive-behavioural work.

Course

The disorder often persists for years, and may continue into adult life, sometimes combined with depression.

Social anxiety disorder and social phobia

ICD-10 has a category called *social anxiety disorder of childhood* that has no exact counterpart in DSM-IV, though there was an equivalent category called *avoidant disorder* in DSM-III-R. What this category describes is an exaggerated and persistent version of the normal developmental phase of stranger anxiety that is commonly prominent up to the age of 30 months in ordinary children. Affected children have good social relationships with family members and other familiar individuals but show marked avoidance of contact with unfamiliar people, resulting in social impairment (for example, in peer relationships). They may remain unassertive and socially impaired into adolescence, or they may improve spontaneously. It is not clear how useful it is to think of these children as having an anxiety disorder as opposed to extremely shy personalities. In practice, many affected children also meet the criteria for other anxiety disorders, most commonly generalised anxiety disorder.

The sort of social anxiety described in the previous paragraph is clearly not exactly the same condition as *social phobia*, with the latter typically starting in the mid-teens and involving fear of public scrutiny and humiliation. Nevertheless, social phobia can arise from a background of long-standing childhood shyness and inhibition. Thus the distinction between early-onset social anxiety and later-onset social phobia may not be clear-cut. The relationship with avoidant personality disorder in adulthood is unknown.

Panic disorder

The key feature of panic disorder, which may or may not be accompanied by agoraphobia, is the presence of discrete panic attacks, at least some of which occur unexpectedly without any obvious precipitant. The peak age of onset is 15–19 years. Panic attacks are rare or non-existent in prepubertal children. During an attack, the individual experiences an intense fear of impending danger, disaster or death, accompanied by a mixture of somatic symptoms such as sweatiness, a racing heart, or hyperventilation. Treatment options include cognitive therapy and tricyclic antidepressants.

Subject review

Pine DS, Klein RG. (2008) Anxiety disorders. *In*: Rutter M *et al.* (eds) *Rutter's Child and Adolescent Psychiatry*, 5th edn. Wiley-Blackwell, Chichester, pp. 628–647.

Further reading

Barrett PM. (1998) Evaluation of cognitive-behavioural group treatments for childhood anxiety disorders. *Journal of Clinical Child Psychology* **27**, 459–468.

Biederman J *et al.* (1993) A three-year follow-up of children with and without behavioral inhibition. *Journal of the American Academy of Child and Adolescent Psychiatry* **32**, 814–821. (This examines the extent to which childhood anxiety disorders are in continuity with one of the most widely studied traits of early childhood.)

Compton SN *et al.* (2004) Cognitive-behavioral psychotherapy for anxiety and depressive disorders in children and adolescents. *Journal of the American Academy of Child and Adolescent Psychiatry* **43**, 930–959.

Lewinsohn PM *et al.* (2008) Separation anxiety disorder in childhood as a risk factor for future mental illness. *Journal of the American Academy of Child and Adolescent Psychiatry* **47**, 548–555.

CHAPTER 10
Depression

To avoid confusion, it is useful to distinguish between three distinct meanings of the term 'depression'. It can refer to:

- a single symptom;
- a symptom cluster;
- a disorder.

Depression as a single symptom

Epidemiological studies show that many children and adolescents are miserable. In the Isle of Wight studies, about 10% of 10-year-olds were miserable according to their parents, and over 40% of 14-year-olds were miserable by their own account (with almost 15% being observably sad at interview). Among children and adolescents with psychiatric disorders, the symptom of misery is commoner still (being common among those with behavioural as well as emotional disorders). It is uncertain whether the symptom of depression differs from ordinary sadness in kind or just in degree. Possible features distinguishing abnormal depression from normal sadness include greater severity, longer persistence and the individual describing the mood as qualitatively different from ordinary sadness.

Depression as a symptom cluster

Just as in adults, the symptom of depression in children and adolescents is sometimes part of a wider constellation of affective, cognitive and behavioural symptoms. Associated symptoms include: reduction or loss of ability to experience pleasure (anhedonia); low self-esteem; self-blame; guilt; helplessness; hopelessness; suicidal thoughts and acts; loss of energy; poor concentration; restlessness; and changes in appetite, weight and

Child and Adolescent Psychiatry, Third Edition. Robert Goodman and Stephen Scott.
© 2012 Robert Goodman and Stephen Scott. Published 2012 by John Wiley & Sons, Ltd.

sleep. The symptom cluster of depression is not necessarily abnormal: it can, for example, be a part of normal grief.

Depression as a disorder

When should someone with the symptom cluster of depression be described as experiencing a depressive disorder? The criteria have become less stringent over the past two decades, so that rates of diagnosed depression have risen dramatically. DSM-IV and the research version of ICD-10 both specify that symptoms must persist for at least two weeks to constitute a depressive episode, and core symptoms have to be present for most of the day for the majority of these days. Some definitions state that a disorder is only present if the depressive symptoms result in social incapacity as well as distress: an additional criterion that has the advantage of sharpening the distinction between normality and abnormality, but the disadvantage of excluding children who manage to continue with their everyday lives even though their depressive symptoms cause them much suffering. Some children and adolescents who do not meet the full diagnostic criteria for a depressive disorder do have depressive symptoms as part of a relatively undifferentiated emotional disorder that also involves symptoms of anxiety, fearfulness or obsession. Such undifferentiated disorders are common but are not well handled by the current diagnostic systems. By convention, depressive disorders are not diagnosed if an individual also meets criteria for schizophrenia.

Features of depression at different ages

Children under 5 who are separated from their attachment figures will often go through a phase of despair, but it is unclear whether this despair is equivalent to depression. From roughly the age of 8, however, some children do experience depressive disorders that are phenomenologically very similar to adult depressive disorders. This similarity enables depressive disorders to be diagnosed in children and adolescents using unmodified (or only slightly modified) adult criteria. Sleep and appetite disturbance seem less common than in adults. Guilt and hopelessness are probably less common in depressed children than in depressed adolescents and adults (perhaps reflecting the cognitive sophistication needed to experience guilt or hopelessness). The suicidal plans of depressed children are typically less lethal than the plans of depressed adolescents or adults. For example, depressed children may try to drown themselves by putting their head under water in the bath. The constellation of depressive symptoms may include refusal or reluctance to attend school, irritability, abdominal pain and headache. Indeed, somatic complaints should always be asked about;

they are probably the rule rather than the exception and they are not simply due to co-existing anxiety.

Depressive equivalents

It has been suggested that many psychiatric disorders, ranging from enuresis to behavioural disorders, are the childhood equivalents of adult depression even if the children do not appear miserable. There is no good evidence for this view, and children should not be diagnosed as depressed in the absence of clear affective symptoms.

Epidemiology

The recent British national surveys cited in Chapter 3 found that around 0.2% of 5–10-year-olds were depressed, as were around 2% of 11–15-year-olds. The rise in adolescence seems to be more closely linked to pubertal status than to chronological age. Studies that rely primarily on informants (parents and teachers) report lower rates of depression than studies that rely primarily on the self-reports of children and adolescents. The long-term significance of inner misery that is not apparent to parents and teachers is still uncertain. The female preponderance seen in adult depression is evident from middle or late adolescence. Before puberty, by contrast, the sex ratio is equal or there may even be a male preponderance. A link with social disadvantage has been suggested but the evidence is contradictory. Over recent decades, the evidence suggests that the prevalence of depression in children and adolescents has risen and the average age of onset has fallen. These trends are probably real and not just a reflection of improving recognition or less stringent diagnostic criteria.

Classification

Children and adolescents who have enough persistent symptoms of depression to meet the criteria for a depressive episode can be assigned one of several diagnoses, depending on how many episodes they have had and whether they have also had any manic, hypomanic or mixed episodes (see Chapter 11). Thus, an individual who has experienced two or more major depressive episodes but no manic, hypomanic or mixed episodes can be classified under DSM-IV as having 'major depressive disorder, recurrent'. Those with milder symptoms may meet the diagnostic criteria for dysthymia or adjustment disorder with depressed mood. Dysthymia involves chronic mild symptoms for at least one year (as opposed to the two years stipulated for adults). An adjustment disorder can be diagnosed if the symptoms occur shortly after an identifiable stressor (within one month according to ICD-10 and within three months according to DSM-IV) and do not outlast the stressor by more than six months.

Associated features

1 *Comorbidity*. Over 50% of depressed children in epidemiological samples have at least one other psychiatric disorder as well (typically an anxiety or disruptive behavioural disorder), and the rate of comorbidity is often even higher in clinic samples.
2 *Friendship difficulties* are common during depressed episodes, and may precede (and possibly precipitate) these episodes.
3 *Biological features*. A variety of neuroendocrine abnormalities such as raised cortisol levels have been described, though none are sufficiently consistent or marked to be useful diagnostic tests in everyday practice. Sleep studies do not consistently show the sorts of abnormalities described in adults (but these abnormalities are less marked in young adults too).

Differential diagnosis

1 Normal sadness, including normal bereavement reactions. It is worth noting, though, that bereavement and depression can co-exist. DSM-IV allows a depressive episode to be diagnosed if a depressive symptom cluster persists for more than two months after a major bereavement or is particularly severe, for example, with suicidal ideation, psychotic symptoms or marked functional impairment.
2 Misery can occur as just one feature of another psychiatric disorder, without the additional affective, cognitive and behavioural features needed to diagnose a true depressive disorder. But remember that just because a child or adolescent has some other disorder, this does not mean that he or she cannot have depression too.

Causation

Depression runs in families. Depressed children are more likely than children with other psychiatric disorders to have parents or siblings who are themselves depressed. Conversely, parents with depression are more likely to have depressed children. The relative importance of genetic and environmental transmission is uncertain: twin studies suggest moderate heritability, but this has not been replicated in adoption studies. There is preliminary evidence that a genetic loading for depression may sometimes act by increasing a young person's vulnerability to adverse life events – if so, this is an example of a gene–environment interaction.

Treatment

Family therapy, school liaison, and supportive individual therapy are commonly used to tackle depression by reducing stress levels. For example, if a bullied child becomes depressed, then tackling the bullying may be enough to cure the depression as well. In other cases, however, it is necessary to treat the depression itself, either because it is not possible to identify and abolish key stresses, or because the original stressor has triggered off a vicious cycle that needs to be interrupted. The best researched psychological treatments for depression are cognitive-behavioural therapy (CBT) and interpersonal therapy (IPT). These have a moderate effect size and are discussed in Chapter 40. The *cognitive restructuring* component of CBT is designed to alter negative cognitions, improve self-esteem and enhance coping skills. The equally important *behavioural activation* component is designed to increase involvement in normal and rewarding activities. Social skills training, problem solving treatment and remedial help with specific learning problems may also be offered.

The role of medication is controversial. It is clear that practically any medication, including placebo, can have a large effect – but less clear which medication performs better than placebo. Meta-analyses of controlled trials of tricyclic antidepressants suggest that they are little or no better than placebos for children and adolescents. By contrast, there is evidence that serotonin reuptake inhibitors (SSRIs), particularly fluoxetine, are better than placebos at treating child and adolescent depression (especially severe depression). Fluoxetine is the only antidepressant approved by the US Food and Drug Administration (FDA) for the treatment of depression in children. However, there are also concerns that SSRIs increase the risk of self-harm or suicide. Analyses of reported adverse effects do suggest an increase in suicidal ideation and threats, with few attempts and no completed suicides. In the light of reported levels of adverse effects with different SSRIs, the British Government guidelines do not support the use of SSRIs other than fluoxetine for depressed children or adolescents.

Given current uncertainties about the psychological and pharmacological treatments for depression, how should clinicians manage depressed children and adolescents? The best plan probably depends on the severity of the depression:

In *mild* depression, support and stress reduction are often sufficient.

In *moderate* depression, a three-step plan can be helpful:

1 Try support and stress reduction.
2 If this fails, try CBT or IPT.
3 If this fails, consider a trial of fluoxetine.

In *severe* depression, some clinicians prefer to combine stress reduction, CBT (or IPT) and perhaps fluoxetine from the outset. Others advise jumping straight to fluoxetine by itself, with some trial evidence suggesting that this can be as effective as combined pharmacological and psychological treatment (and more cost-effective). Admission to an in-patient unit is indicated when there is severe suicidality, psychotic symptoms, or refusal to eat and drink.

Except for very mild depression, it may be advisable to continue successful therapy (whether psychological or pharmacological) for about six months after symptomatic remission in order to prevent early relapse.

Pharmacological treatment of depression occurring in the context of a known bipolar disorder poses additional challenges. Treatment resistance is common, and SSRIs can trigger mania. Neuroleptics may be useful, for example, quetiapine alone, or olanzepine combined with fluoxetine. There may be a role for mood stabilisers such as lithium or carbamazepine.

While resistant depression is sometimes treated with combinations of different medications or ECT, these are techniques that should probably only be used in specialist centres.

Prognosis

1 *Likelihood of recurrence.* An adjustment disorder with depressed mood usually lasts a few months and does not typically recur. Major depressive episodes often last six to nine months and commonly recur. Dysthymia typically persists for several years; dysthymic individuals are at a high risk of major depressive episodes. Someone with 'double depression' (that is, major depressive episodes superimposed on dysthymia) is particularly likely to experience recurrent major episodes.
2 *Adult outcome.* Depression occurring in adolescence is often followed by depression in adult life, and also predicts a roughly six-fold increase in adult suicide rates. Depression occurring before puberty is less likely to lead to adult depression. Whereas 'pure' depression does not increase the risk of adult antisocial outcomes, the mixture of depression and conduct disorder is associated with higher rates of subsequent criminality.

Subject review

Brent D, Weersing VR. (2008) Depressive disorders in childhood and adolescence. *In*: Rutter M *et al.* (eds) *Rutter's Child and Adolescent Psychiatry*, 5th edn. Wiley-Blackwell, Chichester, pp. 587–612.

Further reading

Goodyer I. *et al.* (2007) Selective serotonin reuptake inhibitors (SSRIs) and routine specialist care with and without cognitive behaviour therapy in adolescents with major depression: Randomised controlled trial. *BMJ* **335**, 142–146.

Hazell P. *et al.* (1995) Efficacy of tricyclic drugs in treating child and adolescent depression: a meta-analysis. *BMJ* **310**, 897–901.

March J *et al.* (2004) Fluoxetine, cognitive-behavioral therapy, and their combination for adolescents with depression: Treatment for Adolescents With Depression Study (TADS) randomized controlled trial. *JAMA* **292**, 817–820.

CHAPTER 11
Mania

Are depression and mania the opposite ends of a single mood dimension? Just as depression can be described as 'feeling low', so mania can be described as 'feeling high'. Consequently, the simplest model of mood disorders involves each individual moving up and down a single dimension of mood that ranges from severe depression through normality ('euthymia') to hypomania and on to severe mania (see Box 11.1).

Box 11.1 A schematic one-dimensional model of mood

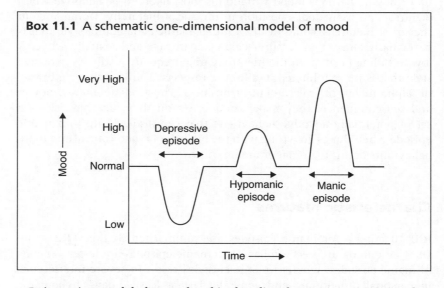

It is a nice model that makes bipolar disorder easy to envisage, but it cannot explain everything. To make things more complicated, there are also *mixed episodes* in which an individual meets the criteria for both major depression and mania almost every day for at least a week. This is challenging to plot on the graph shown in Box 11.1. It cannot simply be that the individual switches rapidly backwards and forwards between pure mania and pure depression because this could not explain how individuals in a mixed episode can display manic and depressive symptoms at the same time, for example, a simultaneous mixture of high energy and low mood.

Child and Adolescent Psychiatry, Third Edition. Robert Goodman and Stephen Scott.
© 2012 Robert Goodman and Stephen Scott. Published 2012 by John Wiley & Sons, Ltd.

How else can we conceptualise two complex mood states (depression and mania) that are normally mutually exclusive, but not always? Perhaps it is like using a car's brake and accelerator at the same time – not an adaptive thing to do, not something we normally do, but not logically impossible either. Or think about the way we spend our lives oscillating from being awake to being asleep. There are intermediate drowsy states, but we would not normally consider it possible to be fully awake and fully asleep at the same time. However, this seems to be exactly what happens in narcolepsy, a sleep disorder described in more detail in Chapter 20. Symptoms such as sleep paralysis, cataplexy and hypnagogic hallucinations reflect being completely awake while also being fully immersed in at least some aspects of dreaming (REM) sleep. Mixed affective episodes may reflect similar pathology in mood regulation, resulting in a combination of mood symptoms that would not normally occur together.

From an evolutionary perspective, it is interesting to wonder about the adaptive purpose of mood variation. When might it be adaptive to be up or down? Perhaps mood variation is most likely to be adaptive when it mirrors an individual's position in the social hierarchy. Dominance in the social hierarchy could justify a rather manic behavioural style that is particularly energetic, pleasure-seeking, aggressive and sexually active. A low or falling position in the hierarchy might equally justify a depressive style that is more inhibited in all these respects. Think of the 'big beasts' or 'alpha males' of government or business. They radiate energy, power and self-confidence, they make conquests, and they take big risks – a set of potentially adaptive behaviours that can also add up to a manic episode when things go wrong with the biology of mood control and these behaviours occur in an inappropriate context.

Characteristic features

ICD-10 criteria for manic episodes are summarised in Box 11.2 – the DSM-IV criteria are very similar. Hypomanic episodes are lesser versions of manic episodes: whereas manic episodes result in severe interference in personal functioning and generally last at least 7 days, hypomanic episodes result in less interference and only need to be present for at least 4 days. Different sorts of episodes – manic, hypomanic, mixed and major depressive episodes – are the building blocks from which bipolar disorders are made. For example, DSM-IV distinguishes between:

- *Bipolar I disorder* which refers to individuals who have experienced at least one manic or mixed episode. There may be episodes of hypomania and depression too.
- *Bipolar II disorder* which refers to individuals who have experienced at least one hypomanic episode and at least one depressive episode. They have not experienced mixed or manic episodes (or they would be classified as Bipolar I).

Box 11.2 A summary of ICD-10* criteria for a manic episode

There is a prominent episode of elevated, expansive or irritable mood that is definitely abnormal for the individual concerned and sustained for at least 7 days (or requires hospitalisation). During the episode of altered mood, at least three of the following symptoms need to have been present, leading to severe interference with personal functioning in daily living. (If the abnormal mood is irritable rather than elevated or expansive, then the minimum requirement is four rather than three symptoms.)

1 Increased purposeful activity (getting more done) or psychomotor agitation.
2 More talkative.
3 Flight of ideas or a subjective sense of accelerated thought.
4 Loss of normal social inhibitions, resulting in behaviour that is inappropriate to the circumstances.
5 Less need for sleep, for example, feeling alert and fully rested after just a few hours sleep per day.
6 Exaggerated self-esteem or grandiosity.
7 Easily distracted by small or unimportant stimuli.
8 Reckless behaviour whose risks the individual does not recognise, for example, spending sprees.
9 Marked sexual energy or sexual indiscretions.

The symptoms are not directly attributable to substance use (for example, cocaine) or a medical illness (for example, hyperthyroidism).

Note: * DSM-IV criteria are generally similar. *The ICD-10 Classification of Mental and Behavioural Disorders: Diagnostic Criteria for Research* (World Health Organization 1993).

In addition, it is worth noting that some depressed individuals experience 'rebound' hypomanic symptoms when treated with antidepressants. This alone is not enough to qualify for Bipolar II (since symptoms are directly attributable to treatment). Individuals who experience an antidepressant-induced rebound may be at increased risk for future bipolar disorder.

A manic episode can potentially be accompanied by the full range of psychotic symptoms described in Box 24.1. It is relatively easy to see that grandiose delusions – involving special powers and high status – are congruent with elevated mood and exaggerated self-esteem. It is a surprise, however, to find that mania can also involve the hard-to-understand psychotic symptoms that many psychiatrists link particularly to schizophrenia. This is potentially a diagnostic trap: a psychotic adolescent with some hard-to-understand hallucinations or delusions may be given a premature diagnosis of schizophrenia that later needs to be changed to bipolar disorder once it becomes clear that there are clear episodes of mania and depression, with good recovery in between. It is worth adding, however, that drawing a sharp distinction between schizophrenia and bipolar disorder may distort what is actually a continuum, both phenomenologically and genetically.

Classical and juvenile-specific criteria for bipolar disorder

In any discussion of bipolar disorder affecting children and adolescents, it is crucial to distinguish between 'classical criteria' for mania and hypomania, on the one hand, and controversial 'juvenile-specific criteria', on the other hand:

1 *Classical* criteria involve episodes of mania or hypomania that fully meet the official ICD-10 or DSM-IV criteria, with these criteria being applied in exactly the same way to children and adolescents as to adults.
2 *Juvenile-specific* criteria involve a wide variety of controversial semi-official or unofficial definitions of manic episodes that have been specially adjusted for use with children and adolescents. There are certainly precedents for adjusting diagnostic criteria for different age ranges. For example, although adults should only be diagnosed with obsessive-compulsive disorder if they resist their obsessions and compulsions, both ICD and DSM drop this requirement for children and adolescents. Similarly, the DSM-IV criteria for major depression in adults stipulate that depressed mood must be present, whereas irritable mood is an acceptable alternative to depressed mood in the case of children and adolescents. Thus the principle that diagnostic criteria can be adjusted for age is not controversial. What is controversial is whether such adjustment is needed in the specific instance of bipolar disorder, and if so, how it should be done. There are many opposing suggestions from different experts – the only certainty is that they cannot all be right. In the rest of this chapter, classically defined bipolar disorder is considered first, turning subsequently to the debate about bipolar disorder diagnosed on the basis of juvenile-specific criteria.

Epidemiology

In adolescence, classically defined bipolar disorder is uncommon until the late teens, with community surveys suggesting a prevalence of between 0.1% and 1% – and a fairly even gender ratio. Mania and depression are probably equally common as first episodes of bipolar disorders in adolescence, with mania being more common thereafter. Bipolar disorder that begins in childhood or adolescence rather than adulthood seems to be associated with a particularly high rate of mixed episodes and rapid cycling (i.e. four or more episodes per year).

Clinical reports make it clear that classically defined bipolar disorder does also occur in prepubertal children, but only rarely. Why might prepubertal mania be rare? Perhaps the neural substrate for going high is particularly late to mature – something that could make evolutionary sense if mania-like behaviours are usually only adaptive in dominant adults (see above).

A possible hint in that direction is that prepubertal children do not have a euphoric response when given amphetamines or related stimulants.

Causation

Bipolar disorder runs in families – mainly as a result of shared genes rather than shared environments. The heritability of bipolar disorder is around 60%. Both population and molecular genetics indicate that there is a substantial genetic overlap between bipolar disorder and schizophrenia. Whereas the average IQ is below average in schizophrenia, it is average in bipolar disorder. Indeed, there is a link with above-average school performance. A longitudinal study of almost a million Swedish 15–16-year-olds showed that excellent school grades predicted a fourfold increase in the risk of later bipolar disorder. Perhaps this reflects the potential advantages of mild mania-like symptoms such as greater energy and creativity – advantages that could explain why genes for mania persist in the population despite the devastating effects of severe bipolar disorder.

Treatment

Acute mania usually needs urgent pharmacotherapy. On the basis of the relatively limited number of relevant trials involving adolescents, plus extrapolation from the more extensive adult literature, the treatment of choice in the acute phase is usually an atypical neuroleptic such as quetiapine, olanzepine, and risperidone; lithium is second choice; and an antiepileptic drug such as carbamazepine or valproate is third choice.

In the longer term, lithium – or antiepileptic drugs such as carbamazepine, valproate or lamotrigine – can be used to reduce the risk of recurrence (see Chapter 38).

Bipolar disorder diagnosed with juvenile-specific criteria

While children and younger adolescents rarely experience classically defined manic or hypomanic episodes, it is fairly common for them to experience:

1 *Short-lived episodes of elevated mood*. These episodes mostly last minutes or hours – far less than the minimum of 4 or 7 days needed to meet ICD-10 and DSM-IV criteria for hypomania and mania respectively. Various experts have adjusted the duration requirement to classify these episodes as manic. This is achieved in a variety of ways, including: setting lower thresholds; letting the duration of brief episodes accumulate until the total meets the classical threshold; or counting x days with multiple

short episodes every day ('ultradian cycling') as an episode that had lasted x days.

2 *Chronic irritability*. The classical ICD-10 and DSM-IV definitions of mania accept irritability as an alternative to elevated or expansive mood, but specify that the altered mood must occur in distinctive episodes that clearly differ from the individual's normal state. Some assert that the requirement for episodicity (non-chronicity) can be dropped for children and adolescents. Others agree that chronic irritability is a significant problem – possibly to be included in DSM-V as *Disruptive Mood Dysregulation Disorder* – but demonstrate that it differs in so many ways from classically defined bipolar disorder that the two should not be grouped together.

Is there a case for accepting juvenile-specific criteria for bipolar disorder? On the one hand, some people say that it is in the nature of children and adolescents to get over-excited or irritable, and that there is no justification for turning these features into disorders and then treating them. On the other hand, it could be true that individuals who are going to develop a classically defined bipolar disorder as adults pass through a phase of having mania-like episodes in childhood or adolescence that do not meet classical criteria. If so, individuals who meet juvenile-specific criteria for bipolar disorder, sometimes referred to as '*pediatric bipolar disorder*', might do better in the long term if they received early treatment. Overall, the evidence is mixed and generally weak. An alternative view is that the majority with this symptom profile suffer from oppositional-defiant disorder and will do well if managed with parent training, which is likely to make them better over the long term and avoid unpleasant side-effects of medication. The well-worn phrase that "more research is needed" certainly applies here.

One thing that does seem fairly clear is that those individuals who meet juvenile-specific criteria for bipolar disorder also frequently have other disorders, particularly disruptive behavioural disorders and ADHD. This raises a further question as to whether having an externalizing disorder sometimes result in relatively brief episodes of irritability, 'clowning about' or over-excitement that look like mania without actually being mania. If that is the case, they may do best if managed with the sorts of treatment approaches for externalising disorders described in the Chapters 5 and 6. Is pediatric bipolar disorder truly on the bipolar spectrum, or is it not really bipolar at all despite its superficial similarity? The jury is still out.

In the absence of compelling research findings one way or the other, large numbers of clinicians seem to have made up their minds anyway. In many places – starting in the USA but now spreading globally – a growing number of children and adolescents are diagnosed as having pediatric bipolar disorder and many of them, including some preschool children, are then treated with mood stabilisers and neuroleptics. The evidence that this is beneficial is not compelling, while the potential for serious adverse effects is considerable. Many leading US experts have expressed grave reservations about this trend.

Subject review

Leibenluft E, Dickstein DP. (2008) Bipolar disorders in children and adolescents. In: Rutter M *et al.* (eds) *Rutter's Child and Adolescent Psychiatry*,
5th edn. Wiley-Blackwell, Chichester, pp. 613–627.

Further reading

Baroni A. *et al.* (2009) Practitioner review: The assessment of bipolar disorder in children and adolescents, *Journal of Child Psychology and Psychiatry*
50, 203–215.

Lichtenstein P. (2009) Common genetic determinants of schizophrenia
and bipolar disorder in Swedish families: A population-based study,
Lancet **373**, 234–239.

MacCabe JH *et al.* (2010) Excellent school performance at age 16 and
risk of adult bipolar disorder: National cohort study. *British Journal of
Psychiatry* **196**, 109–115.

Stringaris A *et al.* (2010) Youth meeting symptom and impairment criteria
for mania-like episodes lasting less than four days: An epidemiological
enquiry, *Journal of Child Psychology and Psychiatry* **51**, 31–38. (Classical
bipolar is rare in 8–19-year-olds. By contrast, brief episodes of mania-
like symptoms are relatively common and impairing – but it is unclear if
these are related to classical mania, or just superficially similar.)

Zammit S. (2004) A longitudinal study of premorbid IQ score and risk of
developing schizophrenia, bipolar disorder, severe depression, and other
nonaffective psychoses. *Archives of General Psychiatry* **61**, 354–360.

CHAPTER 12

Suicide and Deliberate Self-harm

Completed suicide

Epidemiology

Completed suicide is very rare under the age of 12 and becomes progressively more common thereafter, with peak rates in the elderly. In the United Kingdom, there are roughly five suicides (including definite suicides and the more common 'undetermined deaths', which are very often suicides) per million children aged 5–14 per year. The rate rises to roughly 45 suicides per million for 15–19-year-olds, which is still substantially lower than rates in older age bands. There is a male excess at all ages, partly reflecting the male predilection for violent and more lethal methods (hanging, shooting, electrocution), as opposed to the female predilection for poisoning (mostly with analgesics and antidepressants). Rates vary by country and ethnicity, for example, being higher in the USA, where the rate in Whites is about 50% higher than in Blacks. Since the mid-1990s, suicide rates in the UK and the USA have declined by around 20% in both males and females. Whether this welcome trend is due to improved treatment of teenage depression, as some have suggested, is far from certain.

What protects younger children?

Though children commonly believe that death is reversible, the claim that it is this belief that inhibits suicidal ideas or acts seems implausible. More plausible protective factors include: the relative rarity of severe depressive disorders and substance abuse problems before puberty; the lack of sufficient cognitive maturity to experience profound hopelessness or plan a successful suicide; restricted access to lethal methods; and the presence of a supportive network of relationships at home or school.

Child and Adolescent Psychiatry, Third Edition. Robert Goodman and Stephen Scott.
© 2012 Robert Goodman and Stephen Scott. Published 2012 by John Wiley & Sons, Ltd.

Background factors

1 *Disrupted home circumstances*, for example, abuse, marital discord, broken home, deaths.
2 *Family members with a psychiatric history*, mainly relating to:
   (a) alcohol and drug abuse;
   (b) depression and other emotional disorders;
   (c) suicide and self-harm.
3 *Psychiatric disorder in the individual.* Among adolescents and young adults, retrospective assessments by means of 'psychological autopsies' suggest that around 60% had some psychiatric disorder, with affective disorders being especially common in both sexes, and with substance abuse and conduct disorder also being common, especially in males. The link between depression and suicidal ideation may be mediated by lack of hope about the future. Up to half of those who kill themselves have been in contact with professionals for their mental health problems. The proportion with a psychiatric disorder is probably somewhat lower in younger teenagers, who are correspondingly more likely to be responding to a recent upset or an impending threat, for example, being left by a boy/girlfriend, or the imminent arrival of a bad school report.
4 *Models of successful or attempted suicide.* These include family, friends, and the media, particularly television.
5 *One or more previous episodes of deliberate self-harm* in about 40% of cases. In addition, many have made suicidal threats or shown suicidal behaviour in the 24 hours prior to the suicidal act.
6 *Availability of highly lethal means.* For example, guns that have not been adequately locked away are the most commonly used means in the USA, but are relatively rare means in the UK, where far fewer families possess guns.

Precipitating factors and motivation

Few adolescent suicides are carefully planned long in advance: most are impulsive responses to a precipitating stress. For younger teenagers, the commonest precipitant is a disciplinary crisis, with the individual having got into trouble with the school or the police, and the parents being about to find out. Other precipitants include problems with a psychotic parent or rows with parents, friends, or boy/girlfriend. Adolescents who are out of school at the time may be at particular risk because of lack of social support. Judging from suicide notes, the desire to escape from a recent crisis is a common motivation, with expressed anger more often being directed outwards towards other people or adverse circumstances than inwards towards the self.

Biological risk

Adoptees who kill themselves are more likely to have biological relatives who have killed themselves. This suggests that the clustering of suicides within families may be at least partly genetic. Some of this may be mediated by the known heritability of depression, substance use and other psychiatric disorders, but impulsive aggression is a heritable trait that also seems to be important. Various studies of people who have killed themselves suggest that abnormalities in serotonergic neurotransmission might have contributed to increased impulsiveness in response to stress.

Management

Where a current or former patient commits suicide this is likely to be very distressing for the family and often very unsettling for the clinical team too. There may be lot of guilt and 'if only we had . . .' talk. Families may need repeated meetings over time to begin to come to terms with an act that profoundly breaks the rules of the living and may be highly wounding for the surviving family and loved ones.

Deliberate self-harm (DSH)

DSH (attempted suicide, parasuicide) refers to any sort of deliberate non-fatal self-inflicted injury or poisoning, irrespective of the individual's motivation or desire to die. It is roughly a thousand times commoner than completed suicide in childhood or adolescence. Roughly 15–20% of adolescents in the UK and the USA report that they have considered suicide in the previous 12 months, while 3–7% have deliberately harmed themselves in the last year, of whom only a minority received medical attention as a result (with contact being much more for likely for self-poisoning than for cutting). Under the age of 12, DSH is commoner among boys than girls. The ratio reverses dramatically during the teenage years, with females predominating by at least 2:1 (much higher in clinical studies). Self-poisoning is by far the most common form of DSH, particularly among females. Rates of DSH have declined steadily since a peak in the 1980s.

Background factors

1 *Lack of supportive family relationships*. Associated with 'broken homes', placement in residential care, and family environments with low warmth, high conflict and poor communication. Conflict with parents often centres on roles, responsibilities and restriction.
2 *Family members with a psychiatric disorder*. Alcohol abuse is common in parents, particularly fathers.
3 *Most have a current or recent history of psychiatric disorders*, of which the commonest are depression, anxiety disorders, substance use disorders and disruptive behavioural disorders. However, the majority do not have a severe enduring depression.
4 *A history of physical or sexual abuse*. Children from abusing backgrounds may be particularly liable to hate themselves.
5 *School or work problems are common*. Academic attainments are typically below average, and there have commonly been problems relating to

teachers and peers. *Being bullied and bullying others are both more likely.* Unemployment is common among older teenagers.

6 *Family members, friends, or media reports may have provided models for imitation.* Contagion within adolescent units is well described. There is concern, but little hard evidence, on the role of the internet and social networking sites.

7 Roughly 10–20% have made a previous attempt.

8 Since most DSH is on the spur of the moment, *impulses* are more likely to be acted on when there is immediate access to prescribed or over-the-counter medication.

Precipitating factors

A clear precipitant in the two days before DSH can be identified in about two-thirds of cases; psychiatric disorder is more likely when there is no identifiable precipitant. In many cases, a relatively minor additional stress seems to be the 'last straw' for an individual who has been rendered vulnerable by a multiplicity of prior and concurrent adversities. Acute precipitants sometimes trigger DSH in young people who are otherwise well adjusted. The commonest precipitants are rows with family, friends, or boy/girlfriend. An episode of physical or sexual abuse may also precipitate DSH.

Motivation

At the time they harm themselves, young people commonly feel angry with someone, or feel lonely and unwanted. Worry about the future is more prominent in older teenagers. Hopelessness is prominent only in the severely depressed minority. DSH typically reflects a desire for temporary respite from distressing circumstances (functioning rather like getting drunk), or a wish to influence family and friends. It is rarely a 'cry for help' directed at professionals (which is one reason why offers of help from professionals are commonly rejected). The circumstances of the DSH do not usually suggest a serious intent to die or advanced planning. DSH is usually impulsive: roughly half of the young people have contemplated it for less than 15 minutes before carrying it out. At the other extreme, only 10–15% have thought about self-harm for more than a day.

Assessment

It is widely held that all children and adolescents who harm themselves should have a mental health and psychosocial assessment – a view that owes more to commonsense and prudence than to hard evidence that universal rather than selective assessment reduces subsequent recurrence rates or fatality. Assessment may involve a child and adolescent psychiatrist, but can equally involve a suitably trained social worker, nurse or other mental health professional. Informants can be interviewed at once, but assessment of the child or adolescent may need to wait until toxic

> **Box 12.1** Characteristics suggesting serious suicidal intent
>
> 1 Carried out in isolation.
> 2 Timed so that intervention unlikely.
> 3 Precautions taken to avoid discovery.
> 4 Preparations made in anticipation of death.
> 5 Other people informed beforehand of the individual's intention.
> 6 Extensive premeditation.
> 7 Suicide note left.
> 8 Failure to alert other people following the episode.

effects of the overdose have worn off. The assessment should cover the following areas:

1 The circumstances of the self-harm and the degree of suicidal intent (see Box 12.1).
2 Possible precipitating factors in the preceding days.
3 Predisposing factors: previous and current life circumstances, family history, models for suicidal behaviour.
4 History and mental state examination to evaluate current psychiatric state and suicide risk. Have suicidal talk or behaviour been escalating progressively?
5 Was the episode of self-harm typical of a long-standing difficulty in coping with stress or obtaining support in a more adaptive way?
6 Attitude of individual and family to professional help.

Management

Parents should be advised to lock away potentially poisonous medicines and guns, and to limit the individual's access to alcohol and drugs. When DSH is an out-of-character response to acute stress in an otherwise well-adjusted individual, referral back to the family doctor is usually all that is necessary. At the other extreme, psychiatric admission is occasionally necessary for further assessment, for treatment of a major psychiatric disorder, or because of continuing high suicide risk. Between these two extremes, people who have harmed themselves are commonly offered out-patient treatment, though many never turn up. Associated psychiatric disorders, such as depression and conduct disorder, can be treated in the normal way, as described elsewhere in this book.

As regards the self-harm itself, there is no strong evidence that any intervention makes a significant difference to recurrence rates or long-term psychosocial adjustment. Nevertheless, many clinicians feel the need to administer something. A family approach may seem indicated, though the families are usually difficult to engage or change. Some families dismiss the episode as trivial; they should be encouraged to regard the episode as a serious challenge to solve problems or reduce stresses. Brief individual therapy may be helpful, particularly if it is focused on improving the individual's capacity to solve problems and handle stresses in a more adaptive way. Occasionally this sort of crisis intervention will lead on to longer-term psychotherapy. Individuals and families are more likely to accept treatment when there is continuity of care between the assessment and treatment phases. Engagement is more likely if the initial assessment includes some time exploring what the child or adolescent would find helpful – and ideally provides an immediate advance instalment so as to make it seem worth returning.

Since selective serotonin reuptake inhibitors (SSRIs) may be prescribed when a child or adolescent has deliberately harmed themselves in the context of low mood, it is important to note two points covered in Chapter 10. Firstly, the evidence for the efficacy of SSRIs in adolescent depression is weak as far as mild or moderate depression is concerned, but is stronger for severe depression. Secondly, there is some evidence that SSRIs can increase suicidal ideation. The case for giving rather than withholding SSRIs clearly needs careful reflection.

A number of trials of preventive programmes are emerging, usually delivered in secondary schools, but so far results have been disappointing. While some show a reduction in *ideas* of self-harm, none has yet proven to reduce *acts* of self harm.

Prognosis

There are relatively few high-quality follow-up studies of young people who have harmed themselves, in large part because of the difficulties involved in tracing and recruiting subjects. One month later, the overall adjustment is generally better than at the time of DSH, but a substantial minority are still experiencing considerable adjustment problems a year later. Continuing difficulties are predicted by co-existent antisocial traits. Individuals who harm themselves during an acute crisis but who were previously well adjusted have a particularly good prognosis. Roughly 10% of young people who harm themselves do so again within the next year. Predictors of repetition include male sex, more than one previous episode of DSH, extensive family psychopathology, poor social adjustment and a psychiatric disorder (including substance abuse). Subsequent episodes may be fatal, either by design or because the individual underestimates the lethality of what was intended to be a non-fatal overdose or injury. Roughly 1% of young people who harm themselves do subsequently kill themselves, usually within the next two years. Factors that increase the risk of eventual suicide are male sex, being an older adolescent, the presence of a psychiatric disorder and use in the initial episode of active rather than passive means (for example, hanging rather than an overdose).

Subject review

Hawton K, Fortune S. (2008) Suicidal behavior and deliberate self-harm. *In*: Rutter M *et al.* (eds) *Rutter's Child and Adolescent Psychiatry*, 5th edn. Wiley-Blackwell, Chichester, pp. 648–669.

Further reading

Brent DA, Mann JJ (2005) Family genetic studies, suicide, and suicidal behavior. *American Journal of Medical Genetics Part C: Seminars in Medical Genetics* **133C**, 13–24.

Shaffer D. (1974) Suicide in childhood and early adolescence. *Journal of Child Psychology and Psychiatry* **15**, 275–291. (Though old, this is an excellent descriptive study of completed suicide in 12–14-year-olds; most other studies focus on older teenagers.)

CHAPTER 13

Stress Disorders

This chapter is primarily concerned with diagnosable disorders that arise after discrete major shocks such as being trapped in a burning building, being raped, or seeing your mother held up at gunpoint. These are the sorts of shocks that can potentially trigger a post-traumatic stress disorder. This chapter is not about the damage caused by less intense but longer-term stresses such as having a disabling illness, being bullied, or living with parents who constantly fight or suffer from serious mental disorders. These adversities and related coping processes are discussed in Chapter 34, which should be read in conjunction with this chapter.

DSM-IV and ICD-10 include three disorders that can result from discrete shocks:

1 *Post-Traumatic Stress Disorder* (PTSD) has a precisely defined symptom profile that needs to have been present for at least a month. It is a response to an event that would have distressed almost anyone. That being so, some experts question whether labelling this understandable distress as a disorder is an unwarranted medicalisation of the human condition. This is a reasonable concern but there are possible counter-arguments:

   (a) While distress after a serious shock is understandable, some of the symptoms of PTSD – such as flashbacks – are not part of normal distress.

   (b) When many individuals are exposed to the same catastrophe, some develop relatively mild self-limiting symptoms while others develop severe persistent symptoms. Thus a prolonged adverse reaction is far from inevitable.

   (c) Prolonged reactions can cause severe impairment in everyday activities.

   (d) Recovery can be hastened by the recognition of PTSD and the administration of relatively specific treatments.

2 *Acute stress disorder*, like PTSD, is triggered by an event that would have distressed almost anyone, but differs from PTSD in lasting under a month and having a slightly wider symptom profile.

Child and Adolescent Psychiatry, Third Edition. Robert Goodman and Stephen Scott.
© 2012 Robert Goodman and Stephen Scott. Published 2012 by John Wiley & Sons, Ltd.

3 *Adjustment disorder* differs from PTSD and acute stress disorder in that it involves a less severe shock and the response triggered by this shock is greater than would be expected for most people. It involves a very wide range of possible symptoms that are not marked enough to meet criteria of any specific disorder, and these symptoms may continue for up to six months after the upsetting event has ceased. Bereavement, which is not allowed to be coded as an adjustment disorder in DSM-IV, is discussed separately.

Assessment

Until the 1970s some textbooks of child and adolescent psychiatry stated that children showed few reactions to acute stress. This view was based, in part, on an approach to assessment that only gathered information from adult informants without asking children about their own experiences. It has since become clear that it is vital to carry out a careful appraisal of stressed children's emotions, cognitions and behaviour. It is often possible to get useful accounts from children as young as 3 years of age. Thus even with young children, it is important not to rely exclusively on interviewing parents and getting teacher reports.

It is now recognised that a comprehensive assessment needs to consider specific circumscribed fears and not just general fearfulness; to enquire about intrusive thoughts and images; and to ask about avoidance. Children will often reveal these when asked sympathetically, and may say they hadn't previously told their parents about these symptoms because they hadn't wanted to upset them. It is also important to consider any effect on psychosocial functioning as seen in friendships and schoolwork.

General screening measure of child and adolescent symptoms, such as the SDQ or CBCL, will pick up indications of serious problems in most children and adolescents with PTSD – but a significant minority will be missed. This is particularly a problem if the screening measure is only administered to adult informants – preoccupied and numbed children may seem particularly well behaved to teachers or parents. When filled in by the stressed children or adolescents themselves, general screening measures will usually pick up associated anxiety, misery and impact – but they cannot detect PTSD-specific symptoms because they do not ask about them. When assessing victims of severe traumas, routine screening measures clearly need to be supplemented by specific enquiries about PTSD symptoms. It is sometimes helpful to use a structured measure such as the Impact of Events Scale.

Post-traumatic stress disorder (PTSD)

PTSD was first recognised as a disorder by the American Psychiatric Association in 1980 in DSM-III. This was the result of accumulating experience with Vietnam War veterans who presented with the characteristic triad of:

intrusive thoughts of the trauma; emotional numbing and avoidance of reminders of the trauma; and physiological hyperarousal.

It was subsequently recognised that PTSD also occurred in children and adolescents in a broadly similar form, though modified criteria are needed with very young children, for example, repetitive, intrusive thoughts about the trauma may be more evident from young children's drawings and play than from anything they say. As well as occurring after experiencing or witnessing disasters and gross violence, PTSD can also occur after sexual or physical abuse, life-threatening illnesses, medical procedures and road traffic accidents. Children and adolescents also commonly witness serious domestic violence; it has been estimated, for example, that they witness 10–20% of murders (the majority of murders arise out of domestic disputes). Those in hospital with serious injuries or illnesses are also at higher risk, as are refugees from war-torn countries. Within these various groups, a substantial minority or even a majority develop PTSD. In many cases, the PTSD goes unrecognised and untreated. The first step is to recognise the PTSD. The second step is to formulate a broad management plan the not only treats the PTSD symptoms but also takes adequate account of broader difficulties in the child and family's life – a plan in which education and social services may play larger roles than health services.

Diagnostic criteria for PTSD

The criteria differ slightly between DSM-IV and ICD-10, but both stipulate that in the aftermath of an event that would have distressed almost anyone, the person (there are no specific child or adolescent criteria) experiences for at least a month symptoms in each of the following three groups:

1 The traumatic event is persistently re-experienced, leading, for example, to intrusive images, traumatic dreams, repetitive re-enactment in play, or distress at reminders.
2 There is either continued avoidance of stimuli associated with the trauma or numbing of responsiveness, as indicated by: avoidance of thoughts, feelings, locations, situations; feelings of being alone or detached, reduced interests and restricted emotional range; poor memory for important aspects of the trauma; and loss of confidence in the future, for example, leading some affected individuals to feel that they should live one day at a time and not plan ahead.
3 There are new symptoms of increased arousal. These can include: sleep disturbance; irritability; poor concentration; memory problems in learning new material and in recalling previously learned facts and skills; hypervigilance and alertness to any perceived danger; and an exaggerated startle response.

Clinical manifestations

In addition to the symptoms covered by the PTSD criteria themselves, separation difficulties are frequent and children may want to sleep with their parents. Panic attacks occur not infrequently. Increased irritability can lead to angry outbursts against family and friends. In disasters where friends or family have been killed or injured, it is common for surviving children and adolescents to experience 'survivor guilt' because they lived while others died, because of what they did to survive, or because they did not do enough to aid others.

The degree of exposure to the trauma influences the extent of symptoms, with those directly experiencing pain or coming very close to death tending to be the worst affected. There is typically marked fear and avoidance of objects or events directly connected to the trauma, and lesser fear and avoidance of tangentially related stimuli. For example, children who have been on a sinking ship are subsequently likely to have marked fears related to boats, and may also have lesser fears relating to travel by train or plane; they are no more likely than other children to fear objects or events unrelated to the disaster. While general anxiety and depression tends to wane over time, specific fears and avoidance can be remarkably persistent. The symptoms are often accompanied by ongoing physiological effects. For example, five years after an Armenian earthquake, those with symptoms of intrusive re-experiencing of the trauma still had elevated resting cortisol levels.

Moderating variables

Both in childhood and adulthood, apparently similar traumas can have extremely different effects on different individuals. In part, this may reflect differences in temperament, personality or genetic liability to specific disorders. Some cognitive attributes, such as good problem-solving skills, may also be relevant. It also seems likely from the literature on resilience that affected children and adolescents will be better able to buffer stress if they have a good relationship with at least one parent, a cohesive and harmonious family and support from a wider social network of peers and teachers. Conversely, family dysfunction, peer problems and severe social disadvantage are all likely to impair resilience. These factors are more fully discussed in Chapter 34.

Epidemiology

Community studies of older adolescents have reported that around 6–10% have experienced PTSD *at some point in their lives* (lifetime prevalence). The British survey described in Box 3.1 (Chapter 3) showed that *at the time of the survey*, roughly 0.4% of 11–15-year-olds met criteria for PTSD (point prevalence), with girls being affected twice as often as boys. A point prevalence will obviously be lower than a lifetime prevalence – but the difference between 0.4% and 10% is so great that other factors are probably also relevant, for example, variation in the sensitivity of different assessment tools.

Physiological changes

In the short term, stress leads to activation of the sympathetic nervous system (SNS) resulting in higher heart rate, arousal and alertness – the well-known 'flight or fight' response. There is also immediate activation of the hypothalamic–pituitary–adrenal (HPA) axis, leading to an outpouring of cortisol into the bloodstream. In the longer term, the SPS remains hypersensitive, responding more vigorously than normal to further stressors. The long-term effect on the HPA seems more complex, with generally below-normal blood cortisol levels (reflecting down-regulation as a result of chronic over-stimulation), plus a tendency to over-secrete cortisol in response to new stressors.

Treatment

Many traumatised children and adolescents have never had the opportunity to talk freely about their experiences to a sympathetic and informed adult. They may have feared that they were going mad when they began to experience intrusive thoughts, and may have been very frightened by what seemed to them to be inexplicable panic attacks. Hearing that these are normal responses to abnormal experiences can help such children and adolescents to make sense of their world and so begin to be reassured.

Parents and teachers may also need to be helped to acknowledge what has happened and comfort the affected individual. When adults feel that the trauma and its aftermath should not be talked about 'so as not to make things worse', or because they are frightened about what they might hear, children and adolescents often read the signs and keep obligingly quiet.

Cognitive-behavioural therapy (CBT) approaches have been effective for adults with CBT, and there are some randomised controlled trials showing the same for children and adolescents. Current cognitive models of PTSD suggest that trauma memories differ from ordinary memories in being *situationally accessible* (triggered by trauma-related reminders and then re-experienced in the present in a vivid but fragmentary way) rather than *verbally accessible* (deliberately retrieved from memory, more coherent, less vivid, more clearly part of the past). Part of the therapeutic challenge is to shift the balance towards verbally accessible memories that can then be worked through. It is also important to tackle children and adolescents' fears that experiencing situationally accessible memories shows that they are going mad, or that the immediacy of these memories means that the world continues to be very dangerous or that their life has been ruined forever. Attempts to suppress intrusive thoughts and images make things worse. So too may rumination. At a practical level, triggers for anxiety attacks can be identified and then addressed by teaching relaxation and other anxiety-reducing techniques. These can then be followed by graded exposure to the distressing scene; exposure generally needs to be vivid and long to overcome avoidance. Other cognitive techniques include challenging maladaptive thoughts and using guided imagery to gain mastery over distressing feelings. Group discussions with fellow victims and their parents can be helpful, but need to go beyond the expression of feelings (which may only renew anxiety) and take a more therapeutic approach.

Narrative exposure therapy is a relatively brief treatment for survivors of multiple traumas. Based on the principles of cognitive-behavioural exposure therapy, it was developed for use in low-resource countries affected by crises and conflict. Intensively trained local lay therapists work with individuals to recreate a detailed narrative of their whole life from birth up to the present situation, particularly focusing on obtaining detailed reports of the traumatic experiences. The aims are to habituate the exaggerated emotional response to trauma-related reminders and to build up a non-fragmented autobiographical memory. Initial data from randomised controlled trials are encouraging. For example, an 8-session treatment by local lay therapists resulted in substantially greater reduction in PTSD symptoms among former child soldiers in Uganda than did either of two control conditions: being on a waiting list; or an academic catch-up program with elements of supportive counselling.

Eye movement desensitisation and reprocessing (EMDR) is a method developed in the early 1990s in which affected individuals are asked to conjure up an image of the traumatic event while simultaneously moving their eyes to follow the therapist's hand, which travels widely across the visual fields. Unlike cognitive-behavioural approaches, few verbal interventions or interpretations are offered. In some cases, the images lose their anxiety-provoking qualities and substantial improvement is seen. In adults, the effectiveness of EMDR has been convincingly demonstrated – the evidence that it works in children and adolescents is less conclusive, but it is widely used in clinical practice.

Difficulty getting to sleep may be helped by simple techniques such as listening to a music or story tape when in bed to help banish unpleasant intrusive thoughts. Bad dreams can be retold during the day with the affected individual giving them a happy ending. In addition to treating the specific symptoms of PTSD, it may be necessary to address wider issues. For example, when children have lost their parents in the disaster, it may be vital to help them and their new caregivers adjust to one another's needs. They may need help to distinguish grief from fear aroused by the incident.

Prevention

Prevention of PTSD through debriefing early (within a fortnight) after a traumatic event is controversial since in adults several randomised controlled trials have been carried out and these do not show unequivocal benefit, and some suggest that early debriefing may be harmful. It could be that focusing early on symptoms interrupts normal healthy processing. However, leaflets that alert young people and their parents to possible emotional sequelae are likely to be helpful and are increasingly available from charities such as the Child Accident Prevention Trust.

Acute stress disorder

This diagnosis is applied when a range of symptoms are present for at least two days, but under a month, following a traumatic event that involved or threatened death or severe injury. The reaction has to include intense fear, helplessness or horror. In addition to the type of re-experiencing, avoidance, and arousal symptoms seen in PTSD, dissociative symptoms are present, such as emotional numbness, reduced awareness of surroundings ('being in a daze'), derealisation, depersonalisation, denial or amnesia. There are few studies of Acute Stress Reactions in childhood. The symptoms tend to be seen as likely precursors of PTSD and handled accordingly.

Adjustment disorder

This term is used to denote a wide range of symptoms that do not meet full criteria for any other disorder, but that appear to be excessive in relation to how upsetting the event was. Impairment is an important criterion in making the diagnosis. Although symptoms characteristic of most common disorders can occur, the commonest presentations are with depression alone, or with a mixture of anxiety and depression; children and adolescents who suffer adverse life events are about five times more likely to suffer from these disorders. Excessive reactions to acute stress are far commoner when the individual is already experiencing several ongoing adversities – they are 'the straw that broke the camel's back'. Underlying mechanisms are more fully discussed in Chapter 34.

Treatment should help the individual understand and cope with the stress. In addition, it is often important to attempt to reduce the ongoing adversities, for example, by pointing parents towards couple therapy to reduce their discord, contacting teachers to tackle bullying, and encouraging moving out of a dangerous area. Promoting protective factors can help considerably, for example, by encouraging a child to join a sports team or a dance class so that skills, self- confidence and positive peer relations can be fostered.

Bereavement

Three main stages of grief in children were described by writers such as Anna Freud and John Bowlby; empirical observations have broadly confirmed these. First, there is an initial crisis response with shock, denial and disbelief, emotional numbness and feelings of detachment; thoughts and behaviour are mainly directed towards the lost one. Emotional disorganisation follows, with sadness and crying, anger and resentment, feelings of despair, disappointment, hopelessness and worthlessness, poor sleep and appetite, and sometimes guilt or self-blame. Adjustment to the loss is eventually evident in reduced anxiety, increased enjoyment of life, greater engagement in everyday activities and the formation of new attachments. These stages merge into each other and may co-exist. The rate of progress from one stage to another is very variable, and transitions are not irreversible – the child may temporarily go back a stage when stressed again.

As a group, bereaved children have higher rates of psychopathology than control children for the year following the loss. In a sense, bereavement reactions are an inevitable corollary of attachment relationships. However, when there are long-term harmful sequelae, they usually arise not because of the psychological impact of the loss, but because there has also been disruption of good quality emotional and general care, loss of activities, change of schooling, poorer living conditions, and so on. Psychiatric assessment may be indicated where children are under 10 years old, have intellectual disabilities, have suffered previous losses, where there is a personal or family history of psychiatric disorder, where death is sudden or otherwise traumatic, where there are multiple adversities; and where the surviving parent is failing in the care of their child. Intervention includes supporting the parent to look after their child sensitively, and helping the child or adolescent to understand the loss, visit the grave and mark anniversaries, thus sharing the mourning. Trials of such interventions show they reduce psychopathology and improve functioning.

Subject review

Black D. (2002) Bereavement. In: Rutter M, Taylor E (eds) *Child and Adolescent Psychiatry*. 4th edn. Blackwell Science, Oxford, pp. 299–308. (This masterly summary has no equivalent in the 5th edition and is still well worth reading for its clinical wisdom.)

Yule W, Smith P. (2008) Post-traumatic stress disorder. *In*: Rutter M *et al.* (eds) *Rutter's Child and Adolescent Psychiatry*, 5th edn. Wiley-Blackwell, Chichester, pp. 686–697.

Further reading

Ertl V *et al.* (2011) Community-implemented trauma therapy for former child soldiers in Northern Uganda: A randomized controlled trial. *JAMA* **306**, 503–512.

King NJ *et al.* (2000) Treating sexually abused children with post-traumatic stress symptoms: A randomised clinical trial. *Journal of the American Academy of Child and Adolescent Psychiatry* **39**, 1347–1355.

Smith P *et al.* (2009) *Post Traumatic Stress Disorder*. Routledge, London. (In series on CBT with Children, Adolescents and Families.)

Yule W *et al.* (2000) The long-term psychological effects of a disaster experienced in adolescence. *Journal of Child Psychology and Psychiatry* **41**, 503–511.

CHAPTER 14
Obsessive-compulsive Disorder

Psychiatrists have long been aware that children and adolescents some-times develop troublesome and distressing rituals and ruminations, but until about 30 years ago these were generally considered relatively non-specific symptoms of broad-band emotional disorders. It has since become clear that obsessive-compulsive disorder (OCD) is a relatively distinct sub-group of the emotional disorders in terms of symptomatology, aetiology, treatment and prognosis.

Epidemiology

Roughly a third to a half of adults with OCD have their first symptoms before the age of 15. Epidemiological studies suggest a prevalence of about 0.5%–2% in adolescents. The prevalence is lower in prepubertal children, but typical OCD can occur in children aged 7 or even younger. Males and females are equally commonly affected from adolescence onwards, but males predominate in prepubertal OCD.

Characteristic features

Obsessions are unwanted repetitive or intrusive thoughts. Compulsions are unnecessary repetitive behaviours (or mental activities, such as count-ing). There are surprisingly few differences between the symptoms of a 5-year-old and a 25-year-old with OCD. The most common compulsions involve washing, cleaning, repeating, checking and touching. The most common obsessions focus on contamination, disasters, and symmetry, often have aggressive or sexual themes, and religious obsessions are prominent in some cultures. Most children and adolescents with OCD have both obsessions and compulsions; some have just compulsions; and relatively few have just obsessions. Although resistance to obsessions and compulsions is a diagnostic requirement for adult OCD, both ICD and DSM recognise that this resistance is not always present in children or

Child and Adolescent Psychiatry, Third Edition. Robert Goodman and Stephen Scott.
© 2012 Robert Goodman and Stephen Scott. Published 2012 by John Wiley & Sons, Ltd.

adolescents. It is common for those affected to go to great lengths to hide their symptoms from parents, peers and professionals because of their concern that their symptoms will seem peculiar or 'mad' to others. This is probably one reason why mental health services see children and adolescents with OCD less often than would be expected from the disorder's prevalence in the community.

Associated features

Comorbid anxiety and depressive disorders are common and may be secondary to the OCD. Sometimes it is the anxiety or depression that leads to psychiatric referral and the child or adolescent may not disclose the 'shameful' obsessive-compulsive symptoms unless specific inquiry is made. Parents and siblings may be drawn into rituals and demands for reassurance. About 10% have premorbid obsessive personality. There is no premorbid excess of bedtime rituals, and children and adolescents with OCD can generally distinguish clearly between their obsessive-compulsive symptoms and their ordinary rituals and superstitions.

Differential diagnosis

1 *Normal development.* Bedtime rituals often peak at 2–3 years and rarely persist much beyond 8 years. Rule-bound play increases from 5 years. Collecting often begins around 7. Adolescent 'obsessions' such as with a particular sport or pop idol are culturally sanctioned and aid peer integration. OCD has some resemblance to normal rituals, with a bedtime peak and some common themes, for example, counting and putting things in order. OCD also differs from normal rituals: there is no age trend in OCD rituals, and symptoms interfere with, rather than enhance, socialisation and the growth of independence.
2 *Primary depressive disorders* can result in secondary obsessive-compulsive symptoms. It is important to take a careful history to determine whether depressive symptoms started first.
3 *Undifferentiated emotional disorders.* Children and adolescents (like adults) may present with relatively undifferentiated emotional disorders in which mild obsessive-compulsive symptoms are mixed with fears, worries and misery, with no one element predominating.
4 *Autistic spectrum disorders.* The ritualistic and repetitive behaviours characteristic of autistic spectrum disorders differ in several respects from those seen in OCD:
   (a) They are accompanied by other autistic impairments in communication and social interaction.
   (b) They are often simpler than OCD rituals.
   (c) They are not seen as unwelcome, distressing or alien (ego-dystonic).

However, it is important to remember that children and adolescents with autistic spectrum disorders do sometimes develop an additional OCD that may respond well to behavioural therapy or medication.

5 *Schizophrenia* can be accompanied by obsessions and compulsions. It is important to clarify if an 'obsession' is actually a voice, and if a 'compulsion' is actually a response to a command.

6 *Anorexia nervosa* has obsessive-compulsive qualities relating to food and exercise, but these do not automatically warrant an additional OCD diagnosis. Conversely, OCD may involve avoidance of 'contaminated' food, or compulsive exercising, but this does not warrant a comorbid diagnosis of anorexia nervosa if the child or adolescent has a realistic body image. In some instances, though, OCD and eating disorders do genuinely co-exist.

7 *Tourette syndrome* is commonly accompanied by obsessive-compulsive features, sometimes amounting to OCD (see Chapter 15). Complex tics preceded by an 'urge' are arguably compulsions by a different name. Since family studies suggest that the same genes may increase liability to both tics and OCD, it is less surprising that the phenomenology of tics and OCD also overlaps.

Causation

The disorder often emerges insidiously without any evident precipitant. Even when parents or young people can identify a precipitant, the response is generally disproportionate to the initiating stress. It is likely that constitutional vulnerability is important in many cases. Despite an earlier enthusiasm for psychodynamic explanations, current theories emphasise biological and behavioural explanations. Judging from neurological and neuroimaging studies, OCD involves structural or functional abnormalities affecting the basal ganglia, frontal lobe regions (orbitofrontal and anterior cingulate) and thalamus. From an ethological perspective, compulsions can perhaps be seen as fixed action patterns related to grooming and cleaning that have escaped suppression by 'higher centres' and taken on a life of their own. Once initiated, rituals may persist because of their anxiety-reducing effects.

A positive family history of OCD is fairly common, and twin studies suggest a heritability of around 50%. Several studies support the involvement of a candidate gene (SLC1A1) involved in glutamatergic neurotransmission (which plays a part in cortico-striate connections). Tic disorders and OCD may cluster in the same families, suggesting that these disorders may sometimes reflect the same underlying gene or genes (see Chapter 15). There may be other genes that predispose to OCD but not to tic disorders.

In some instances, OCD has a sudden onset accompanied by other acute symptoms such as tics, emotional lability, disruptive behaviour, attentional difficulties, depression, and sleep disturbance. These are sometimes referred to as childhood acute neuropsychiatric symptoms (CANS) and may have many possible causes. One possible cause that has generated particular interest is a streptococcal infection that initiates an autoimmune response that damages the individual's own basal ganglia – a condition often referred to as PANDAS (**P**aediatric **A**utoimmune **N**europsychiatric **D**isorders **A**ssociated with **S**treptococcal infections). Though PANDAS is a relatively new label and the source of some controversy, the association between post-streptococcal conditions and obsessive-compulsive symptoms has long been recognised in Sydenham chorea, the neurological manifestation of rheumatic fever.

Treatment

Given widespread misunderstanding of OCD, it is vital to educate affected individuals – along with their parents, teachers and classmates – about the disorder. As regards specific therapy, both cognitive-behavioural therapy and medication can be very effective in children and adolescents.

Psychological management of compulsions often begins with an initial period of diary keeping. The child or adolescent then helps to draw up a hierarchy of compulsions, ranging from the easiest to tackle to the hardest (most anxiety-provoking). Starting with the easiest, the affected individual is encouraged and helped to avoid carrying out the compulsion. When all goes well, this 'exposure with response prevention' only leads to a temporary surge of anxiety, followed by a more lasting reduction in the compulsive drive. Obsessions that have no obvious behavioural accompaniment (ruminations) may be harder to tackle using behavioural approaches, but can usually be treated in the same way as there is almost always an associated avoidance, even if there is no clear compulsion. Family work can be particularly helpful when family members are being drawn into the rituals.

Medication has an important role in many cases, whether as an adjunct or an alternative to psychological approaches. Selective serotonin reuptake inhibitors (SSRIs) or clomipramine are particularly effective, and are generally well tolerated even by children as young as 6 years old. They should be started at low doses and slowly titrated upwards. Long-term maintenance medication may be needed, particularly if previous discontinuation has led to relapses despite adequate psychological therapy directed to relapse prevention. Immunotherapy, including plasma exchange, has been used to treat acute-onset OCD after a streptococcal infection; though some dramatic responses have been reported, it is still too early to recommend this as standard treatment.

Prognosis

Unlike some other emotional disorders of childhood and adolescence, OCD seems to be remarkably persistent; even years later, only a minority have recovered fully without treatment. Even with optimal treatment, a substantial number of affected individuals continue to have OCD or at least some troublesome symptoms.

Subject review

Rapoport J, Shaw P. (2008) Obsessive-compulsive disorder. *In*: Rutter M *et al.* (eds) *Rutter's Child and Adolescent Psychiatry*, 5th edn. Wiley-Blackwell, Chichester, pp. 698–718.

Further reading

Bolton D *et al.* (2011) Randomised controlled trial of full and brief cognitive-behaviour therapy and wait-list for paediatric obsessive-compulsive disorder. *Journal of Child Psychology and Psychiatry* **52**, 1261–1268.

Kreb G, Heyman I. (2010) Treatment-resistant obsessive compulsive disorder in young people: Assessment and treatment strategies. *Child and Adolescent Mental Health* **15**, 2–11.

Nakatani E. *et al.* (2011) Children with very early onset obsessive-compulsive disorder: clinical features and treatment outcome. *Journal of Child Psychology and Psychiatry* **52**, 1251–1260.

Singer HS *et al.* (2012) Moving from PANDAS to CANS. *Journal of Pediatrics* **160**, 725–731.

Swedo SE, Grant PJ. (2005) PANDAS: A model for human autoimmune disease. *Journal of Child Psychology and Psychiatry* **46**, 227–234.

Walitza S *et al.* (2010) Genetics of early-onset obsessive–compulsive disorder. *European Child and Adolescent Psychiatry* **19**, 227–235.

CHAPTER 15

Tourette Syndrome and Other Tic Disorders

Tics are sudden, repetitive, stereotyped movements (motor tics) or utterances (phonic or vocal tics). They are either involuntary or partly voluntary in response to a premonitory 'urge'. Simple motor tics (such as blinks, grimaces or shrugs) and simple phonic tics (such as grunts, sniffs or barks) are clearly purposeless. Complex motor tics (such as brushing hair back, spinning round, touching things) and complex phonic tics (such as words or phrases) may seem more purposeful but are out of context. Tics commonly occur in bouts and characteristically vary in intensity from week to week and from month to month. They can briefly be suppressed, are often better during sleep or an absorbing activity, and usually worsen with either stress or relaxation. The stress of being teased or stared at because of tics can make the tics worse, setting up a vicious cycle.

Classification

While tics can be transient and all of the same type, Tourette syndrome involves chronic motor and vocal tics: more than one type of motor tic plus at least one type of phonic tic, lasting for over a year and starting before 21 years of age. Other disorders recognised by DSM-IV and ICD-10 are 'chronic motor or vocal tic disorder' and 'transient tic disorder'.

Most child and adolescent psychiatric disorders can only be diagnosed when the characteristic symptoms result in significant distress or social impairment – a useful way of distinguishing between normal variation and disorders likely to require clinical services. The 'distress or impairment' requirement was present in the DSM-IV definition of tic disorders but is absent from both DSM-IV-R and ICD-10. A disadvantage of this omission is that many individuals can be diagnosed as having tic disorders even though they have no need for services.

Child and Adolescent Psychiatry, Third Edition. Robert Goodman and Stephen Scott.
© 2012 Robert Goodman and Stephen Scott. Published 2012 by John Wiley & Sons, Ltd.

Epidemiology

Most estimates of the prevalence of Tourette syndrome are in the region of 3–10 per 10,000 children and adolescents – but some estimates are much higher. The ratio of males to females is at least 3:1. Chronic motor tics are probably at least three times commoner than Tourette syndrome. Transient tics are much commoner still, reportedly affecting up to 4–16% of young people at some stage (but these rates are based on parent reports and may be overestimates due to misidentification).

Characteristic features

The average age of onset of motor tics is 7 years, with onset being rare before two or after 15. The commonest motor tics are simple motor tics involving eyes, face, head or neck. Complex motor tics are rarer and emerge later. Phonic tics usually start a year or two after motor tics. Simple phonic tics are commoner than complex phonic tics. Complex phonic tics involving obscene speech (coprolalia) only occur in a minority, starting about four to eight years after onset. It is a mistake, therefore, to rule out the diagnosis of Tourette syndrome on the basis that the famous symptom of coprolalia is absent. Echoed speech (echolalia), echoed actions (echopraxia), and obscene actions or gestures (copropraxia) may also occur.

Associated features

1 Obsessive-compulsive symptoms (sometimes amounting to an obsessive compulsive disorder (OCD)) occur in a third to two-thirds of individuals with Tourette syndrome, particularly among older subjects. 'Evening up', counting and ritualistic touching are particularly common, though the checking and contamination concerns of 'ordinary' OCD may also occur.

2 Inattention and hyperactivity symptoms (sometimes amounting to ADHD) occur in 25–50%, typically emerging before the onset of tics themselves. It is probably comorbid ADHD rather than the presence of tics per se that best predicts difficulties with behaviour, peer relationships and learning.

3 Many other less common associations have been described, including self-injury, failure to inhibit aggression, sleep problems, affective disorders, anxiety disorders, schizotypal personality, intellectual disability, specific learning difficulties and autistic spectrum disorders.

Differential diagnosis

1 Other dyskinesias may resemble simple tics, but they all differ from tics in some respects (for example, not increased by relaxation).

2 The stereotypies that are commonly seen in severe intellectual disability and autistic spectrum disorders may look like complex motor tics, but it is very rare to have complex tics without some simple tics too.

3 Compulsions cannot clearly be distinguished from complex tics preceded by 'urges', but the latter are nearly always accompanied by simple tics too.

Causation

Tourette syndrome, chronic tics and OCD often run together in families: male relatives are more likely to have tic disorders than OCD, while the reverse is true for female relatives. Not much progress has yet been made in identifying the relevant genes at a molecular level, but ongoing genome-wide searches may be more successful. Neuroimaging and neuropathology studies have provided suggestive evidence for an imbalance between the direct (excitatory) and indirect (inhibitory) pathways within the cortico-striato-thalamo-cortical circuits.

While there is strong evidence for the involvement of striatal dopaminergic systems in Tourette syndrome, there is less consistent support for specific hypotheses linking tics to an excess of dopamine or increased sensitivity of dopamine D2 receptors. In addition, there are many plausible but unproven theories linking tics to imbalance in other neurotransmitter systems, including cholinergic, noradrenergic, serotonergic, glutaminergic or GABAergic systems.

Streptococcal infections have been associated with some cases of sudden-onset tic disorders accompanied by other acute neuropsychiatric symptoms such as obsessions, compulsions, emotional lability, disruptive behaviour, attentional difficulties, depression, and sleep disturbance. This has been designated PANDAS syndrome (**P**aediatric **A**utoimmune **N**europsychiatric **D**isorders **A**ssociated with **S**treptococcal infections) and is described in more detail in Chapter 14.

Treatment

It is essential to explain to everyone involved – the affected family and school as well as the affected individual – that Tourette syndrome is a medical disorder. It is not deliberate disruptiveness or possession by evil spirits. Mild tics may need no specific treatment. There is increasing evidence that psychological treatments such as habit reversal may help some children and adolescents. This may be an appropriate first line of treatment for individuals with relatively mild tic disorders. It may also be appropriate for individuals with more severe tic disorders who are strongly motivated to try psychological approaches before considering medication.

The best established pharmacological approach to treating tics involves neuroleptics, a family of drugs that are also sometimes described as 'antipsychotics' – an unfortunate name that could potentially give families the misleading impression that tics are somehow psychotic. Neuroleptics can generally reduce tic severity by about two-thirds, although sometimes at a price. Complete abolition of tics is often not possible without pushing neuroleptics to levels that result in unacceptable side effects. Historically, haloperidol and pimozide have been the most widely used *typical* neuroleptics, but concerns about adverse effects such as extra-pyramidal symptoms have prompted some to switch to *atypical* neuroleptics such as risperidone – though atypicals can have different but equally important adverse effects of their own, including rapid weight gain and its metabolic complications. The dosage needs to be titrated against clinical need in order to ensure that the child or adolescent is always treated with the lowest possible dose compatible with adequate (rather than total) tic control. Clonidine or guanfacine can be used instead of neuroleptics: they cause fewer adverse effects, but their corresponding disadvantage is lower efficacy – tic severity is generally reduced by about one-third instead of two-thirds.

Associated obsessions and compulsions may be helped by behaviour therapy or medication: usually a selective serotonin reuptake inhibitor (SSRI) or clomipramine, augmented, if necessary, by a neuroleptic. When a child or adolescent with a tic disorder also has a significant problem with inattention and restlessness, the use of stimulants is controversial since they may aggravate tics. However, several large trials of children with ADHD and tics have shown on average that tics do not worsen, and stimulants remain the most effective treatment for ADHD. Alternatives to stimulants include clonidine, atomoxetine, guanfacine, buproprion and tricyclics such as desipramine.

Prognosis of Tourette syndrome

Complete or partial resolution is common in late teens or early twenties. Tourette syndrome may persist throughout adulthood, but if it does, the severity gradually wanes.

Subject review

Leckman JF, Bloch MH. (2008) Tic disorders. *In*: Rutter M *et al*. (eds) *Rutter's Child and Adolescent Psychiatry*, 5th edn. Wiley-Blackwell, Chichester, pp. 719–736.

Further reading

Bloch MH *et al*. (2009) Meta-analysis: Treatment of attention-deficit/hyperactivity disorder in children with comorbid tic disorders.

Journal of the American Academy of Child and Adolescent Psychiatry **48**, 884–893.

Piacentini J *et al.* (2010) Behavior therapy for children with Tourette disorder: A randomized controlled trial. *JAMA* **303**, 1929–1937.

Roessner V *et al.* (2011) European clinical guidelines for Tourette syndrome and other tic disorders. Part II: Pharmacological treatment. *European Child and Adolescent Psychiatry* **20**, 173–196.

CHAPTER 16
Selective Mutism

Selective mutism affects children and generally resolves well before adolescence. Children with selective mutism are able to understand what other people say, but restrict their own speech to a small group of very familiar people in specific circumstances. Typically, the child talks freely to parents and siblings at home, but does not speak to classmates or teachers at school. Much more rarely, the child speaks at school but not at home. Mutism usually develops at about 3–5 years of age. However, it does not usually lead to specialist referral while the child is at playgroup; referral is more often made after the start of formal schooling. Many clinicians only make the diagnosis if the period of mutism exceeds six months, though DSM-IV and ICD-10 only stipulate a period of one month (not counting the first month at school).

Epidemiology

Refusal to speak at school is relatively common during the first few months after school entry, affecting almost 1% of children in one study (with higher rates among the children of immigrants). These problems are nearly all short-lived. By the age of 6 or 7, the reported rates range from 3–18 per 10,000 (roughly a tenth as common as autistic spectrum disorders). Whereas boys are more prone than girls to developmental language disorders, selective mutism is probably more common in girls. There is no clear association with socio-economic status, family size, or birth order.

Associated features

1 *Other psychiatric problems.* Increased rates of anxiety, depression, enuresis, encopresis, hyperactivity and tics have all been described. Recent studies have particularly emphasised the high rate of social anxiety, with

---

Child and Adolescent Psychiatry, Third Edition. Robert Goodman and Stephen Scott.
© 2012 Robert Goodman and Stephen Scott. Published 2012 by John Wiley & Sons, Ltd.

most children meeting diagnostic criteria for social phobia (DSM-IV) or social anxiety disorder of childhood (ICD-10). Indeed, some argue that selective mutism should be seen simply as a symptom of a social anxiety disorder rather than as a distinct diagnostic syndrome.

2 *Language problems.* By definition, the child must be able to chat fairly normally in some situations, but there is often a history of somewhat delayed speech milestones, or continuing minor problems with articulation. This has implications for assessment. Since selectively mute children are unlikely to talk to the assessor, it is important to assess the child's articulation and language level in some other way, for example, by listening to an audio recording of the child chatting at home, or asking to see written work. Despite this limitation, a formal assessment of language level by a psychologist or speech and language therapist can sometimes be very helpful. It is possible to screen for receptive language problems by using a picture vocabulary test – this assessor reads out words and asks the child to point to the picture that best illustrates each word.

3 *Intelligence.* This obviously needs to be assessed using tests that do not require the child to speak, for example, using the visuospatial subtests from wide-ranging intelligence tests. The average non-verbal IQ in selective mutism was 85 in one study, but ranged from above 100 to under 70. Selective mutism can occur in children with mild or severe intellectual disability.

4 *Relationships.* Most children have been noted to be markedly shy from the preschool years onwards, and are withdrawn both with children and adults.

5 *Personality.* An unshakeable determination not to speak in some settings is often accompanied by other evidence of a strong will. Some children are sulky with strangers and aggressive at home; other children are shy with strangers and submissive at home; and yet other children are sensitive and easily distressed both at home and elsewhere. Mixtures of these personality styles are common.

6 *Family factors.* There is often a history of social anxiety or selective mutism in a parent or sibling. Maternal over-protectiveness is commonly described, as is an association with marital discord (but not marital breakdown), parental mental illness (anxiety and depression), and parental personality problems (marked aggression or shyness).

7 *Traumatic experiences.* Although studies of selective mutism have generally emphasised personality factors rather than specific traumas, there is some evidence that selectively mute children are more likely than classroom controls, or children with developmental speech or language problems, to have suffered definite or probable abuse, usually sexual abuse. The role of abuse and other traumatic experiences has yet to be confirmed.

Differential diagnosis

1 *Normality*. Young children vary markedly in how forthcoming they are in unfamiliar situations. Is transient mutism at school entry an exaggeration of normal shyness? Is persistent mutism also on the same continuum, or is it qualitatively distinct? There are no definitive answers yet.

2 *Serious developmental or acquired language disorders* can only be ruled out when there is convincing evidence that the child's language is fairly normal in some settings.

3 *Autistic spectrum disorders* are ruled out by evidence from reports or direct observations that the child not only has fairly normal language in some settings, but can also engage in imaginative play; has normal social interactions with family members or friends; and is free from marked ritualistic or repetitive behaviours, or restricted interests.

4 *Hysterical muteness* generally involves loss of speech in all settings. It is usually sudden in onset (sometimes following a definite stress), and is not typically preceded by marked lifelong shyness.

Causation

Selective mutism may result from a combination of constitutional and environmental factors. Perhaps marked constitutional shyness is exacerbated by stress at home, by immigrant status, or by self-consciousness about relatively minor articulation difficulties or cognitive problems. The mutism may be rewarded by extra attention and affection at home and at school. Without twin or adoption studies, it is impossible to determine whether family clustering points to genetic transmission or social modelling. Do anxious and over-protective parents fill their children with social anxieties? Or do the same genes that predispose parents to be anxious and over-protective also predispose their children to be anxious and selectively mute? Or do constitutionally sensitive children evoke greater protectiveness from their parents?

Treatment

Behavioural techniques may be helpful, for example, desensitising the child to speaking in large groups by starting with just one familiar person and gradually increasing the size of the group. It is obviously essential to ensure that the rewards for speaking are greater than the rewards for not speaking (in terms of attention, for example). Since selective mutism is usually a school-based problem, teachers and classroom assistants are often the most appropriate 'front line' behaviour therapists, advised by clinicians or educational psychologists. Speech therapy can be used to tackle articulation problems and thereby reduce the children's embarrassment about speaking in front of others. Social skills training and family therapy can be included in the therapeutic package to tackle associated problems with social relationships.

Selective serotonin reuptake inhibitors (SSRIs) have been advocated when both social phobia and selective mutism are present. Several small studies provide suggestive but not conclusive evidence for their utility. It would seem prudent not to try medication until a thorough course of behavioural treatment has been given and failed. When medication is used and works, it should subsequently be withdrawn gradually.

Prognosis

Although mutism at school entry is usually transient, the likelihood of resolution drops dramatically once the mutism has persisted for at least 6–12 months. One study of established cases found that half showed little or no improvement five to ten years later. Improvement is most likely to occur in the early school years, but may occur at a later stage. Resolution of the mutism is usually, but not always, accompanied by improved relationships too. As adults, those who have recovered from earlier selective mutism have a higher rate of phobic disorders.

Subject review

Standard S, Le Couteur A. (2003) The quiet child: A literature review of selective mutism. *Child and Adolescent Mental Health*, **8**, 154–160.

Further reading

Kearney, C (2010). *Helping Children with Selective Mutism and Their Parents: A Guide for School-Based Professionals*. Oxford University Press, Oxford.

Kristensen H. (2000) Selective mutism and comorbidity with developmental disorder/delay, anxiety disorder, and elimination disorder. *Journal of the American Academy of Child and Adolescent Psychiatry* **39**, 249–256.

MacGregor R *et al.* (1994) Silent at school – elective mutism and abuse. *Archives of Disease in Childhood* **70**, 540–541.

Steinhausen HC *et al.* (2006) A long-term outcome study of selective mutism in childhood. *Journal of Child Psychology and Psychiatry* **47**, 751–756.

CHAPTER 17

Attachment Disorders

Children's pattern of attachment to their parents and other caregivers is of great developmental importance, with the quality of these selective attachments being predictive of their subsequent development. As discussed in Chapter 32, about a third of children display an insecure attachment pattern, and they tend to fare worse than securely attached children in many aspects of their psychological and social development. An insecure attachment pattern is best seen as a risk factor for psychosocial maladjustment rather than as a disorder in itself; many insecurely attached children are well adapted to their environment and do not develop any psychiatric problems. In contrast, there are a few children who, following severe deprivation (usually in institutions), do not display anything close to selective security-seeking behaviour with any attachment figure. These children's behaviour is pervasive across all their relationships, and is associated with marked distress or social impairment; they are deemed to have an attachment *disorder*. This is in contrast to children with insecure attachment *patterns*, who may function well, without distress, and may get on perfectly satisfactorily in a range of relationships.

Varieties of attachment disorder

Both ICD-10 and DSM-IV recognise two varieties of attachment disorder:

1 *Disinhibited*. This relatively well-defined clinical picture is called 'disinhibited attachment disorder' by ICD-10 and 'reactive attachment disorder, disinhibited type' by DSM-IV. The child does seek comfort when distressed, but lacks the normal degree of selectivity in the people from whom comfort is sought. Social interactions with unfamiliar people are poorly modulated with generally clinging behaviour in infancy or attention-seeking and indiscriminately friendly behaviour in early or middle childhood. There is accumulating research evidence for the validity of disinhibited attachment disorders, which are typically linked to repeated changes in caregiver in the early years of life, including

Child and Adolescent Psychiatry, Third Edition. Robert Goodman and Stephen Scott.
© 2012 Robert Goodman and Stephen Scott. Published 2012 by John Wiley & Sons, Ltd.

frequent changes in foster placement, or rearing in a group home with a high turnover of staff.

2 *Inhibited*. This clinical picture is called 'reactive attachment disorder' by ICD-10 and 'reactive attachment disorder, inhibited type' by DSM-IV. Core features include lack of social and emotional responses, an absence of attachment behaviours even in times of stress, and marked problems with emotional regulation. There is a striking lack of positive emotional responses. In contrast, negative emotional reactions, especially fear and irritability are frequently seen, despite there being no or only minimal discernible triggers. Social and emotional reciprocal interactions are almost totally absent. Inhibited attachment disorders are usually associated with either severe abuse in the first years of life, or with being raised in institutions. It is worth remembering, however, that most children who are severely abused and the majority raised in institutions do not develop an inhibited attachment disorder. Whether it arises from an interaction between pathogenic care and, for example, a neurodevelopmental predisposition remains to be discovered. The fact that the disinhibited type responds less well to intervention (see below) and is less associated with pathogenic care at a critical, early period has led some to suggest it is a form of neurodevelopmental disorder.

Diagnosis

According to the ICD-10 and DSM-IV classifications, the following diagnostic criteria are relevant:

1 *Severity*. The children are not attached in any meaningful sense. They do not have enduring relationships with people who provide them with a 'secure base' and a 'safe haven'.

2 *Pervasiveness*. A seriously troubled relationship with one particular parent or other caregiver is insufficient. The attachment problems must be evident across a number of different caregivers.

3 *Distress or disability*. Attachment disorders cause the child persistent distress or social disability, partly as a consequence of the lack of normal attachment relationships, and partly as a consequence of a wider range of associated social difficulties (for example, with poor peer relationships).

4 *Onset before the age of 5 years*. Along with autism, it is one of the psychiatric disorders that is often first diagnosed in a child of 3 or under.

5 *Not autistic*. The child's impaired social relationships are not attributable to an autistic spectrum disorder (see Chapter 4). Relevant evidence is the lack of other autistic impairments, such as ritualistic and repetitive behaviours, or communication difficulties. In addition, some capacity for social reciprocity and responsiveness is usually evident in interactions with normal adults. In extreme cases, though, the child's social potential may not be apparent for as long as he or she lives in adverse social circumstances. The response to a more favourable caregiving environment is then of diagnostic value. For example, the rapid emergence

of social responsiveness and reciprocity in a foster placement points to an attachment disorder rather than an autistic disorder.

6 *Mental age over 10–12 months.* Children with severe intellectual disability may lack selective attachments simply because they have not yet reached a mental age when these would normally emerge. This does not warrant an additional diagnosis of an attachment disorder.

7 *Pathogenic care.* DSM-IV criteria require an abnormal caregiving context, involving either repeated changes of primary caregiver, preventing the formation of stable attachments, or persistent disregard of the child's basic emotional or physical needs. ICD-10 also makes it clear that an attachment disorder is usually associated with pathogenic care but does not make this a diagnostic requirement. This allows the diagnosis to be made in those transnationally adopted children who meet all the other criteria without much being known of their care history.

Differential diagnosis

Disinhibition and indiscriminate friendliness can also be seen in ADHD, mania and after frontal lobe damage, for example, following severe closed head injuries. Inhibition can also be seen in social phobia and shyness – while it is usually evident that shy or socially anxious children are attached to their parents, this can be hard to establish in the presence of severe intellectual disability.

Attachment disorders v. insecure attachment

Attachment has been one of the key themes in developmental research for decades, with much being written about secure and insecure attachment patterns (see Chapter 32). How do attachment disorders differ from insecure attachment patterns? First, the rates are dramatically different, with about 40% of children being classified as insecurely attached, whereas attachment disorders appear to be rare. Second, a child may be insecurely attached to one key caregiver (for example, the mother) but not to others (for example, the father), whereas attachment disorders involve problems that are pervasive as well as severe. Third, an insecure attachment pattern does not necessarily result in distress or social impairment, whereas an attachment disorder does. Finally, the characteristic symptoms of attachment disorders (particularly disinhibited attachment disorders) do not correspond to any of the recognised subtypes of insecure attachment, including insecure-disorganised attachment (type D).

Assessment of the child

When evaluating a child who may have an attachment disorder, it is not sufficient to carry out one of the standard assessments of attachment security, such as the Ainsworth Strange Situation Procedure (see Chapter 32), which is only reliable under the age of 2 years anyway. It is important to take a careful history from multiple informants and observe the child in several settings. It may also help to get the carer to keep a diary of the child's behaviour, especially focusing on times of stress when a child might be expected to turn to their attachment figure, for example, when very tired, ill, upset or frightened. The main focus is on various aspects of attachment:

1 *A safe haven?* Does the child have a narrow range of people to turn to in times of distress, in order to obtain comfort and renew confidence? Children with an attachment disorder may not seek comfort, or may seek it from whoever is around at the time (disinhibited type), or may seek comfort in obviously odd ways, for example, by backing into the caregiver rather than walking forward and making eye contact.
2 *A secure base?* Can the child venture out to explore the world, returning to the attachment figure for security when necessary? The child with an attachment disorder may be excessively inhibited about exploring, or may be a disinhibited explorer without due regard for his or her own safety.
3 *An affectionate bond?* The child with an attachment disorder may show a lack of affection or promiscuous affection.
4 *Selectivity?* Does the child make use of fairly unfamiliar adults as attachment figures, turning to them for comfort, clinging to them, or showing them inappropriate affection? Does the child become over-familiar with strange adults, for example, sitting on their lap at first meeting?

A full assessment also needs to determine the age of onset of problems and establish the type and quality of current and previous caregiving. Wider social impairments also need to be considered. For example, how well does the child relate to other children? Does he or she tend to ignore or attack other children when they are distressed? It is also essential to look for evidence of autistic impairments and severe intellectual disability. These are possible differential diagnoses and need to be excluded if the diagnostic criteria for an attachment disorder are to be met. ADHD or brain injury may also need to be considered as an alternative explanation for over-familiarity with adults, disinhibited exploration and poor peer relationships. However, neither ADHD nor brain injury would account for failure to seek comfort from attachment figures when distressed.

Assessment of the care received

A careful history should be taken from birth onwards. The focus should be on the constancy of the chief caregivers versus the number of changes, and on the quality of care given, including warmth, emotional availability, neglect, and hostility or abuse. Informants who know the child well should be questioned closely. These may include health visitors and relatives as well as the immediate caregivers. Direct observation of the interaction between the child and his or her current caregiver should be carried out, looking for insensitive and inappropriate responding and unusual child behaviours.

Management

The principal objective of management is to improve the children's care-giving environment. The main contribution of child and adolescent mental health professionals is often to provide appropriate advice on this to social services and the courts. If a child is currently being maltreated, an alternative placement is obviously needed if the current caregivers cannot be helped to change. If the child has passed through a succession of brief foster placements or has grown up in an institution with rapidly changing staff, he or she needs to be given the opportunity to form lasting attachments, ideally with permanent foster or adoptive parents. Though attachment-based interventions have been developed for the treatment of a variety of severe relationship difficulties and have proved to be moderately successful at reducing insecure patterns of attachment in infancy, there is less evidence whether these approaches benefit children with attachment disorders. Two observational studies of young children adopted from severely depriving Romanian orphanages (one to parents in Canada, one to England) converge in suggesting that while symptoms of both the inhibited and disinhibited type reduced as the children grew up into late middle childhood and the teenage years, they persisted to a marked degree in around half. One study of children in depriving Hungarian institutions randomised the children to continuing care in the institution or foster care. Those remaining in the institution continued to show both types of disorder, whereas those allocated to foster care showed virtual elimination of the inhibited type of disorder and reduction but not elimination of the disinhibited type.

In conclusion, on both theoretical grounds and on practical empirical evidence, the best treatment for attachment disorders is long-term good-quality parental-type care with sensitive responding to the child's needs. This needs emphasising as fosterers and adopters of maltreated children with attachment problems or disorders may get desperate and instead of seeking sensible advice from a skilled child and adolescent mental health professional, may fall into the hands of eccentric and potentially dangerous practitioners. Controversial therapies include: regression therapy; holding therapy; rebirthing therapy; corrective attachment therapy; holding time and rage-reduction therapy. The names change frequently and carers do not know if their attachment therapy is 'controversial'.

Course and prognosis

A number of cohorts of children raised in depriving circumstances have now been followed-up over the longer term. In general, early attachment disorders seem particularly likely to interfere with friendships and intimate relationships; somewhat less likely to result in behavioural problems; and least likely to affect cognitive development. The impact of early attachment difficulties is lessened but not abolished when children's social circumstances change for the better, as noted above. Those who were removed earlier, and had fewer symptoms at the time of removal, do better.

Subject review

Zeanah CH, Smyke AT. (2008) Attachment disorders in relation to deprivation. *In*: Rutter M et al. (eds) *Rutter's Child and Adolescent Psychiatry*, 5th edn. Wiley-Blackwell, Chichester, pp. 906–915.

Further reading

Chaffin M *et al*. (2006) Report of the American Professional Society on the Abuse of Children Task Force on Attachment Therapy, Reactive Attachment Disorder, and Attachment Problems. *Child Maltreatment* **11**, 76–89. (A review of what is sensible in treatment of attachment problems and disorders and a strong call to avoid controversial therapies.)

Gleason M *et al*. (2011) Validity of evidence-derived criteria for reactive attachment disorder: Indiscriminately social/disinhibited and emotionally withdrawn/inhibited types. *Journal of the American Academy of Child and Adolescent Psychiatry* **50**, 216–231.

Rutter M *et al*. (2009) Attachment insecurity, disinhibited attachment, and attachment disorders: Where do research findings leave the concepts? *Journal of Child Psychology and Psychiatry* **50**, 529–543.

Zeanah C *et al*. (2009) Practitioner review: Clinical applications of attachment theory and research for infants and young children. *Journal of Child Psychology and Psychiatry* **52**, 819–833.

CHAPTER 18

Enuresis

Though enuresis is sometimes considered a psychiatric disorder, with some parents imagining that it is due to deep-seated emotional problems, it is more often a habit or developmental problem than a mental health problem. Though children and adolescents with enuresis do still get referred to mental health specialists who are familiar with behavioural approaches, it is worth remembering that these same behavioural approaches can often be applied equally effectively by other professionals, for example, specialist health visitors.

It is important to distinguish between *nocturnal enuresis* (bed wetting) and *diurnal enuresis* (daytime wetting). Nocturnal and diurnal enuresis differ in several respects and examination questions often seem to be designed to catch out people who confuse the two. Boys are more prone to nocturnal enuresis, while girls are more prone to diurnal enuresis. Nocturnal enuresis is commoner than diurnal enuresis (see Box 18.1) and it is less likely to be associated with urinary tract infections or psychiatric disorders.

Box 18.1 Overlap and relative prevalence of nocturnal and diurnal enuresis

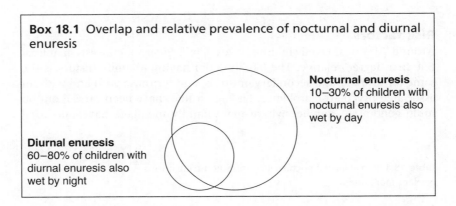

Nocturnal enuresis
10–30% of children with nocturnal enuresis also wet by day

Diurnal enuresis
60–80% of children with diurnal enuresis also wet by night

Child and Adolescent Psychiatry, Third Edition. Robert Goodman and Stephen Scott.
© 2012 Robert Goodman and Stephen Scott. Published 2012 by John Wiley & Sons, Ltd.

Nocturnal enuresis

Primary and secondary

Children and adolescents are said to have primary enuresis when they have never acquired normal bladder control. By contrast, someone who acquires bladder control for at least six months and then loses it again is said to have secondary enuresis. This sort of relapse is most likely at the age of 5 or 6 and is rare after the age of 11. Primary and secondary enuresis are equally likely to be associated with a positive family history, but do differ in other ways: secondary enuresis has a worse prognosis and is probably associated with a higher likelihood of psychiatric disorder.

Prevalence

Table 18.1 shows the prevalence of nocturnal enuresis occurring at least once a week in the Isle of Wight study. The current DSM-IV threshold for nocturnal enuresis is set higher – at twice a week or more – resulting in a lower prevalence, for example, 2.6% at 7 in the English ALSPAC study (1.6% in girls, 3.6% in boys). The emergence of a male preponderance reflects two processes:

1 Males are slower to achieve dryness (that is, slower resolution of primary enuresis).
2 Males are more likely to relapse (that is, more liable to secondary enuresis).

After the age of 7, secondary nocturnal enuresis is commoner than primary nocturnal enuresis.

Risk factors

Around 70% of affected children have a *family history* of enuresis in at least one first degree relative. The likelihood of having a family history is the same for primary and secondary enuresis, and for those with and without associated psychiatric problems. Linkage studies have been carried out on multi-generation families where many family members have nocturnal

Table 18.1 Prevalence of nocturnal enuresis occurring once a week or more often

Age	Prevalence (%)	Male:female ratio
5	13	1:1
7	5	1.4:1
9	2.5	1.6:1
14	0.8	1.8:1

Source: (Rutter *et al.*, 1970).

enuresis; these studies have implicated different chromosomal sites in different families. This may reflect the existence of many relevant genes, each of which is rare but potentially powerful.

Environmental factors also seem to play a part.

1 Enuresis is associated with *urinary tract infections* (UTIs), particularly in girls. Thus in 5-year-old girls, asymptomatic UTIs are present in about 5% of those with enuresis, as opposed to about 1% of those without. The likelihood of associated UTIs is even higher if the enuresis is diurnal or particularly frequent.

2 *Stressful life events* at the age of 3–4 are associated with twice the risk of enuresis. Relevant events include family break-up, separation from parents, moving house, the birth of a sibling, admission to hospital and accidents. Recurrent hospital admission is particularly associated with bed-wetting. Sexual abuse is associated with secondary enuresis.

3 Enuresis is associated with several indicators of *social disadvantage*: lower socio-economic status, an overcrowded home and institutional care.

4 Starting *toilet training* after 20 months is associated with a higher rate of subsequent enuresis. Otherwise, the role of specific toilet training practices is unclear. Harsh training seems undesirable since it is more upsetting for the child, but there is no evidence that it results in more enuresis.

Pathophysiology

1 Two-thirds of nocturnal enuresis involves some combination of two underlying problems:

(a) In most children and adolescents, the rate of urine production falls at night as a result of increased nocturnal secretion of antidiuretic hormone. This can reduce the quantity of urine that accumulates in the bladder overnight to an amount that the individual can hold in their bladder without waking or wetting themselves. Nocturnal enuresis is associated with a high rate of urine production at night – either they secrete unusually little antidiuretic hormone levels at night or their kidneys are resistant. As a result, bladder capacity is reached rapidly. Pointers to this pattern of nocturnal enuresis include large wet patches and the first episode of wetting occurring fairly soon after going to sleep. A lack of antidiuretic hormone at night can be treated by taking desmopressin (an artificial equivalent of antidiuretic hormone) before sleep (see below).

(b) Reaching bladder capacity would not result in bed wetting if the individual woke up and went to the toilet. However, enuresis is also associated with a reduced likelihood of waking up in response to the sensation of a full bladder. Contrary to what many families suspect, this is not due to sleeping unusually deeply. Enuresis can occur at any stage of sleep and individuals with enuresis do not sleep more deeply than other people. An enuresis alarm can help the individual to learn to wake up in response to a full bladder (see below).

2 One third of nocturnal enuresis involves bladder over-activity or in-stability. Pointers to this include: small wet patches; daytime urgency; frequent daytime urination (over seven times per day); or daytime wetting. Bladder training and anticholinergic medication may reduce excessive and unstable activity of the bladder wall (see below).

3 Though an epileptic seizure may involve urinary incontinence, there is no evidence that ordinary enuresis is an *epileptic equivalent*. Children with enuresis are no more likely than other children to have an abnormal EEG.

Assessment

It is always necessary to obtain a detailed history of the wetting and any other urological symptoms. Urine testing is indicated when the onset of the enuresis is recent or combined with daytime urinary problems. Physical examination and urological investigation are not necessary if straightforward enuresis is unaccompanied by any other urological symptom. Ask about any associated psychiatric problems, and remember to ask specifically about faecal soiling. It is important to enquire about factors that may influence choice of treatment. What has the family already tried? How motivated is the child or adolescent to get dry? Are the parents motivated to participate in treatment, for example, getting up in the middle of the night to supervise their child changing sheets and resetting an enuresis alarm? Is the main concern about nights spent away from home? If so, temporary suppression of enuresis (with medication) may be all that is needed.

Prognosis

Continuing nocturnal enuresis is predicted by: male sex, low socio-economic status, secondary rather than primary enuresis, and wetting the bed every night. The prevalence of enuresis is still 2–5% at the onset of puberty and continues to drop thereafter, leaving some 1–3% of adults with intractable enuresis.

Treatment

Since uncomplicated enuresis is best seen as a developmental rather than a mental disorder, it is entirely appropriate that professional help usually comes from health visitors, general practitioners and paediatricians rather than from child mental health professionals. Whichever professional is involved, if the child is under the age of 5 or 6, it is often sufficient to reassure the parents that nocturnal enuresis is common and usually outgrown.

Parents have often tried 'common-sense' measures such as taking their still-sleeping or half-awake child to use the toilet in the late evening or restricting fluids before bedtime. It is not clear, though, whether these measures help or hinder: lifting could be seen as a way of training the child to urinate while asleep or half asleep (exactly what you don't want!) and fluid restriction may promote bladder over-activity.

Behavioural measures

Rewards

It is important that parents do not inadvertently reward and thereby reinforce enuresis, for example, by letting their child sleep in the parents' bed once the child's own bed is wet. The emphasis should be on praise, attention and other rewards for dry nights rather than on criticism and punishment for wet nights. Keeping a wall chart of wet and dry nights for a month (with the child marking each dry night with a star) is quite often all that is needed to cure the enuresis.

Enuresis alarm

If enuresis persists and the family are sufficiently motivated, the most successful behavioural technique for bringing about a lasting cure is an enuresis alarm. Urination activates an alarm that wakes the child. Modern devices use a small pad in the child's pyjamas or underpants, with the alarm being carried in a pocket or on a wristband. When the alarm goes off, the child is expected to get up, go to the toilet, and change pyjamas and sheets as necessary (with parental help if needed). Cure rates of 60–80% are often reported, with children typically achieving 14 consecutive dry nights in the second month of treatment (though children with intellectual disability may take up to six months). The likelihood of cure is unaffected by whether or not the enuresis is primary or secondary, or by the presence or absence of a family history. The cure rate is lower when there is a high level of family stress, when the child wets several times a night, also wets by day, has a psychiatric disorder, or is unconcerned about the enuresis. Roughly a third of those who become dry while using the alarm subsequently resume wetting the bed again in the year after treatment is stopped. There is some evidence that the relapse rate can be significantly reduced by an 'over-learning' technique: once the child has learned to be dry at night, he or she is encouraged to drink a large quantity of fluids before bedtime, and the enuresis alarm is continued until the child is dry despite the fluid loading. However, there are also concerns that a process that initially worsens wetting may be demoralising.

Why, in behavioural terms, does the enuresis alarm work? There are elements of classical conditioning: the sound of the buzzer (the unconditioned stimulus) leads to waking, and eventually the sensation of a full bladder (the conditioned stimulus) leads to waking too. There are elements of operant conditioning too: the sound of the buzzer is a somewhat aversive stimulus and the child learns to avoid it by not wetting the bed. Finally, social learning theorists might add that the use of the bell and pad helps the family to notice dry nights and to make more of a fuss of the child after dry nights.

If the enuresis alarm does not work, it may be sensible to try the combination of enuresis alarm and desmopressin (see below); or to switch to medication alone, aiming for symptomatic relief rather than for a cure; or to give up for a year or so before trying again. Another option for older and highly motivated children is dry-bed training, which is an intensive form of behavioural therapy that involves hourly waking on the first night, high fluid intake and frequent behavioural rehearsal of proper toileting. Though reportedly successful for some otherwise resistant cases, the technique is not suitable for young and poorly motivated children, who are likely to see it as a torture.

Bladder training

This involves regular fluid intake and toileting during the day, thereby increasing the individual's opportunities for learning normal bladder control. Children and adolescents who experience urinary urgency are taught to go to the toilet immediately if the sensation persists. There is some evidence that this sort of daytime training can promote a switch from unstable to stable bladder function at night.

Medication

The first choice should usually be *desmopressin* (DDAVP), a synthetic analogue of antidiuretic hormone that is probably best reserved for those aged 7 or more (and is inappropriate for children under the age of 5). The medication is generally very safe, though it is important to warn families of the need to avoid large fluid intakes in the evenings in order to reduce the small risk of water intoxication. Given before bedtime, desmopressin stops bed-wetting in roughly 20% of users and reduces the frequency of bed-wetting in many others. In many instances, though, relapse occurs as soon as the medication is stopped. Despite this reversibility, desmopressin is still a valuable symptomatic treatment that may enable a child or adolescent to go on school trips or stay overnight with friends without having to face the embarrassment of a wet bed. In addition, the combination of desmopressin and an enuresis alarm may be more successful than an alarm alone, resulting in a higher long-term cure rate. This is particularly true for those with severe wetting or associated behavioural and family problems.

Tricyclic antidepressants in relatively low doses (for example, 25–75 mg of imipramine at bedtime) have also been shown to perform better than placebo in the symptomatic treatments for nocturnal enuresis. The effect is evident within the first week, and does not seem to be due to the antidepressant, anticholinergic or sleep-altering properties of tricyclics. Tolerance may emerge after two to six weeks on medication, and immediate or delayed relapse on withdrawal of medication is very common. Since tricyclics are no more effective than desmopressin but are considerably more toxic in overdose, they should seldom be used nowadays.

Anticholinergic medications such as oxybutynin may be of some use in relaxing the bladder wall and increasing bladder capacity. There is weak evidence that this may be helpful when the pattern of nocturnal enuresis suggests bladder over-activity or instability (see above).

Diurnal enuresis

As already noted, diurnal enuresis is rarer than nocturnal enuresis. In the Isle of Wight study, 2% of 5-year-olds experienced diurnal enuresis at least once a week. There is a female excess at all ages. The most common form involves the sort of bladder over-activity or instability that is also seen in a minority of those with nocturnal enuresis (see above). There is often urge incontinence, with wetting of small volumes, and frequent daytime urination (over seven times per day). Bladder training and anticholinergic medication may be helpful. It is good practice to test routinely for urinary infections.

A less common form of diurnal enuresis that affects more boys than girls involves children postponing urination because they are too busy doing other interesting things to notice (or choose to pay attention to) the fact that they have a full bladder. They wet large volumes. Regular reminders to use the toilet may help, and this is less likely to be resented as nagging if the reminders can be delivered automatically via a watch or mobile phone rather than by a parent or teacher.

The link with psychiatric problems

Since an association between enuresis and psychiatric problems has been well demonstrated in epidemiological samples, the link cannot simply be an artefact of referral bias. Although the rate of psychiatric disorder is roughly two to six times higher in those with enuresis than in controls, it is important to remember that over half of all those with enuresis have no psychiatric disorder. The presence of a psychiatric disorder is more likely to occur in girls, when the enuresis is diurnal rather than nocturnal, and when there are associated developmental problems. It is probably more likely when the enuresis is secondary rather than primary. It is unrelated to the frequency of wetting, or to the presence or absence of a family history. Among those with both enuresis and a psychiatric disorder, the type of disorder is not specific: behavioural and emotional disorders predominate just as they do in the general population. The link between enuresis and psychiatric disorder could reflect three sorts of causal mechanism:

1 Both enuresis and psychiatric problems result from the *operation of a third factor*, for example, social disadvantage or biological-developmental problems. Overall, this is the best supported causal mechanism, though the other two probably are important for some children.
2 *Psychiatric problems cause enuresis.* There are some children who are more likely to wet the bed when they are anxious, for example, after first starting school. One prospective study has shown that children who developed secondary enuresis were more likely than controls to have had emotional or behavioural problems before the enuresis began.

3 *Enuresis causes psychiatric problems.* Several studies have shown that successful treatment or natural remission of enuresis is accompanied by a decrease in the rate of psychiatric problems. However, children whose enuresis has resolved still have a higher rate of psychiatric problems than controls.

Subject review

Butler RJ. (2008) Wetting and soiling. *In*: Rutter M *et al.* (eds) *Rutter's Child and Adolescent Psychiatry*, 5th edn. Wiley-Blackwell, Chichester, pp. 916–929.

Further reading

Butler RJ *et al.* (2005) Nocturnal enuresis at 7.5 years old: Prevalence and analysis of clinical signs. *BJU International* **96**, 404–410.

Nunes VD *et al.* (2010) Management of bedwetting in children and young people: Summary of NICE guidance. *BMJ* **341**, c5399 – print edition of 30 October.

Rutter M *et al.* (1970) *Education, Health and Behaviour*. Longman, London.

CHAPTER 19
Faecal Soiling

Children have normally acquired reliable bowel control by the age of 3 or 4, though they may still have the occasional accident after that. When soiling occurs more than once a month after the age of 4 years, this is generally regarded as an elimination disorder. For children with intellectual disability, however, the cut-off should probably be at a mental rather than a chronological age of 4 years. Soiling occurs more than once a month in roughly 5% of 4-year-olds, falling to 1–2% of 7-year-olds, and under 1% of 11-year-olds. By the age of 16, the prevalence of soiling is practically zero. Both epidemiological and clinic series show that soiling is roughly three times commoner in boys than girls.

Faecal soiling can be divided into five types:

- constipation with overflow;
- failed toilet training;
- toilet phobia;
- stress-induced loss of control;
- provocative soiling.

Each of these has specific implications for treatment. The term encopresis may be used to refer to all types of faecal soiling, or may be used more narrowly to refer to the passage of relatively normal stools in inappropriate places, including underclothing. On the basis of a careful history and physical examination, it is usually possible to identify the type (or types) of soiling and so formulate an appropriate management plan.

Types of soiling and their management

The five types of soiling do not always occur in isolation. Children seen clinically commonly have hybrid presentations, showing some of the features of more than one type of soiling. For such children, the different components of their soiling each need to be addressed by the overall management plan. When the symptoms are severe or complicated, or when the soiling does not respond to standard treatment, it will be important for both paediatricians and child mental health workers to be

Child and Adolescent Psychiatry, Third Edition. Robert Goodman and Stephen Scott.
© 2012 Robert Goodman and Stephen Scott. Published 2012 by John Wiley & Sons, Ltd.

involved, since (unlike enuresis) there is a high chance that psychological problems have either contributed to the soiling or resulted from it.

Constipation with overflow

Children can become constipated for many reasons. A constitutional liability combined with a low-fibre diet is important in some cases. In other instances, an episode of constipation may be initiated by deliberate retention on the part of the child, perhaps because an anal lesion (such as a fissure) makes defecation painful, or perhaps because of a 'battle of wills' over toilet training. Whatever the initiating process, constipation can become self-perpetuating. A large faecal plug is hard to pass and the child may give up for fear of the consequences, promoting further retention. In addition, as the rectum becomes increasingly distended, 'rectal inertia' may set in, with loss of the stretch response that normally results in a sensation of fullness and desire to defecate. Eventually, liquid or semi-liquid faeces may leak round the blockage and overflow.

The appropriate management is to unblock the bowel and re-establish a normal toilet routine. From the outset, the child and family's anxiety and anger need to be defused by adequate explanations of the underlying physiology. Recovery is best promoted by a calm family atmosphere with positive expectations. Clearing the bowel may be possible by using a stimulant laxative, such as senna, in combination with a stool softener such as lactulose; microenemas or phosphate enemas may be needed initially; bowel washouts are only rarely required. A star chart or similar behavioural programme is used to reward the return to a normal toilet routine. Laxatives are replaced as soon as possible by a high-fibre diet.

Failed toilet training

Some children have never learned bowel control. This can be referred to as primary faecal soiling, by analogy with primary enuresis. Though sometimes associated with neurological problems, developmental delays, and intellectual disability, primary faecal soiling may also reflect incon-sistent, insensitive or neglectful toilet training, usually in the context of multiple social and family disadvantages. Suboptimal training may have a particularly marked impact if the child is exposed to chronic psychological stresses during the toddler years when bowel control is usually acquired. Behavioural treatments based on careful record keeping, realistic targets, star charts and appropriate rewards are generally suitable. The most challenging task is often to 'sell' the behavioural package to the family and then ensure that it is correctly and consistently carried out.

Toilet phobia

Some children are scared of the toilet, for example, fearing that monsters live there, or that a hand will reach up and grab them. Parents are only sometimes aware of these fears, so it is important to explore possible anxieties through conversation, play and drawing, usually with the child on his or her own. The family can then be helped to discuss the child's fears openly and sympathetically, without ridicule. The fears themselves can be addressed through appropriate reassurance and graded exposure with rewards. Shy children may be afraid to use the toilets at school, or of having to ask a teacher's permission to go to the toilet during class time. Bullied children may reasonably fear unsupervised encounters with bullies in the school toilets.

Stress-induced loss of control

Some children acquire bowel control normally but then lose it again after a significant stress, such as a traumatic hospital admission, marked family discord or disruption, or an episode of sexual abuse. If the child is handled sympathetically, bowel control is usually rapidly regained once the stress is reduced. The primary emphasis of management, therefore, should be on reducing stress and making the child feel safe again.

Provocative soiling

Some children's pattern of soiling seems designed to irritate those around them. For example, they may deliberately defecate into baths or onto furniture, or may smear faeces on walls – subsequently denying that they were responsible for these acts. This covert aggression is often also evident in other aspects of these children's relationships with parents and siblings. Indeed, provocative soiling is usually a marker for multiple problems in the child and family. The child commonly has additional emotional and behavioural problems, and the family as a whole is often severely dysfunctional, failing to meet the child's most basic social and emotional needs. These children and families need help on many fronts, often from social services and education, as well as from child mental health professionals.

Prognosis of soiling

Whatever type of soiling is involved, persistence into adulthood is very unusual. Resolution is generally more rapid when soiling is the only problem. The prognosis is worse when there is coexistent ADHD or when the soiling happens at night. A chronic course seems particularly likely when there is a poor compliance with treatment and when soiling is accompanied by other problems: behavioural, developmental, scholastic, family and social.

Associated psychiatric disorders

Many studies have shown that a substantial minority of children who soil also have one or more psychiatric disorders. For example, in a nationally representative British sample, the rate of psychiatric disorder was found to be over 30%. What could account for this strong association? Logically, there are three possibilities. First, psychiatric disorders could lead on to soiling, though follow-up studies provide no evidence for this. Second, soiling could result in psychiatric disorder, perhaps by evoking criticism and teasing from parents, teachers and peers. Third, soiling and psychiatric disorders may co-occur because of shared risk factors such as neglect, abuse developmental immaturity or neurological disorder.

Subject review

Butler RJ. (2008) Wetting and soiling. *In*: Rutter M *et al.* (eds) *Rutter's Child and Adolescent Psychiatry*, 5th edn. Wiley-Blackwell, Chichester, pp. 916–929.

Further reading

Buchanan, A. in collaboration with Clayden, G. (1992) *Children Who Soil: Assessment and Treatment.* Wiley, Chichester.
Sourander A. (2011) Time-trend changes and psychological risk factors for soiling: Findings from the Finnish 16-year time-trend study. *Acta Paediatrica* **100**, 1276–1280.

CHAPTER 20
Sleep Disorders

Sleep problems are relevant to child and adolescent mental health professionals because there is a complex relationship between sleep disorders and psychiatric disorders:

- Psychiatric disorders can cause sleep problems. For example, difficulties getting to sleep or staying asleep are common in anxiety and depressive disorders, while nightmares can be a prominent feature of post-traumatic stress disorder.
- Conversely, sleep disorders may cause, mimic or aggravate psychiatric disorders. For instance, sleep deprivation in a 6-year-old may result in over-activity, poor concentration, impulsiveness and irritability, that is, features that are normally part of ADHD and disruptive behavioural disorders.
- It may be hard to distinguish between sleep disorders and psychiatric disorders, for example, nocturnal panic attacks can be mistaken for nightmares or night terrors, or vice versa.
- Psychotropic medication (or its withdrawal) may induce sleep problems, for example, difficulty getting to sleep when taking methylphenidate, or nightmares following the abrupt withdrawal of antidepressants.
- A single risk factor may predispose a child to both sleep problems and psychiatric difficulties. For example, children growing up in chaotic household without routines or consistently enforced rules are more likely to develop both disruptive behavioural problems and difficulties getting a regular night's sleep.

Normal sleep

The structure of a normal night's sleep is shown schematically in Box 20.1, along with accompanying notes. Daytime sleepiness tends to peak in the afternoon – different cultures have different expectations as to when (if ever) children should cease having an afternoon nap/siesta. The pineal hormone, melatonin, helps coordinate the sleep–wake cycle with the 24 hour dark–light cycle. Just as good and bad hygiene alter the risks

Child and Adolescent Psychiatry, Third Edition. Robert Goodman and Stephen Scott.

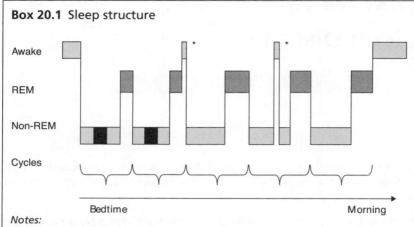

Box 20.1 Sleep structure

Notes:

- REM = Rapid Eye Movement: the phase of sleep when most dreaming occurs and muscle tone is at its lowest. Makes up about 25% of sleep and is commonest towards the end of the night.
- Non-REM: the deepest non-REM sleep (stages 3 and 4, shown in black) mostly occurs in the first two cycles.
- Brief awakenings are normal at all ages, and can occur from either REM or light non-REM (shown as * in diagram).
- After early infancy, falling asleep is a transition to non-REM sleep.
- Sleep cycles last about 50–60 minutes in childhood, increasing to 90–100 minutes in adolescents and adults.
- Total sleep declines from an average of 12 hours per day in 4-year-olds to an average of 8 hours per day by late adolescence.

of infectious diseases, so good and bad 'sleep hygiene' alter the risks of sleep problems. Box 20.2 lists some of the key components of good sleep hygiene.

Epidemiology of sleep problems

Very severe sleep disorders are rare, for example, narcolepsy affects fewer than 1 in a thousand children and adolescents, while some degree of obstructive sleep apnoea affects 2% of children and adolescents. Less severe sleep problems are much commoner, for example, about a quarter of preschool children have significant problems getting to sleep or staying asleep, while up to 15% of adolescents have an erratic or delayed sleep–wake cycle. Sleep problems are particularly common among children and adolescents with intellectual disability and are also linked to physical disabilities (for example, cerebral palsy), sensory impairments (for example, blindness), psychiatric disorders (for example, generalised anxiety), and physical disorders that worsen at night (for example, asthma) or that cause night-time discomfort (for example, itching due to eczema).

Box 20.2 Good sleep hygiene

Daytime
- Avoid naps, particularly late in the day.
- Regular exercise (but not too close to bedtime).
- Resolve worries and make plans for the next day (so these aren't left for bedtime).
- Restrict caffeine-containing drinks (coffee, cola), particularly late in the day.
- Tobacco, alcohol and drugs can also disrupt sleep, and may be used by adolescents without their parents knowing.

Approaching bedtime
- Finish any homework well before bedtime.
- Gradual winding down without over-stimulation.
- Avoid large meals late at night.

Choice of bedtime
- Duration from bedtime to wake-up time should provide enough sleep for the individual's age and constitution.
- Sending children or adolescents to bed too early conditions them to associate lying in bed with being awake rather than asleep.

Go to bed
- At a fairly consistent time.
- When sufficiently tired to fall asleep relatively rapidly.
- Without repeatedly getting out of bed again.
- With soothing routines, for example, with a story or a tape; avoid frightening stories or exciting TV while in bed.
- Phasing out the need for a parent to be present equips an individual to get to sleep (and get back to sleep) when alone.

Bedroom
- Comfortable bed.
- Temperature, light and noise controlled.
- Neither aversive nor too exciting.

Wake-up
- At a fairly consistent time (long lie-ins can reset the sleep–wake cycle).
- Do not reward waking up too early, for example, by providing wonderful videos.

Presentation

Sleep problems typically present in one (or more) of three ways:

- problems getting to sleep or staying asleep;
- excessive daytime sleepiness;
- episodic disturbance at night, for example, nightmares, night terrors.

These are presentations, not diagnoses. Making a diagnosis requires a detailed clinical history and may also require special investigations, for example, polysomnography, involving simultaneous recordings of brain activity (EEG), muscle movements and eye movements during sleep.

Specific types of sleep disturbance

The sleep problems that are most relevant to child mental health practitioners are discussed below.

Difficulty getting to sleep or staying asleep

This is the commonest sleep problem from infancy to old age, but is particularly common among preschool children. The problem can usually be tackled successfully by improving sleep hygiene (see Box 20.2) and phasing out rewards for not being asleep. When children need parental attention to get back to sleep after waking in the middle of the night, this is often because they haven't learned the skill of getting to sleep by themselves. The easiest way to teach them this skill is by practising at bed time. If parents progressively fade themselves out at bedtime (for example, leaving the bedroom before the child is asleep), children learn how to get to sleep by themselves, and can usually then do so in the middle of the night too. Sometimes, children are kept awake by fears and worries that need to be tackled in their own right (see Chapter 9).

Circadian sleep–wake cycle disorder

If you move from London to New York or vice versa, your body clock and sleep–wake cycle adjust. Imagine what would happen if your sleep–wake cycle didn't adjust. The Londoner in New York would always go to sleep before everyone else, and then wake ridiculously early (advanced sleep phase syndrome). Conversely, the New Yorker in London would get up very late each day and not go to sleep until the early hours of the morning (delayed sleep phase syndrome). This sort of problem with being 'stuck in the wrong time zone' is exactly what happens to some children and more adolescents. Advanced sleep phase syndrome is relatively unusual, and is usually due to parents putting children to bed too soon, with the result that they habitually wake too early and disturb the rest of the family.

Delayed sleep phase syndrome is far commoner, particularly among teenagers. They stay up late (TV, homework, parties) and then sleep in late whenever they can. It is hard to wake them for school, and the principal complaint is often of deteriorating school performance (and behaviour) because of daytime sleepiness. Once the sleep phase has shifted, having an early night no longer helps but just condemns the teenager to lying awake for hours before finally falling asleep in the early hours 'as normal'.

Reprogramming the sleep phase is possible with patience, effort and motivation (and some adolescents are not motivated to change). When the sleep phase is only two or three hours delayed, it is possible to let the adolescent sleep in for a few days and then move wake-up time about 15 minutes earlier per day – bedtime will naturally move earlier too. When sleep phase is delayed by three or four hours or more, it is usually better to push it even later, with the adolescent staying awake an extra two or three hours each night until the normal phase is re-established, for example, moving forward 18 hours over a week instead of trying to move backwards six hours. The shift is aided by bright lights while awake and darkness while asleep. High levels of parental input and motivation are essential.

Obstructive sleep apnoea

Muscle tone in the upper airways decreases during sleep, so if the airways are already partly blocked, sleep can lead to under-ventilation. Whereas most adults with this condition are obese, the same only applies to about 20% of affected children. The commonest cause in childhood is enlargement of tonsils and adenoids. Children with Down syndrome are also at high risk.

There is chronic loud snoring and parents may notice cyclical obstruction, involving repeated episodes when the child stops breathing or struggles for breath. The child may wake up distressed after obstructive episodes, or there may be frequent brief arousals that disrupt sleep quality without parents noticing. Even when the child sleeps a normal number of hours, the poor quality of sleep can lead to daytime sleepiness (or hyperactivity, poor concentration, impulsiveness and irritability). Treatment options include surgical removal of enlarged tonsils and adenoids, or weight loss if obese. Tricyclic medication is sometimes used for adults with obstructive sleep apnoea, but does not appear to be effective for children.

Night terrors, sleepwalking and confusional arousals

These all involve partial arousal (without waking) out of deep non-REM sleep (see Box 20.1). They are therefore most likely to occur in the first couple of hours of sleep when deep non-REM is concentrated (see Box 20.1). They may occur more commonly when the child or adolescent is living with anxiety, for example, after a break-in to the house.

- *Confusional arousals* are common among infants and toddlers: the child cries, calls out or thrashes around, and does not respond when talked to. If left alone, the child calms down and resumes peaceful sleep after about 5–15 minutes. Trying to wake the child generally increases agitation and prolongs the episode.
- *Sleepwalking* occurs in up to 17% of children, with 4–8 years being the peak age. For up to ten minutes or so, the child wanders around with eyes wide open and a glassy stare, and may then return to bed or sleep elsewhere. Urination may occur in inappropriate places. There is a significant risk of injury, for example, falling down stairs. The environment needs to be made as safe as possible. Trying to restrain or wake the child generally make things worse.

• *Night terrors* affect about 3% of children, mainly in the 6–12 year age range but they can start at any age including adulthood. Parents are woken by a sudden scream and find their child looking terrified: sweaty, with a rapid pulse, eyes wide open, calling out or crying. The child may get out of bed and rush around in an agitated state (perhaps sustaining injuries). After just a few minutes, the child resumes peaceful sleep, and often doesn't remember anything of the episode in the morning. If they happen to wake after an episode, they may describe an intense but non-specific sense of danger or impending doom, but they don't describe the sort of elaborate plot of a typical nightmare. The main differential diagnoses are nightmares (vividly remembered and mostly happening in the second half of the night) and some types of nocturnal seizures.

When night terrors (or sleepwalking or confusional arousals) are happening frequently and at a regular time, they can sometimes be prevented by 'scheduled awakenings'. These involve gently waking the child up 15–30 minutes before the episode is due and then letting the child go rapidly back to sleep. If the arousals have failed to respond to scheduled awakenings, and if they are exposing the child to danger, medication should be considered. Benzodiazepines can be effective, but should only be given short term under specialist supervision.

Nightmares

These are very common and arise from REM sleep. The individual wakes up, frightened and alert, and remembers all too clearly what was going on in the dream. The fear takes a while to subside enough for the individual to go back to sleep. Parental reassurance and comforting usually help. Nightmares are more likely to occur when the child or adolescent is stressed or ill. Post-traumatic stress disorder often results in prominent nightmares related to the trauma. REM sleep is suppressed by alcohol and many medications (most antidepressants, benzodiazepines, stimulants). Sudden withdrawal of any REM-suppressing substance can lead to nightmares as part of the REM rebound.

Rhythmic movement disorder

This involves head banging, head rolling or body rocking at the onset of sleep (and sometimes during nocturnal awakenings or at the end of sleep). Episodes can last up to 15 minutes or more. It is common in infancy, nearly always ending by the age of 3 or 4. Whereas head banging while awake is often associated with severe intellectual disability or major psychiatric difficulties, head banging while asleep is generally benign. All that is needed in most cases is reassurance for the parents and padding for the cot sides.

Narcolepsy and related symptoms

About 1 in every 3,000 individuals has narcolepsy, with males and females equally affected and with most having had their first symptoms in adolescence or even childhood (around 5% before 5 years old). The symptoms involve elements of REM sleep intruding into wakefulness:

1 *Sleep attacks*: sudden onset of sleep even during activities such as meals.
2 *Cataplexy*: sudden loss of muscle tone, leading to collapse without loss of consciousness. This is often precipitated by strong emotion such as anger or amusement.
3 *Sleep paralysis*: loss of ability to move or speak while awake, either just before going to sleep, or just after waking up.
4 *Hallucinations* on falling asleep (hypnagogic hallucinations) or waking up (hypnopompic hallucinations). These are effectively waking dreams.

These four features occurring together make up the classical narcolepsy tetrad. It is even commoner to get just one, two or three of these features. When cataplexy is present, the cause is generally loss of the hypothalamic neurones that produce hypocretins (also known as orexins). These are excitatory neuropeptides that play a central role in the regulation of wakefulness, while also influencing food intake and energy expenditure. The neuronal loss is probably due to an autoimmune process that is more likely to occur in genetically predisposed individuals, possibly triggered by streptococcal or viral infections.

Methylphenidate is often useful for sleep attacks (in combination with good sleep hygiene and planned naps). Various types of antidepressants – including tricyclics and selective serotonin or noradrenaline reuptake inhibitors – can reduce or prevent cataplexy. Sleep paralysis and hallucinations can also be helped by antidepressants, though reassurance is often enough.

Kleine-Levin syndrome

This rare syndrome typically affects adolescent males. It involves episodes of excessive sleep, overeating and sexually disinhibited behaviour, sometimes accompanied by mood disorder, restlessness and bizarre behaviour. The episodes can last hours, days or weeks, and recur every few weeks or months. Hypothalamic abnormalities have been suspected but not proven. Adolescents and their parents and teachers can be reassured that this is a recognised condition that is neither wilful nor psychotic. Tricyclics or lithium may reduce recurrence. It usually remits spontaneously in later adolescence or early adulthood.

Medication

Education, reassurance and management advice are the main treatments for sleep disorders in childhood and adolescence. As described above, there are some indications for medication. However, it is important to stress that hypnotics should seldom be used. Although effective in the short term for common problems with getting to sleep or staying asleep, hypnotics are far less effective (and potentially more hazardous) than psychological approaches in the long term. It is generally a mistake to use benzodiazepines for more than a week or two since they lose effectiveness, induce dependence, and often result in 'rebound' worsening of sleep problems when they are finally discontinued. Sedating antihistamines are commonly prescribed, but without good evidence that they do more good than harm. There has been considerable interest in the use of melatonin: it is not a cure-all but probably does have a useful, though limited, role in the treatment of circadian rhythm disorders in some children with autism (where several trials have proven its usefulness) and severe intellectual disability. However, meta-analyses of trials in normal IQ adults with circadian rhythm disorders do not suggest any benefits, so prescribing melatonin in most children as a 'sleeping pill' should probably be avoided, despite its increasing popularity.

Further reading

Buscemi, N. *et al.* (2006) Efficacy and safety of exogenous melatonin for secondary sleep disorders and sleep disorders accompanying sleep restriction: Meta-analysis. *BMJ* **332**, 385–393.

Hill, C. (2011) Practitioner review: Effective treatment of behavioural insomnia in children. *Journal of Child Psychology and Psychiatry* **52**, 731–740.

Owens, J.A. (2009) Pharmacotherapy of pediatric insomnia. *Journal of the American Academy of Child and Adolescent Psychiatry* **48**, 99–107.

Rossignol D, Frye R. (2011) Melatonin in autism spectrum disorders: A systematic review and meta-analysis. *Developmental Medicine & Child Neurology* **53**, 783–792.

Stores, G. (2001) *A Clinical Guide to Sleep Disorders in Children and Adolescents.* Cambridge University Press, Cambridge.

van Geijlswijk, I *et al.* (2010) Dose finding of melatonin for chronic idiopathic childhood sleep onset insomnia: An RCT. *Psychopharmacologia* **212**, 379–391.

CHAPTER 21
Psychosomatics

Splitting off the mind as a completely separate entity from the body is often lamented in contemporary times, and its start is attributed to the dualism of Descartes (seventeenth century). In fact, Plato (fourth century BC) said. 'This is the great error of our day, that physicians separate the mind from the body.'

Nowadays most paediatricians and child and adolescent psychiatrists accept the need for a holistic approach, recognising that the physical disorders described in paediatric texts have psychological dimensions, just as the psychological disorders described in this book have physical dimensions. Paediatrics should no more be mindless than child and adolescent psychiatry should be disembodied!

A list of all the disorders that involve both body and mind would potentially include the whole of medicine. In some instances the direction of effect is primarily somatopsychic, with physical antecedents leading on to psychological consequences. For example, chronic illnesses often have considerable psychological consequences. In other instances, the direction of effect is primarily from psychological antecedents to physical consequences; this is what most people mean by psychosomatic. Such presentations may be called 'medically unexplained symptoms', 'functional', or 'psychogenic'. Distinguishing categorically between conditions that are and are not psychosomatic is bound to be arbitrary and leads, predictably enough, to boundary disputes. In the case of asthma, for example, although it is clear that psychological stress can induce or intensify attacks of wheezing in some predisposed individuals, many people would resist calling asthma a psychosomatic disorder since stress is just one precipitant among many. More people would agree that headaches or stomach-aches are often psychosomatic conditions, and yet this may partly reflect our current ignorance of physical predisposing and precipitating factors. It is probably best to speak instead of a psychosomatic approach that is potentially relevant to some extent to any condition.

In this chapter, a general introduction to the psychosomatic approach is followed by sections on three illustrative disorders: recurrent abdominal pain, chronic fatigue syndrome and conversion disorder. Somatopsychic

Child and Adolescent Psychiatry, Third Edition. Robert Goodman and Stephen Scott.
© 2012 Robert Goodman and Stephen Scott. Published 2012 by John Wiley & Sons, Ltd.

links are the focus of Chapter 29, which describes the common psychological complications of children and adolescents' brain disorders.

Some general principles

Stress and anxiety can initiate and amplify somatic symptoms

Most readers will know from personal experience or direct observation that stress can induce a variety of somatic symptoms, including headaches, nausea, abdominal pains, diarrhoea and urinary frequency. It is also common knowledge that an anxious focus on a symptom often makes the symptom seem worse, resulting in increased anxiety, even greater fixation on the symptom, and so on. In addition, a child or adolescent's anxiety and distress can make the parents feel helpless and panic-stricken. If the parents are unable to hide this, this further fuels their child's anxiety. These vicious cycles, and some of the factors moderating or triggering them, are shown in Box 21.1. Family beliefs about illness play a key role. People differ in the extent to which they make 'normalising' or 'pathologising' attributions about the causes of somatic symptoms: normalising attributions relate the symptoms to environmental or psychological factors (for example, 'I have a headache because I am under stress and stayed up too late last night'), whereas pathologising attributions focus on organic or pathological causes (for example, 'perhaps it's a brain tumour'). Normalising attributions are reassuring and can prevent anxiety-related vicious cycles from taking over. Within any one family, the balance of normalising and pathologising attributions will vary over time and according to the nature of the symptom. For example, family stresses may undermine normalising attributions, and having a relative who has recently died of a

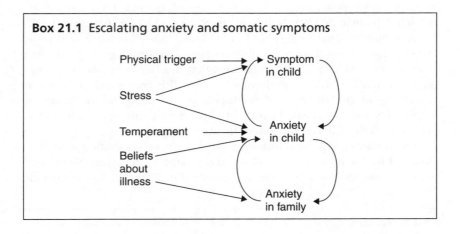

Box 21.1 Escalating anxiety and somatic symptoms

brain tumour may sensitise all family members to possible organic causes of headache. In many instances, anxiety-driven cycles can be interrupted by the reassurance of a trusted doctor who has carried out an adequate investigation. Occasionally, however, doctors are themselves drawn into the vicious cycles of panic and pathologising, with ever more specialist investigations and second opinions reinforcing the family's view that there must be something serious to worry about.

Somatic symptoms can sometimes be a 'mask'

Distress occasioned by psychological or social factors can sometimes be displaced onto a somatic symptom. A particularly transparent version of this can often be witnessed in young children. Thus, a child may fight back tears after a quarrel with a friend but then cry inconsolably after a minor fall a short while later. Obtaining relief or sympathy in this way, by focusing on an 'acceptable' somatic symptom such as physical pain, may have the undesirable long-term effect of training the child to somatise psychological distress in future too (Box 21.2). Sensitive parenting can help children and adolescents learn to disclose their psychological distress without needing to mask it with somatic symptoms (Box 21.3). For both parents and professionals, however, there is also a danger in going to the opposite extreme; psychological probing and psychologising of somatic symptoms can be overdone.

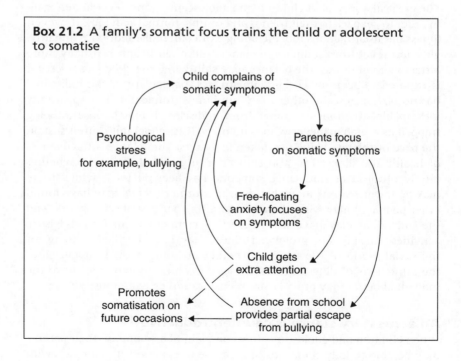

Box 21.2 A family's somatic focus trains the child or adolescent to somatise

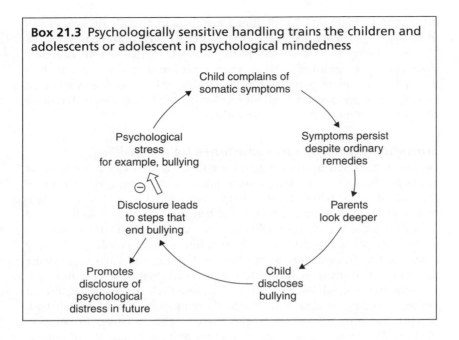

Box 21.3 Psychologically sensitive handling trains the children and adolescents or adolescent in psychological mindedness

Health and illness can each be self-perpetuating

The great majority of ill children and adolescents want to get better again in order to get back to their friends and resume normal activities. However, illness has its attractions too, including extra parental attention, sympathy, gifts and relief from ordinary demands. Although health is usually more attractive than illness, the balance may shift when the child or adolescent is exposed to acute or chronic life stresses, particularly if the individual has no obvious escape other than into illness. Intolerable but apparently inescapable situations can range from undisclosed sexual abuse to being trapped as a high achiever who is doing well at school but cannot sustain the pace or tolerate being overtaken by others. The relative attractiveness of health and illness can also shift after any period of illness, whether purely physical or not. Once someone has been ill for a while, there may be fewer reasons to get better again: former friends may have found other people to play with, there is a daunting backlog of schoolwork, and the individual may have lost interest or competence in former leisure activities. In addition, prolonged illness may have instilled a liking for the social world of the patient, whether at home or in hospital. Once the attractions of illness exceed those of health, any move to make the individual better may provoke an intensification of symptoms.

An accusatory stance is counterproductive

When children and adolescents first complain of a symptom, their parents may be able to jolly them out of it or use a 'come off it' approach with success. However, by the time their symptoms are being presented to health professionals, the child or adolescent would lose face if they got better in response to being told that they were putting it on, or making a mountain out of a molehill, and parents would probably feel foolish and angry too, for having been taken in. Predictably enough, 'pull yourself together and stop wasting our time' suggestions may lead to persistence or worsening of symptoms as the individual demonstrates that he or she really is ill. Indeed, it is not just explicitly critical comments that can be counterproductive; any hint that professionals are being dismissive or condemnatory can have a negative effect.

Factors in the child or adolescent

Children and adolescents with psychosomatic disorders are commonly described as conscientious, obsessional, sensitive, insecure or anxious; these are best seen as personality traits rather than as disorders. Affected individuals may be temperamentally predisposed to withdraw from new situations, and have sometimes had problems with peer relationships. Only a minority have a co-existent psychiatric disorder, and it is difficult to know how often this is a consequence rather than a cause of their somatic complaints: 'Of course, I'm depressed, doctor. Wouldn't you be if you had my symptoms?'

Factors in the family

Family members with somatic symptoms may provide models – in terms of the symptoms themselves, and also in terms of coping style. If relatives have stomach complaints, headaches or seizures, this may sensitise children and adolescents to these problems or even provide them with a model for conscious or unconscious imitation. If adults in the family typically respond anxiously to their own somatic symptoms, assuming that something beyond their control is seriously wrong, this may well foster anxiety, 'pathologising' attributions, and an external locus of control in children and adolescents too.

Although family stresses may initiate or aggravate ill health, there is no convincing evidence that specific types of family stresses are linked with specific types of ill health. 'Psychosomatic' families are sometimes characterised as close families who find it hard to express psychological concerns directly, seeking and providing attention and reassurance through the currency of somatic concern. Other family characteristics that have been said to predispose to psychosomatic disorders are:

- one over-involved parent, with the other distant;
- parental disharmony;
- parental overprotection;
- a rigid or disorganised set of rules rather than a stable and flexible set;
- dysfunctional communication without conflict resolution.

Favourable characteristics are said to include warmth, cohesion and satisfactory adaptation to the realities of the family situation. While these suggested risk and protective factors are certainly plausible, they derive primarily from clinical impressions (a potentially fallible guide) rather than from empirical studies.

External stressors

Both chronic adversities and acute life events can play a part. Abuse only seems relevant in a small minority of cases; bullying and academic stresses are probably more common contributors.

Approach to management

Children and adolescents with somatic symptoms have often been referred to paediatricians in the first instance. An organic cause will not have been found – a correct term is 'medically unexplained symptoms'. Families may be better able to accept a psychosomatic approach to assessment and treatment when their family doctor and paediatrician have taken a holistic approach from the outset, considering the interplay of biological and psychological factors from the first assessment onwards. Involving mental health professionals is then just a change in emphasis rather than a complete switch of direction that carries the implicit message: 'We have completed our investigations and there is nothing really wrong with your child, so you had better see the psychiatrists instead.'

The family need to hear from their doctor that the assessment so far has ruled out the dreadful organic diseases that they were worried about (tumours, ulcers, blockages, or whatever). This does not mean that the symptoms are unimportant; it simply means that effective symptomatic treatments can now be deployed without having to worry that there is something more sinister in the background. This message, which helps de-escalate anxious fixation on symptoms, is undermined if physical investigations continue 'just in case'.

There is little to gain and much to lose from trying to force the family to be more psychologically minded than they want to be. If the family continues to feel that physical factors are important, remember that they may be right: current medical views on body and mind will probably seem ridiculously primitive to future generations. It can be useful to emphasise the value of 'mind over matter' and graded rehabilitation approaches. Psychological and behavioural methods can work even when symptoms have a physical cause, which is why these methods are used to help children and adolescents cope with painful medical procedures or chronic physical symptoms of known organic origin. It is often helpful to teach techniques such as 'self-hypnosis' or relaxation therapy. These can make affected individuals (and their parents) feel more in control of symptoms. This is treatment for the present episode and prophylactic medicine for the future too. The more psychologically minded families may agree from the outset that psychological stresses could have played a part and need to be explored further. Less psychologically minded families can find this too challenging at the outset, but are sometimes more receptive when 'mind over matter' techniques have started to pay dividends. Children and adolescents who have a psychiatric disorder, such as depression, in addition to their somatic symptoms, may need to have their psychiatric disorder treated in its own right if it does not resolve as a result of the other psychological interventions.

Recurrent abdominal pain (RAP)

This affects some 10–25% of children and adolescents, with peak prevalence between the ages of 3 and 9 years. Most parents recognise links between the episodes of pain and psychological stresses and provide psychosomatic management without the need for any medical input. Nevertheless, the minority of cases that do get referred on for specialist opinions are sufficiently numerous to account for about 10% of all new paediatric out-patient visits. Even in tertiary paediatric centres, less than 10% of RAP proves to be associated with a serious organic disorder. Though there is suggestive evidence that some children and adolescents are physically predisposed to RAP, psychological stresses are thought to play major roles as precipitating and perpetuating factors.

Factors in the children and adolescents
Most children and adolescents with RAP are psychiatrically normal; the slightly elevated rate of psychiatric problems is comparable to that of children and adolescents with chronic abdominal pain of known organic aetiology. Affected individuals are often described as timid, high-strung, over-conscientious, or particularly keen on adult approval. Some withdraw from new challenges and others tend to become awkward and irritable when stressed.

Factors in the family
Clinical descriptions of the families emphasise their closeness, their high expectations, and the high level of parental concern about their children. Family members have an elevated rate both of emotional symptoms and of somatic complaints, particularly gastrointestinal complaints, some with known organic bases and some not. It has yet to be established whether this familial aggregation reflects modelling, genetic transmission, or shared exposure to adverse environments.

External stressors
There is an association with life events. Most stresses are of an 'everyday' variety, such as a change in school or an impending examination. It is distinctly unusual for children and adolescents suffering from sexual abuse to present with RAP without other symptoms of more widespread disturbance.

Natural history

The great majority of children and adolescents grow out of RAP; very few turn out to have missed organic disorders. In a proportion, it may be a precursor of the irritable bowel syndrome in adulthood.

Treatment

The family need convincing medical reassurance based on an appropriate assessment. It is often helpful to involve the affected individual and his or her family in systematic monitoring and recording of symptoms, antecedents and consequences is often helpful; this may make the relationship with psychosocial stressors clearer to all concerned. The child or adolescent can be taught techniques to control symptoms: guided imagery, self-hypnosis, or relaxation techniques. The affected individual should be encouraged to resume normal activities despite any residual pain; parents need to reinforce these activities through praise and attention, simultaneously reducing the extent to which symptoms are rewarded by extra attention. Using these approaches, pain usually disappears or becomes easier to live with if it persists or recurs.

Chronic fatigue syndrome (CFS)

Best known in adults, CFS does also occur in children and adolescents, affecting between 0.4 and 2 children and adolescents per thousand, according to one British study. CFS is usually defined on the basis of disabling physical fatigue of over six months duration that is unexplained by primary physical or psychiatric causes. It is often accompanied by mental fatigue and by other physical symptoms, without a demonstrable organic basis. Low mood is common, with the family considering this to be a consequence rather than a cause of the CFS. This low mood is not often associated with self-blame or feelings of worthlessness; a depressive disorder is only diagnosable in roughly a third of cases. As for adult CFS, the evidence for an organic aetiology is weak and inconsistent, but absence of proof is not proof of absence.

This is a disorder where a debate between doctor and family about the relative importance of physical and psychological factors is particularly likely to generate heat rather than light. It is best to remain agnostic, to refuse to be drawn into debates that cannot be resolved on the basis of current evidence, and to get on with treatment. It is helpful to motivate the affected individual and the family to beat the problem by harnessing the 'power of positive thinking' and graded rehabilitation approaches. Working with the family, it is usually possible to get the child or adolescent to do a bit more every day, with a graded return to normal physical activities, leisure pursuits and school. It is worth emphasising that these cognitive-behavioural approaches do help, but that their success does not prove that the disorder was 'all in the mind' in the first place.

Conversion disorders

Conversion disorders involve the presence of symptoms or deficits that affect voluntary motor or sensory functioning; these symptoms or deficits suggest an organic disorder but there is no evidence for organic causation and there is positive evidence for psychological causation. These children and adolescents usually present with a bizarre gait, weakness or paralysis of the legs, funny turns or total incapacitation. Symptoms correspond to the patient's idea of what an illness should look like, only partially matching a doctor's idea; it is these discrepancies that often suggest that the illness is 'hysterical'.

The diagnosis of conversion disorders is fraught with difficulties. A proportion of diagnosed children and adolescents do eventually turn out to have an organic disease accounting for their symptoms. Apparently bizarre symptoms may prove to be recognised features of a rare disorder that the diagnosing doctor had never considered. Alternatively, the children and adolescents may have an unusual presentation of a more common disorder. To make matters even more complicated, organic factors may still be important even if psychological factors are indeed responsible for some symptoms. Children and adolescents whose physical symptoms are not believed may then exaggerate the symptoms in order to be taken seriously. In addition, children and adolescents may mimic their own episodic disorders, so the fact that a child or adolescent sometimes has 'pseudoseizures' does not rule out co-existent true epileptic seizures as well.

Despite all these diagnostic pitfalls, most clinicians are convinced that conversion disorder does exist. It can be seen as an (unconscious) enactment of illness in response to an unbearable predicament. Some children and adolescents respond to stress by acting tough, or grown-up, or pathetic; others respond by acting ill. Doctors need to ensure that they do not make these children and adolescents worse by initiating a protracted series of investigations and second opinions; they also need to help affected individuals find more adaptive ways of dealing with whatever stresses precipitated the episode.

Conversion disorders are relatively rare in high-income countries, accounting for roughly 1% of psychiatric in-patients – though the proportion is probably higher among out-patients, particularly those referred by paediatricians. These disorders are rare before the age of 5 and mostly affect children and adolescents over the age of 10. Postpubertal girls may be particularly susceptible. The rate of conversion disorders may be higher in low- and middle-income countries.

The children and adolescents

Premorbid adjustment has often been normal; some have been particularly perfectionist or conscientious students. Only a minority have another psychiatric diagnosis in addition to the conversion disorder.

The family

The family seems normal in most instances; only about a fifth are grossly abnormal. They are usually convinced that the disorder is organic, wanting further physical assessment and resisting psychiatric referral. There is often a family history of physical or psychiatric disorder.

The context and outcome

The child or adolescent is often stuck in an intolerable predicament, ranging from undisclosed sexual abuse to unsustainably high expectations. The disorder may be precipitated by an adverse life event or by a minor physical illness, although there is sometimes no clear antecedent. In 80% of cases it is possible to identify a model for the symptoms that are enacted: similar illnesses in the family or the wider social circle, or illnesses that the individual has previously had. Most conversion disorders recover fully, but a minority run a very chronic course.

Treatment

Physical investigations need to stop. An initial focus on the symptoms rather than on possible psychological stressors may help the family engage. This is a process that may be slow and cannot easily be hurried. A mixture of physical rehabilitation and training in 'mind over matter' techniques provides the child or adolescent with a way out with honour. The affected individual needs to obtain greater rewards by getting better than by staying sick. This can sometimes be done by altering the family's behaviour, but may sometimes need an in-patient admission. When a child or adolescent is stuck in an intolerable predicament, this needs to be recognised and addressed. In the longer term, the individual needs to learn more adaptive ways of dealing with stresses.

Subject review

Husain K *et al.* (2007) A review of psychological models and interventions for medically unexplained symptoms in children. *Children and Adolescents and Adolescent Mental Health* **12**, 2–7.

Sandberg S, Stevenson J. (2008) Psychiatric aspects of somatic disease. *In*: Rutter M *et al.* (eds) *Rutter's Child and Adolescent Psychiatry*, 5th edn. Wiley-Blackwell, Chichester, pp. 930–944.

Further reading

Chalder T *et al.* (2003) Epidemiology of chronic fatigue syndrome and self reported myalgic encephalomyelitis in 5–15-year-olds: cross-sectional study. *BMJ* **327**, 654–655.

Edwards M, Titman P. (2010) *Promoting Psychological Wellbeing in Children with Acute and Chronic Illness*. London: Jessica Kingsley. (A short, readable book that has many helpful strategies for helping children and adolescents with a variety of illnesses, and for those with medically unexplained symptoms.)

Garralda ME, Chalder T. (2005) Chronic fatigue syndrome in childhood. *Journal of Child Psychology and Psychiatry* **46**, 1143–51.

NICE (2007) *Chronic Fatigue Syndrome/Myalgic Encephalitis: Diagnosis and Management*. London: National Institute for Health and Clinical Excellence. (This includes information and recommendations for children and adolescents.)

White P *et al.* (2011) Comparison of adaptive pacing therapy, cognitive behaviour therapy, graded exercise therapy, and specialist medical care for chronic fatigue syndrome (PACE): a randomised trial. *Lancet* **377**, 823–836. (Although the patients were adults, this thorough trial showed that either CBT or graded exercise [they were not tested in combination] were superior to ordinary specialist medical care or adaptive pacing, whereby the patient dictates the pace of recovery. Sadly the trial led to death threats to some of the authors from an angry minority of CFS sufferers, who appeared to be very concerned by the prospect of being told they might get better.)

CHAPTER 22

Preschool Problems

Many children under the age of 5 years have attentional, emotional or behavioural problems, including the well-recognised disorders described elsewhere in this book, for example, autism or a disinhibited attachment disorder. In other instances, however, the preschool child has just one area of problems (for example, faddy eating) or a few problems that do not add up to any recognised diagnosis. In these instances, the assessment generates a list of problem areas rather than a specific diagnosis.

Common problems

The classic community study of preschool problems and their consequences is the Preschool to School study (see Box 22.1). Preschool children can present with the same sorts of symptoms that commonly bring older children to psychiatric attention: worries, fears, misery, aggression, tantrums, over-activity, inattention, and so on. As shown in Box 22.1, age trends differ by symptom. Thus, as children mature, over-activity and fears become less common while worries become more common – and the number of 'hard to manage' children stays fairly constant.

Developmental or habit problems are particularly common among preschool children. Delays in toilet training are very frequent, as are comfort habits such as rocking, thumb sucking, head banging, masturbation or hair sucking. Other common difficulties include poor appetite, faddy eating, difficulty settling to sleep at night and frequent night wakening. As shown in Box 21.1, maturation leads to the resolution of many developmental and habit problems. Once parents know this, they are often willing to wait for their child to grow out of these behaviours. If the family do want help, then advice on behavioural management is often the answer. This advice may come from a health visitor, a family doctor, a paediatrician or a mental health professional.

Child and Adolescent Psychiatry, Third Edition. Robert Goodman and Stephen Scott.
© 2012 Robert Goodman and Stephen Scott. Published 2012 by John Wiley & Sons, Ltd.

Box 22.1 The Preschool to School Study (Richman *et al.*, 1982)

Method
This study is a random 1 in 4 sample of 3-year-olds from an outer London borough. A two-stage design (see Chapter 3) involved an initial screening interview, followed by detailed assessments at 3, 4 and 8 years of age for all 'screen positive' children and a matched sample of 'screen negative' children.

Main findings at age 3
Moderate or severe problems were present in 7%, with mild problems in a further 15%. There was a slight male excess. Boys were more hyperactive; girls were more fearful. Psychiatric problems were commoner in the presence of specific language delay or adverse social and family factors, including marital discord, low warmth, high criticism, maternal depression, large family size and high-rise housing.

Main findings at age 8
Of the 3-year-olds with problems, 73% of boys still had problems five years later as did 48% of girls. Over-activity and low intelligence predicted persistence in boys, but not in girls. Over-activity predicted disruptive behavioural disorders while fearfulness predicted emotional disorders. Adverse family factors were more relevant as predisposing than as maintaining causes, that is, they predicted the onset of new problems but were not good at predicting whether established problems would persist of not.

Percentage with marked problems definitely present at different ages

	3 years	4 years	8 years
Fears	10	12	2
Overactive, restless	17	13	11
Tempers	5	6	9
Worries	4	10	21
Hard to manage	11	10	11
Soiling at least once a week	16	3	4
Many comfort habits	17	14	1
Waking at night at least 3 times a week	14	12	3

Outcome in later childhood

Though some preschool problems are transient, others persist. The chronicity of some preschool problems is evident both prospectively and retrospectively. Prospectively, follow-up studies such as the Preschool to School study have shown that a substantial proportion of severely troubled preschoolers do develop clear-cut ADHD, disruptive behavioural disorders, and emotional disorders as they grow older. Retrospectively, this continuity is often evident when assessing the psychiatric problems of schoolchildren, with parental accounts making it clear that the problems go back to the preschool years. Many children with oppositional-defiant disorder have always been irritable and prone to temper tantrums; many children with separation anxiety disorder have always been very clingy and fearful; and many children with ADHD have always been over-active and inattentive.

Why, then, have clinicians often found it hard to diagnose ADHD, conduct and emotional disorders with confidence in 3-year-olds? In part, it is because the tools for the job were not available until recently – the sorts of high-quality structured diagnostic assessments that have been widely deployed in research and clinical assessments of school-age children did not extend down to preschool children. This is now changing, at least for the assessment of 2–4-year-olds. However, there is still a signal-to-noise problem. For example, although many 3-year-olds are very active and find it hard to settle to tasks, most of them develop adequate attention and activity control by the time they start school; only a small minority have persistent problems that eventually warrant a diagnosis of ADHD. Detecting early ADHD (the 'signal') is harder when there is so much background 'noise' in the form of self-limiting over-activity and inattention. As assessment techniques improve, it should be possible to predict more accurately which preschool problems are the first signs of chronic disorders. If so, these children could potentially be targeted for continuing extra help before they run into serious problems. By contrast, reassurance or a brief intervention may be all that is needed for preschool problems that are likely to be outgrown.

Outcome in adulthood

The Preschool to School sample was followed up again, in what could have been called the 'Preschool to Court' study, since the only outcome measure obtained in young adult life was whether the individual had a criminal record. Perhaps the single most important finding is that it is not possible to predict accurately which 3-year-olds will turn out to be law-breakers – a finding that will be a relief to many, though a disappointment to some. Nevertheless, even after allowing for gender, social background and developmental delay, some preschool problems were modestly predictive of adult criminality. Thus, 3-year-olds who were markedly over-active or hard to manage were roughly twice as likely to commit adult offences, while 3-year-olds with marked temper tantrums were about four times as likely to commit violent adult offences. These findings add to the case for providing parents of oppositional-defiant preschoolers with effective help (see Chapter 6) and not simply assuming that they will 'grow out of it'.

Treatment

When preschool children have one of the psychiatric syndromes covered elsewhere in this book, treatment generally follows the standard lines discussed in the relevant chapter. Liaison with the education authority is particularly important for children with chronic disorders such as autism, since it is often helpful for the education authority to know in advance about children with emotional, behavioural and learning problems that are likely to require special educational provision. Early warning may also allow the child to be placed in an appropriate playgroup or nursery school, which will often help not only the child but also the worn-out parents.

If the assessment identifies one or more problem areas rather than a specific diagnosis, management strategies need to be considered for each problem. In some instances, parents may not feel that any treatment is necessary once they have been reassured that a problem is common and likely to be short-lived (and told how and when to get back in touch in the event that the problem does persist). When treatment is indicated, behavioural approaches are often particularly valuable. For example, if temper tantrums or night wakening are being reinforced by parental attention, the solution may be to pay less attention to the problem. The behavioural programme needs to be tailored to the characteristics of the parents as well as those of the child. For example, if parents do not have nerves of steel, they may find it hard to 'extinguish' night wakening by completely ignoring their child's calls or cries in the middle of the night. A more 'softly, softly' approach may suit such parents better, for example, paying progressively less attention each successive night. It is important to remember that a behavioural programme that the parents cannot carry through to completion is worse than nothing, since it demoralises the parents and trains the child to hold out against any subsequent attempt to tackle the problem behaviour.

Subject review

Gardner F, Shaw DS. (2008) Behavioral problems in infancy and preschool children (0–5). *In*: Rutter M *et al.* (eds) *Rutter's Child and Adolescent Psychiatry*, 5th edn. Wiley-Blackwell, Chichester, pp. 882–893.

Further reading

Egger HL, Angold A. (2006) Common emotional and behavioral disorders in preschool children: Presentation, nosology, and epidemiology. *Journal of Child Psychology and Psychiatry* **47**, 313–337.

Richman N *et al.* (1982) *Preschool to School: A Behavioural Study*. Academic Press, London.

Stevenson J, Goodman R. (2001) Association between behaviour at age three years and adult criminality. *British Journal of Psychiatry* **179**, 197–202.

Tremblay RE *et al.* (2004) Physical aggression during early childhood: Trajectories and predictors. *Pediatrics* **114**, e43–e50.

Zeanah CH (2009) *Handbook of Infant Mental Health*, 3rd edn. Guilford Press, New York. (Infancy in this book refers to the period from birth to 3 years.)

CHAPTER 23

Introduction to Adolescence and Its Disorders

Since adolescence falls between childhood and adulthood, it is not surprising that most of the psychiatric disorders of adolescence are either continuations of childhood disorders or early manifestations of adult disorders. But adolescence is not just a blend of childhood and adulthood; it is a stage with unique biological and social characteristics of its own that colour both normal and abnormal behaviour during the teenage years. Before focusing on abnormal behaviour, it is important to consider the uniqueness of the world the adolescent lives in, as well as the processes of internal mental and physical maturation particular to this stage of life. The behavioural problems that peak in the teenage years, such as delinquency, substance abuse, deliberate self-harm and anorexia nervosa, often involve exaggerated and unresolved versions of the ordinary trials and tribulations of adolescence.

A potted history of adolescence

Although puberty is a biological process, adolescence, as we currently know it, is a relatively new social phenomenon. In the developing world, many people leave school and begin work before or during puberty; physical maturity develops in step with economic and social maturity. The same was true in the developed world until fairly recently, when the combination of earlier puberty (reflecting better nutrition and health) and prolonged education resulted in a 'no man's land' opening up between childhood and adulthood. This is the prolonged period when teenagers acquire adult bodies but not adult roles, rights or financial independence. Of course, this is an over-simplification, but it points to the need to think of adolescence (and indeed every other stage of life too) as culturally as well as biologically determined.

Child and Adolescent Psychiatry, Third Edition. Robert Goodman and Stephen Scott.
© 2012 Robert Goodman and Stephen Scott. Published 2012 by John Wiley & Sons, Ltd.

Rules and autonomy

During adolescence there is a shift from accepting rules and boundaries imposed by others to setting them oneself, substituting self-imposed control for externally imposed control. Young people face a demanding task as they try to exercise their growing capacity and desire for self-determination within limits acceptable to their parents and society as a whole. Not surprisingly, surveys confirm that the commonest causes of arguments with parents in this period are issues relating to rules and autonomy. At the more disturbed end of the spectrum, 'out of control' teenagers pursue their own desires while paying little or no heed to society's rules and other people's needs. It is the simultaneous absence of externally imposed and self-imposed control that makes these adolescents particularly difficult to manage for all those involved, including parents, teachers, social workers and psychiatrists. When parents can no longer cope, simply taking these youngsters into care into a foster home may not improve matters, unless the foster carers have better disciplinary skills that the birth parents (which they may do, especially if they have had specific training). Placing them in a children's home may only aggravate the problem, since the lack of containment in many children's homes is reflected in high rates of various 'out of control' activities. These activities can include precocious and unprotected sexual activity, overdoses and wrist cutting, drug taking, running away for days at a time and theft. There is often a frustrating gap in services where all a clinician or parent can do is watch an adolescent decline: out of control but not harming themselves enough to be detained under legislation, or offending sufficiently seriously to be incarcerated in a young offenders' institution (which may not do them much good anyway).

Biological and social influences interact

Biological factors contribute to the pubertal upsurge in sexual and aggressive behaviours in humans as in other animals; the consequences of delayed puberty bear this out. However, different cultures channel these biological predispositions in different ways, amplifying some features and suppressing others. Commonsense notions to the contrary, there is no convincing evidence that hormone levels are abnormally high among extremely aggressive delinquents or multiple sex-offenders, and the efficacy (let alone desirability) of 'chemical castration' in these circumstances remains very dubious. Pathological variations in post-pubertal sexual and aggressive 'drives' seem more related to social and psychological variables than to biological variables.

The interplay of biological and social factors in adolescent development is well illustrated by the findings of a Swedish study of the consequences of early puberty for girls. Roughly 10% of a large and representative sample of girls entered puberty at least two years earlier than average. As adolescents, these early-maturing girls were more likely than their contemporaries to smoke, drink, steal, play truant, disobey their parents, and leave school at the earliest opportunity. These differences stemmed from the tendency of the early-maturing girls to associate with older girls, perhaps particularly with disaffected older girls who were doing poorly at school. A biological difference (early puberty) led on to a social difference (choice of peer group), and it was the social difference that affected adjustment; early-maturing girls without older friends were not at increased risk of norm breaking.

Cognitive development

In many respects, teenagers from the age of 14 or 15 have comparable cognitive capabilities to adults, for example, on tests of abstract reasoning or 'frontal lobe' functions. Conflicts can easily arise from the fact that teenagers are the equals of their parents or teachers in these respects, while differing enormously in experience and power. Adults may underestimate teenagers' ability to think things through for themselves; teenagers may underestimate the value of experience.

Just as people vary considerably in the age at which they reach their adult height, it seems likely that people vary widely in the age at which they reach their adult cognitive potential, with this variation having important consequences for psychosocial adaptation. Some studies of juvenile delinquents indicate that they are behind their peers in the development of conscience and altruism, although this has proved hard to measure.

Identity

In principle, our society offers youngsters a bewildering variety of possible adult roles: 'you can be anything you want if you really work at it'. In practice, many teenagers' options are restricted and unglamorous. This tension adds to the difficulties of adolescence as the young person attempts to work towards a sense of identity that bridges internal aspirations and external realities. A sense of confusion about personal identity can sometimes be so marked that it largely prevents a young person from functioning. DSM-IV provides a coding for Identity Problem under the rubric of other conditions that may be a focus of clinical interest. ICD-10 does not have a comparable category.

There are different risks associated with accepting and rejecting the identities offered by the adult world. Accepting an unglamorous identity that falls well short of previous aspirations may undermine self-esteem and predispose to depression. At the other extreme, some young people seem to define their identity primarily in terms of their rejection of adult

authority and adult norms, predisposing them to delinquency and substance abuse. An identity based on the rejection of adult values sometimes
seems to reflect the cumulative impact of criticism by parents, failure at
school, and subsequent identification with a delinquent peer group.

Sexual identity may not be completely clear to young people; surveys
suggest that while at least 3% are unambiguously homosexual, at least the
same number go through a period of bisexuality, which for the majority is
transient.

Solving problems and weathering stress

Though childhood has its own stresses, the transition to adulthood can
bring on many more: examinations, broken hearts, unemployment, or in-
tensified arguments with parents. Children who have not learned adaptive
ways of relating to others and dealing with crises, perhaps because their
parents also lacked the relevant skills, are likely to find the new stresses of
adolescence particularly hard to cope with. Violence, substance abuse and
self-harm can all be ways of defusing stress or temporarily dealing with
problems that cannot be solved more adaptively.

Epidemiology of adolescent psychiatric disorders

The Isle of Wight study of 14- and 15-year-olds remains the 'classical'
epidemiological investigation of adolescent psychopathology (see Box
23.1). The main conclusions of this study have stood the test of time.
The point prevalence of major depressive episodes in adolescence was
2% on the Isle of Wight 30 years ago – and also 2% in the recent
British national surveys cited in Chapter 3. Other studies have reported
significantly higher prevalence rates for adolescent depression, though it is
not clear if this is because different studies have used different thresholds,
or if rates of depression do indeed vary substantially across space and
time. There is accumulating evidence for a 'two population' model of
adolescent conduct problems, involving a 'hard core' of individuals who
are behaviourally disordered before, during and after adolescence, plus a
larger number of previously well-adjusted individuals who go through a
relatively transient phase of rule breaking and antisocial behaviour during
adolescence.

Emotional and disruptive behavioural disorders are the most common
diagnoses in adolescence, as in middle childhood. These are covered in
the relevant chapters, as are two other problems that peak in adolescence, namely, juvenile delinquency and deliberate self-harm. Chapters
24, 25, 26 are devoted to three conditions that are not covered elsewhere
and that are much more common in adolescence than in childhood:
schizophrenia, eating disorders (anorexia nervosa and bulimia nervosa)
and substance use.

Box 23.1 Isle of Wight follow-up (Rutter *et al.*, 1976)

Method

A total population sample of 2,303 adolescents living on the Isle of Wight were studied using a two-stage design: all subjects were assessed by behavioural screening questionnaires completed by parents and teachers; full psychiatric assessments were carried out on all 'screen positive' individuals and a random sample of 'screen negative' individuals. Most of the subjects had also been studied four years earlier in the original Isle of Wight study, though some were newcomers.

Main findings

1 Judging from the information gathered from parents and teachers, definite psychiatric disorders were present in roughly 10% of the sample – only slightly higher than the rate in middle childhood. In addition, another 10% of adolescents reported marked internal feelings of misery and worthlessness that were not accompanied by significant outward changes. Was this covert depression? Only long-term follow-up can answer the key question as to whether covert adolescent misery is the precursor of overt adult depression.

2 Of the disorders that were evident to informants, most were emotional and conduct disorders. Depressive disorders were commoner than at ten: 2% rather than 0.2%. (Self-reported misery was much commoner still: 48% of girls, 42% of boys.) School refusal was also commoner at age 14 than at age 10, occurring as part of wider anxiety and affective disorders.

3 Just under half of the children with disorders at age 14 had already had a disorder when assessed at age 10. Disorders arising for the first time after the age of 10 differed in three main ways from early-onset disorders: (a) they were not associated with educational difficulties; (b) there was only a slight male excess; and (c) adverse family factors were less often present.

4 Only a minority of adolescents were alienated from their parents (as judged by rows, physical and emotional withdrawal and rejection). Alienation was particularly common when the young person had a psychiatric disorder (especially if this was chronic). Although alienation dating back to middle or early childhood did seem to be linked to psychiatric disorders beginning after the age of 10, alienation beginning in the teenage years was not a common cause of psychiatric disorder.

Further reading

Graham P. (2004) *The End of Adolescence*. Oxford University Press, Oxford. (A leading child and adolescent psychiatrist argues that our society's systematic negative stereotyping of adolescence has contributed to young people being marginalised and disempowered.)

Magnusson E *et al.* (1985) Biological maturation and social development: A longitudinal study of some adjustment processes from mid-adolescence to adulthood. *Journal of Youth and Adolescence* **14**, 267–283. (Investigates the effects of early and late puberty in females.)

Rutter M *et al.* (1976) Adolescent turmoil: fact or fiction? *Journal of Child Psychology and Psychiatry* **17**, 35–56. (This describes the Isle of Wight study of adolescents.)

CHAPTER 24
Schizophrenia

Childhood-onset and adolescent-onset schizophrenia are pretty similar to adult-onset schizophrenia – but are rarer and generally more severe.

Epidemiology

Roughly one in a thousand 12–17-year-olds have experienced a psychotic disorder. Approximately half of these psychotic disorders are schizophrenia, while most of the rest are linked to depression, mania or drugs. Although schizophrenia can occur in children as young as 7, onset is very uncommon before puberty and becomes increasingly common as adolescence progresses, peaking in early adult life. Though males are generally more vulnerable to early-onset schizophrenia, the sex ratio is reversed in the 11–14 age band, perhaps because girls are much more likely than boys to be postpubertal at this age.

Characteristic features

The features of schizophrenia are often divided into *positive* and *negative* symptoms. This terminology is potentially confusing since it could imply that positive symptoms are good and negative symptoms are bad. In fact, 'positive' refer to the *presence* of symptoms that should not normally be there (for example, hallucinations, delusions, thought disorder, motor abnormalities), while 'negative' refers to a *reduction* in characteristics that should normally be there (for example, less speech, sociability, emotional involvement or motivation to do things).

Multivariate analyses suggest that the two-way distinction between positive and negative symptoms should perhaps be replaced by a three-way distinction between negative symptoms, reality distortion (hallucinations and delusions), and disorganisation (thought disorder, bizarre behaviour, inappropriate affect).

Child and Adolescent Psychiatry, Third Edition. Robert Goodman and Stephen Scott.
© 2012 Robert Goodman and Stephen Scott. Published 2012 by John Wiley & Sons, Ltd.

Box 24.1 Some symptoms that can occur in a psychotic episode

Perplexity (typically at the onset of a psychotic episode)
Andrew went through a period of a week or so when he was very upset because he was sure something had gone seriously wrong, but he wasn't sure what. He felt confused for all of this time and nothing seemed right – it was like being trapped in a bad dream for day after day.

Auditory hallucination
Beth hears voices when there is definitely no one around. Sometimes the voices are speaking directly to her ('second person' auditory hallucinations) and sometimes they talk to one another about her ('third person' auditory hallucinations). What they say is mostly critical of her.

Thought insertion
Craig feels strange thoughts being inserted directly into his head. These thoughts are definitely not his own thoughts. Sometimes it seems as if the thoughts are put into his head by laser beams, mobile phone masts, or other special methods.

Thought withdrawal
Daniel sometimes experiences his own thoughts being taken out of his mind or stolen by some strange force.

Delusions of control (passivity phenomena)
At times, Erin feels that her mind has been taken over by a strange force that makes her do things that she did not choose to do – rather as if she had become someone else's robot.

Delusions of reference
Frank experiences a strange force that communicates directly with him by sending special signs or signals that only he can understand. This sometimes happens through the radio or television.

Persecutory delusion
Although her family and friends disagree, Gabrielle is convinced that there is a serious plot against her, involving people who are following her around or who are out to harm or poison her.

Grandiose delusion
Hugh has times when he is sure that he has special powers that make him far better than other people and unbeatable. (Outside these episodes, he realises that he is not very different from most other people of his age.)

Motor abnormalities
Isabel will suddenly bend her trunk forward in a rather uncomfortable way and stay like that for several minutes (posturing). Sometimes she looks upwards and says 'Cancel, cancel' (a mannerism). At other times she repeatedly moves her neck to the right (a stereotypy). Occasionally she freezes (immobility).

Box 24.1 provides examples of some of the symptoms that can occur during a psychotic episode. Schizophrenic symptoms are fairly similar at all ages, though passivity phenomena and poverty of thought are less prominent than in adult-onset schizophrenia. In line with developmental level, delusions in children are generally less complex than in adults, and less likely to have sexual or other adult themes.

Schizophrenia characteristically involves a mixture of psychotic episodes (with prominent positive symptoms) and a progressive accumulation of negative symptoms. In the long term, it is generally the negative symptoms that are more disabling, and more upsetting to relatives. Though DSM-IV and ICD-10 have fairly similar diagnostic criteria for schizophrenia, DSM-IV puts greater weight on the accumulation of negative symptoms, while ICD-10 puts more weight on the episodic psychotic symptoms. On the one hand, this makes the DSM-IV criteria harder to apply in the short term since it takes a while to be sure about the accumulation of negative symptoms. On the other hand, the DSM-IV criteria are more specific in the long term when it comes to distinguishing schizophrenia from affective or drug-induced psychoses. Mania in adolescence can easily be misdiagnosed as schizophrenia in the short term – until it becomes clear that the acute psychotic episodes are linked to mood variation and are not accompanied by accumulating negative symptoms.

Antecedents of schizophrenia

Schizophrenia beginning in childhood or adolescence is particularly likely to be preceded by premorbid abnormalities in development and social adjustment. Neurodevelopmental abnormalities include speech and language delay, clumsiness, inattentiveness, and lowered IQ (mean around 85). The onset of frank psychosis is often preceded by years of poor social adjustment, and sometimes by disturbances of perception and thinking that are milder variants of schizophrenic delusions and hallucinations; sometimes it is preceded by disruptive behaviour disorders. Though this premorbid picture is often clear in retrospect, it is not sufficiently characteristic to permit a confident prospective diagnosis of incipient schizophrenia.

Differential diagnosis

Affective psychoses and drug-induced psychoses are the most likely alternative explanations for a psychotic disorder. In affective psychoses, the psychotic episodes occur during periods of abnormal mood, and full recovery between episodes is more likely and more complete than in schizophrenia – hence the importance of a careful history and mental state examination in making the distinction. It is, however, important to remember that the classical emphasis on there being a clear distinction between schizophrenia and bipolar disorder has turned out to be an over-simplification – they are now seen not as stark alternatives, but as opposite poles of a continuum (with schizoaffective disorders in the middle). Detecting drug-induced psychoses depends on history and drug testing.

In younger and more delayed children, it can be difficult to distinguish delusions and hallucinations from exaggerated age-appropriate fears and fantasies, especially if there is a coexisting language disorder. Rarely, childhood-onset schizophrenia does seem to develop on top of pre-existent autism spectrum disorders. In general, however, the distinction between autism and schizophrenia is straightforward – and since this is a favourite examination topic, we have summarized the key distinguishing features, as well as a couple of points of similarity in Box 24.2.

Box 24.2 Comparing autism and schizophrenia

	Autism	Schizophrenia
Characteristic features	Severe social impairment (aloof or unempathic). Severe communication problems. Rituals and repetitive behaviours.	Hallucinations, delusions, thought disorder, negative symptoms
Onset	Under three years, often from birth	Over seven years, mostly postpubertal ± premorbid developmental abnormalities (milder and less specific than in autism)
Family history	2% of siblings have autism and over 10% have lesser features of autism	Often positive family history of schizophrenia
Intellectual disability	Commonly	Rarely
Course	Non-episodic, chronic, mostly improving somewhat with maturation	Episodic, often with gradually deteriorating social adaptation
Neuroleptics ('Antipsychotics') useful	Rarely	Usually
Severe long-term social impairment	Usually	Usually
Need community care and specialist services	Usually	Usually

Causation

Twin studies suggest that the heritability of schizophrenia is around 80%, that is, genes account for about 80% of the variation between individuals in their liability to schizophrenia (see Chapter 33 for more on behavioural genetics and its limitations). Genetic factors may be even more important in early-onset than adult-onset schizophrenia. Studies using neuroimaging and neuropathology have demonstrated brain abnormalities in schizophrenia such as selective loss of grey matter due to loss of dendritic spines and synapses. Some brain abnormalities seem to precede the onset of psychosis, while others abnormalities may develop subsequently. While there is no doubt that biology plays an important role in the aetiology of schizophrenia, psychosocial stressors such as migration can also increase risk. In some instances, genes and environment seem to interact, for example, adolescent cannabis use may increase the risk of developing schizophrenia subsequently – but only in genetically vulnerable individuals.

In the light of growing evidence that schizophrenia is, at least in part, a neurodevelopmental disorder, why is prepubertal schizophrenia so uncommon? One possible explanation is that although brain abnormalities arise early in development, these are mostly silent until unmasked by *normal* developmental processes such as myelination or the progressive 'weeding out' of excessive synapses – processes that continue into puberty and even beyond. Alternatively, the key neurodevelopmental abnormality in schizophrenia may be *excessive* synaptic elimination occurring during adolescence, perhaps most marked in the prefrontal and temporal regions, resulting in abnormal neuronal connectivity and psychotic symptoms.

Clinical course and treatment

When schizophrenia begins early in life, the onset is often insidious rather than acute. Psychotic episodes commonly involve between one and six months of hallucinations, delusions and thought disorder.

Neuoleptic medications (usually referred to as 'antipsychotics' in this context) often reduce the intensity of positive symptoms but do not necessarily shorten the episode. Many adolescent psychiatrists choose newer 'atypical' antipsychotics such as olanzapine or risperidone as first-line treatment in preference to traditional 'typical' antipsychotics such as haloperidol or chlorpromazine. Head-to-head comparisons of typicals and atypicals suggest that they are roughly equally effective as far as reducing psychotic features are concerned, differing mainly in their adverse effects: typicals are more linked to extrapyramidal side effects (for example, Parkinsonian symptoms) and atypicals to rapid weight gain and its metabolic complications. Clozapine is a special atypical that may be successful when other typical and atypical antipsychotics have failed Patients on clozapine need regular blood monitoring to reduce the risk of serious side effects (for example, agranulocytosis). It is because of these side effects that clozapine should only be used when first-line drugs have failed.

Resolution of positive symptoms is often followed by a recovery phase of several months during which residual negative symptoms partially or fully resolve. As in the case of adult-onset schizophrenia, it is only a small minority who recover completely and have no further episodes. Continuing medication is likely to be needed. Family work will need to address coming to terms with what is often a devastating life-long illness; reducing the young person's exposure to criticism, hostility and other negative emotion may play a part in avoiding relapses. CBT to reduce the impact of residual positive symptoms may be worthwhile but trials in this age group are lacking. Affected individuals may also need special schooling, social skills training, and phased transfer to adult community psychiatric services. Particularly after second and subsequent episodes, recovery is often incomplete and social functioning may gradually deteriorate.

Prognosis

Early onset generally carries a worse prognosis than adult onset. The best predictors of poor long-term outcome are premorbid social and cognitive impairments, a prolonged first psychotic episode, negative symptoms at onset, and a prolonged period without treatment. Is prognosis improved by detecting and treating first episodes of psychosis more rapidly? Unfortunately, there is little evidence that early intervention teams do lead to a long-term improvement in outcome. Perhaps delayed treatment is not damaging in itself – simply a marker for the insidious onset and negative symptoms that confer a worse prognosis even with rapid treatment.

Subject review

Hollis C. (2008) Schizophrenia and allied disorders. *In*: Rutter M *et al.* (eds) *Rutter's Child and Adolescent Psychiatry*, 5th edn. Wiley-Blackwell, Chichester, pp. 737–758.

Further reading

Asarnow JR *et al.* (2004) Childhood-onset schizophrenia: clinical and treatment issues. *Journal of Child Psychology and Psychiatry* **45**, 180–194.

Boeing L *et al.* (2007) Adolescent-onset psychosis: prevalence, needs and service provision. *British Journal of Psychiatry* **190**, 18–26.

CHAPTER 25

Eating Disorders

Anorexia nervosa and bulimia nervosa are the two best-described eating disorders. People affected by these disorders share a strong tendency to judge their own worth largely on the basis of their weight, their shape, and their ability to control that weight and shape. In anorexia, the single-minded pursuit of weight loss is so 'successful' that it undermines physical health and can even result in death. In bulimia, body weight remains in the normal range because the pursuit of weight loss is balanced out by repeated episodes of binge eating in which the individual loses control and consumes a large amount of food. Besides anorexia and bulimia, there are also many variations on similar themes, including partial and hybrid disorders, sometimes lumped together as Eating Disorder Not Otherwise Specified (EDNOS). Although the remainder of this chapter focuses on anorexia and bulimia, readers should not be surprised if they often meet young people whose lives are seriously affected by anorexic and/or bulimic symptoms that do not quite meet the official criteria for either disorder.

Anorexia nervosa

Diagnosis

The main ICD-10 diagnostic criteria for anorexia nervosa are shown in Box 25.1. DSM-IV criteria are similar, with an optional division into two subtypes:

1 The *restricting* type involves weight loss purely via reduced food intake and excessive exercise.
2 The *binge-eating/purging* type involves added features, namely episodes of binge eating that are offset by *purging* (that is, self-induced vomiting or the misuse of laxatives, enemas or diuretics).

Whether these really are two distinct subtypes as opposed to points on a continuum is still in doubt. Depressive and obsessional features are common, sometimes warranting additional diagnoses.

Child and Adolescent Psychiatry, Third Edition. Robert Goodman and Stephen Scott.
© 2012 Robert Goodman and Stephen Scott. Published 2012 by John Wiley & Sons, Ltd.

> **Box 25.1** ICD-10 criteria for anorexia nervosa
>
> 1 Underweight: <85% of expected weight for age and height (due to weight loss or, in children, to lack of expected weight gain).
> 2 Caused by: deliberate dietary restriction, sometimes combined with excessive exercise, appetite suppressants, or purging (i.e. deliberate vomiting or misuse of laxatives, enemas, or diuretics).
> 3 Associated cognitions: intense fear of fatness. Feels fat even when underweight (or only feels about right when very underweight).
> 4 Endocrine consequences: Amenorrhoea in post-menarcheal females, unless on the 'pill'. (Loss of sexual interest and potency in males. Delayed or arrested puberty in early-onset cases.)
>
> *Note: The ICD-10 Classification of Mental and Behavioural Disorders: Diagnostic Criteria for Research* (World Health Organization, 1993).

Epidemiology

Anorexia nervosa has a peak age of onset in the mid-teens and a female:male ratio of up to 10:1. Onset is uncommon before puberty. Prevalence estimates for teenage girls mostly range from 0.1% to 0.7%.

Causation

Twin studies have generated contradictory evidence on the role of genetic predisposition: twins with anorexia are more likely to have affected co-twins than would be expected by chance, but it is still unclear how far this is due to shared genes or shared environment. Perfectionism is a common premorbid trait. Epidemiological studies suggest that social factors can be important. The contemporary western stereotype of female beauty involves a degree of slimness that obliges most adolescent girls to diet. Though most adolescent dieting is benign, social pressures for dieting and slimness may increase the risk of eating disorders. Liability to eating problems is particularly high in careers such as modelling and ballet dancing that particularly emphasise slimness, though it is uncertain whether the careers themselves makes people develop eating disorders, or whether having an eating disorder makes these careers more appealing. Anorexia nervosa is primarily reported in rich countries; in low- and middle-income countries there is some evidence that anorexia nervosa is commoner in the most affluent (and thus most westernised) social strata. There is no specifically 'anorexogenic' family background; the disorder is associated with an increased rate of relatively non-specific problems with family communication and interaction, and also with a higher rate of weight problems, physical illness, depression and alcoholism among relatives.

The predisposing role of specific childhood experiences, including sexual abuse, is uncertain. In many instances, anorexia does seem to have been precipitated by an adverse life event, though the type of life event does not appear to be particularly characteristic. The weight gain and change in body shape due to puberty itself may also contribute to the onset of the disorder, perhaps particularly when the individual is apprehensive about the shift from childhood dependency to sexual maturity and adult independence.

Although it seems natural to assume that anorexic cognitions motivate anorexic behaviour (for example, that a preoccupation with weight leads to excessive dieting), the reverse could also be true. In some circumstances, self-starving behaviour may take on a life of its own. The constipation and delayed gastric emptying associated with starvation can make the affected individual feel full up despite eating little. In addition, starvation may have its own rewards, perhaps in the form of extra attention or a sense of being in control. As starvation reduces thermogenesis and insulation, the compulsion to exercise may automatically increase in order to maintain body temperature, thereby accelerating weight loss. In these sorts of ways, starvation and weight loss may become self-perpetuating, with affected individuals subsequently trying to make sense of their own addiction to starvation by coming up with plausible but irrelevant explanations in terms of feeling too fat. From this perspective, even if weight loss began in response to stress or culturally sanctioned dieting, the process may subsequently become a vicious cycle that is hard to escape.

Treatment

With suitably trained therapists, the treatment of anorexic children and teenagers who live with their families can usually be managed on an out-patient basis. Gradual but steady weight restoration is the first main goal, aiming for an eventual weight within 10% of expected. This is usually accomplished by eating modest meals more often (four to six times per day).

Weight gain is facilitated by some combination of family therapy, behavioural techniques and individual therapy. Family sessions aim to promote a family restructuring that will facilitate recovery, often by putting parents more clearly in charge of dietary intake until normal weight control has been re-established. Evidence from randomised controlled trials suggests that including parents as well as children in the treatment programme is more important than the details of whether parents and children are seen together or separately. There can be advantages to providing group treatments for several affected families at a time. Behavioural techniques can be used to reward adherence to diet and successful weight gain. Individual therapy can provide a mixture of support, cognitive restructuring, education about diet, insight and problem-solving skills. There is no clear role for neuroleptics or appetite stimulants, but antidepressants may have some effect on weight gain and comorbid depression.

Prognosis

Long-term follow-ups of clinic series (almost certainly over-representing severe cases) show that roughly 50% recover, 30% are partly improved and 20% run a chronic course; about a fifth go on to develop affective disorders, and less than half succeed in making a stable long-term intimate relationship. Around 2% die from starvation or suicide. Some individuals start out with the restrictive type of anorexia, change to having the binge-eating/purging type of anorexia, and then make the transition to bulimia nervosa. Factors predicting a poor outcome include greater weight loss, vomiting, binge eating, greater chronicity, prepubertal onset and premorbid abnormalities. Possible indicators of a better outcome include early (but post-pubertal) onset, good parent–child relationships, and rapid detection and treatment.

Bulimia nervosa

Diagnosis

Bulimia nervosa involves frequent episodes of out-of-control overeating in which large amounts of food are consumed in short periods; the disorder should not be diagnosed on the basis of binges that occur exclusively during periods when the individual also meets the criteria for anorexia nervosa. Binges take place against a background of a persistent craving for, or preoccupation with, food. The individual counteracts the fattening effects of binges by means of deliberate vomiting, purging, periods of starvation, or other means. Body weight is usually close to normal, but concern about body weight is heightened.

Epidemiology

The peak age for bulimia is slightly later than for anorexia, but there is a similarly marked excess of females. Though epidemiological studies suggest that bulimia may be more common than anorexia in the general population, bulimia is underrepresented in clinic samples.

Causation

Bulimia may reflect exposure to a combination of risk factors for psychopathology in general (for example, parental neglect, sexual abuse) and risk factors for dieting in particular (for example, premorbid overweight).

Treatment

Most affected individuals can be treated as out-patients with cognitive-behavioural therapy, which is generally the treatment of choice, though there is some evidence for the effectiveness of selective serotonin reuptake inhibitors (SSRIs) such as fluoxetine. In the long term, roughly 50% recover fully, 25% improve, and 25% have a chronic course, often characterised by remissions and relapses. Co-existent or subsequent depression is common and may need treating in its own right.

Binge eating disorder

Though this disorder is being considered for inclusion in forthcoming versions of DSM and ICD, it is less researched than either anorexia or bulimia. In common with bulimia, it involves frequent binge eating with loss of control. In strong contrast to bulimia, however, extreme weight-control behaviours such as vomiting or purging are absent or only occasional, and there is a strong link with obesity. The epidemiology is different from anorexia and bulimia, with less of a female excess and a peak in middle age – though it does occur in adolescence too. It seems more responsive than anorexia and bulimia to treatment, at least in the short term. Cognitive-behavioural and interpersonal therapies seem promising.

Subject review

Fairburn CG. (2008) Eating disorders. *In*: Rutter M *et al.* (eds) *Rutter's Child and Adolescent Psychiatry*, 5th edn. Wiley-Blackwell, Chichester, pp. 670–685.

Further reading

Eddy KT *et al.* (2008) Eating Disorder Not Otherwise Specified in adolescents. *Journal of the American Academy of Child and Adolescent Psychiatry* **47**, 156–164.

Eisler I. *et al.* (2007) Family therapy for adolescent anorexia nervosa: A five year follow-up study of a controlled comparison of two family interventions. *Journal of Child Psychology and Psychiatry* **48**, 552–560.

Le Grange D, Eisler I. (2009) Family interventions in adolescent anorexia nervosa. *Child and Adolescent Psychiatric Clinics of North America* **18**, 159–173.

CHAPTER 26

Substance Use and Abuse

In a society that permits adults to use selected psychoactive substances for pleasure or the relief of stress, it is not surprising that most young people choose to try psychoactive substances, and that many come to consume them regularly, often with major public health consequences. Rates of experimentation and regular use vary by age, gender, country and decade, but it is possible to convey a sense of how common different patterns of use are by using figures from a 2007 survey of British 11–15-year-olds:

- Just over half had consumed at least one alcoholic drink at some point in their lives: ranging from 20% of 11-year-olds to 81% of 15-year-olds. Some 20% of boys and girls reported having drunk in the last week, ranging from 3% of 11-year-olds to 41% of 15-year-olds. Among those who had drunk in the last week, the average consumption was about 13 units (equivalent to nearly one and half bottles of wine or over six pints of normal strength beer).

- A third had tried smoking cigarettes at some point in their lives. Regularly smoking at least once a week ranged in prevalence from 1% of 11-year-olds to 15% of 15-year-olds. The average regular smoker was consuming about six cigarettes per day. Girls were more likely than boys to be regular smokers: 8% vs. 5%.

- A quarter had tried drugs at least once. First drug use was most commonly sniffing volatile substances such as glue, solvents, aerosols or gas (see Box 26.1). Beginning with volatile substances was particularly characteristic of those experimenting early. By contrast, those who first tried drugs at 14 or 15 were most likely to begin with cannabis.

- Overall, 17% reported taking drugs in the previous year, with rates rising from 6% of 11-year-olds to 31% of 15-year-olds. There were similar rates in boys and girls. The most commonly used drug was cannabis, taken by 9% in the previous year. Volatile substances came second, used by 6% in the previous year. Sniffing amyl nitrate ('poppers') came third, with these being used by 5%.

- Drinking, smoking and taking drugs were correlated behaviours – any one form of substance use was associated with higher rates of the other forms of substance use (and also with higher rates of truancy and school exclusion).

Child and Adolescent Psychiatry, Third Edition. Robert Goodman and Stephen Scott.
© 2012 Robert Goodman and Stephen Scott. Published 2012 by John Wiley & Sons, Ltd.

Box 26.1 Volatile substance abuse (VSA)

Inhaling organic solvents, also known as glue sniffing, is a pattern of substance use that is particularly associated with youth and social adversity.

In the UK, VSA peaks in the early teenage years, with roughly 2.5% of British 11–15-year-olds having inhaled solvents in the last month – a figure that applies equally to boys and girls. The prevalence is substantially higher for children from deprived backgrounds.

Elsewhere in the world, VSA is very common among some particularly deprived groups of children, for example, among the millions of street children of Brazil.

For the user, inhaling solvents is attractive as a cheap and readily available means of inducing a 'high', or of escaping from an intolerable situation; the effects are somewhat similar to alcohol but shorter lasting.

Common side effects include nausea, vomiting, headache, tinnitus and abdominal pain. Inhaling solvents from a bag may lead to a rash around the mouth or nose. Rarer side effects include liver and kidney damage, respiratory difficulties and encephalopathy. Death can result from cardiac arrest, inhalation of vomit, or from laryngeal spasm (particularly when lighter fluid or deodorants are sprayed directly into the back of the mouth).

VSA currently accounts for around 0.5% of all deaths in 10–19-year-olds in the UK, sometimes killing children experimenting with solvents for the first time. Though girls are as likely to use volatile substances as boys, around 80% of VSA deaths occur in males, perhaps reflecting sex differences in the pattern of use or choice of solvent.

Though experiments with illicit drugs do not mostly lead to regular use, it is worth remembering that nearly all young adults who are drug abusers first began to use drugs in school, with earlier onset predicting greater persistence. Similarly, the regular use of alcohol and cigarettes tends either to begin in adolescence or not at all – prompting suggestions that adolescence may be a 'sensitive period' when it is particularly easy to become addicted.

While the initiation of substance use typically begins in adolescence, many of the adverse consequences are delayed for years or decades. As a general behavioural principle, even small immediate rewards are often able to reinforce behaviours that may carry a large price in the distant future. Knowing that there is an increased risk of cancer or cirrhosis in several decades time is poor at deterring adolescents from using substances that promise fun, glamour, peer approval or escape from stress right now. Yet not all of the adverse consequences of substance use are delayed – think of the adolescents who kill themselves and other people as a result of driving while drunk; who engage is risky sexual behaviour while disinhibited by alcohol and thereby acquire HIV; who experience drug-induced psychosis; who die from a heroin overdose or from laryngeal spasm after inhaling lighter fluid; or who turn to crime or prostitution to support an expensive drug habit. In addition, there is emerging but still inconclusive evidence that the adolescent brain may be particularly sensitive to repeated alcoholic binges, with hippocampal cell loss, potentially resulting in impaired memory and learning.

Causation

There is no single or simple explanation for the pattern of substance use: price, availability, addictiveness, constitutional predisposition, youth culture, advertising and adult role models all play a part. Prior psychosocial adjustment is one more factor amongst many. Children and adolescent with disruptive behavioural disorders are more liable to become heavy substance users and go on to develop associated complications. The combination of conduct disorder and ADHD carries a particularly high risk. In contrast to this clear link between externalising disorders and substance-related problems, the link between emotional disorders and substance abuse is more complex. Some emotional disorders may predispose adolescents to substance use, as when individuals with social anxiety use alcohol to 'treat' this anxiety. On the other hand, the main link between emotional disorders and substance use is probably in the reverse direction, with established substance abuse being a risk factor for depression.

Substance use disorders

Psychiatric classifications are less concerned with the 'ordinary' use of substances than with the identification of pathological patterns of use that can be classified as a *substance use disorder*. The approach taken by ICD-10 and DSM-IV is ingenious but imperfect. One of the challenges facing any classification of substance use disorders is that there are many relevant substances – and more are being added all the time. If the classification of substance use disorders differed markedly for every single substance, the system could easily end up too complex for most practitioners to understand and remember – and even the best of classifications would be of little value if most people found it too complex to use. To get round this problem, both ICD-10 and DSM-IV apply some broad principles to defining four syndromes that could potentially apply to any substance (though some syndromes are irrelevant to some substances). The four syndromes are:

1 *Dependence*: This syndrome refers to a pattern of repeated use that can lead to tolerance, withdrawal symptoms, and compulsive use. The detailed ICD-10 criteria are shown in Box 26.2.
2 *Harmful use*: The ICD-10 term 'Harmful use' is equivalent to 'Abuse' in DSM-IV. This syndrome refers to individuals who do not meet the full criteria for dependence, but whose pattern of substance use has nevertheless clearly led to physical or psychological harm. The harmful pattern of use needs to have persisted for over a month, or occurred repeatedly within a 12-month period. The harm may have been brought

---

Box 26.2 A summary of ICD-10 criteria for Dependence syndrome*

Three or more of the following have occurred together repeatedly for over a month, or occurred repeatedly within a 12-month period:

1 A strong desire or sense of compulsion to take the substance.
2 Impaired control over substance taking, for example, using larger quantities of the substance or over a longer period than intended, a persistent desire to reduce or control substance use, or unsuccessful efforts to do so.
3 Withdrawal symptoms when cutting down or stopping. This is shown either by the emergence of the characteristic withdrawal syndrome for that substance, or by needing to using the substance (or a closely related substance) with the intention of relieving or avoiding withdrawal symptoms.
4 Evidence of tolerance: either needing much more of the substance to achieve the desired effect, or obtaining a much diminished effect from taking the same amount.
5 Preoccupation with substance use, for example, much time is spent obtaining and using the substance, much less time is devoted to alternative pleasures and interests.
6 Substance use persists despite clear evidence of harmful consequences.

Note: *DSM-IV criteria for Substance Dependence are similar. *The ICD-10 Classification of Mental and Behavioural Disorders: Diagnostic Criteria for Research* (World Health Organization, 1993).

---

about by impaired judgement and dysfunctional behaviour secondary to substance use, for example, causing an accident when driving while drunk. Other common adverse consequences include school drop-out, repeated criminal convictions and disrupted relationships with partners or family members.

3 *Acute intoxication*: The ICD-10 term 'acute intoxication' is equivalent to 'intoxication' in DSM-IV. This syndrome refers to a reversible syndrome of maladaptive behavioural or psychological changes that is characteristic of the relevant substance, and that occurs during or shortly after substance use. Different substances sometimes result in similar intoxication syndromes.

4 *Withdrawal*: This syndrome is triggered by the cessation or reduction of what had previously been heavy and prolonged use. The relevant withdrawal features typically vary according to which substance is involved. For example, the withdrawal syndrome can include: tremor, seizures and hallucinations for alcohol withdrawal; and lethargy, increased appetite and vivid unpleasant dreams for amphetamine withdrawal.

Applying this template to all forms of substance use and abuse is a clever way of bringing out shared features and differences, while also keeping the system simple and memorable enough to be useful. However, it does not solve all problems and may generate some difficulties of its own:

1 The distinction between the dependence syndrome and the harmful use syndrome may be misleading, at least for children and adolescents.

Empirical studies suggest that there is a single dimension of harmful use that encompasses both sorts of symptoms. More broadly, the current focus on present-or-absent categories such as harmful use or dependence may need to give way to a more dimensional approach to classifying patterns of use and abuse.

2 There are some lively controversies as to how best to operationalise concepts such as tolerance or withdrawal symptoms. For example, textbook cases of severe alcohol withdrawal syndrome with full-blown hallucinations and seizures are largely confined to adults. On the other hand, acute withdrawal symptoms after alcoholic binges may be common among children and adolescents, particularly if the symptoms of a hangover are also due to alcohol withdrawal, as some have suggested. Thus 'narrow' and 'broad' interpretations of the same diagnostic criteria can lead to very different estimates of how common substance use disorders are at different ages.

3 Most regular smokers can be classified as having a psychiatric disorder, namely nicotine dependence disorder. Indeed, according to surveys in some countries, this is one of the commonest psychiatric disorders in the general population. There is no doubt that smoking causes enormous damage to the population's physical health and that nicotine is addictive – but does being a regular smoker correspond to what most people would think of as a psychiatric disorder? If so, should mental health professionals be spending much more time tackling cigarette smoking? Or is this a step in the wrong direction, shifting the primary responsibility from more appropriate agencies such as family doctors and schools?

4 If you are concerned about creeping medicalisation (or 'psychiatrisation'), you may be alarmed by a proposed DSM-5 category of 'addiction and related disorders' which will encompass not only substance use disorders but also behavioural addictions such as pathological gambling (and potentially other conditions such as compulsive shopping, internet addiction and videogame addiction). It sounds like a metaphor that has got out of hand, and yet pathological gambling can involve tolerance and withdrawal symptoms, is helped by opiate antagonists; and has been linked in both neuoroimaging and genetic studies to dopaminergic systems. It's certainly an interesting debate.

Treatment

The vast majority of adolescents with substance misuse problems do not come to Child and Adolescent Mental Health Services. For those who do, there is no evidence that general counselling is effective. Some forms of manualised family therapy have shown good effects when delivered by the original programme developers, but have been less successful when delivered in everyday practice. Brief Strategic Family Therapy seems particularly effective when administered by highly skilled therapists, but has much smaller effects with less accomplished therapists.

Prevention

There have been several randomised controlled trials of preventive, educational programmes for adolescents in the USA. However, most only engage about 30% of the 'at risk' population, and have modest effects. Building on these trials is a major public health task.

Subject review

Heath AC. *et al.* (2008) *Substance use and substance use disorder. In*: Rutter M *et al.* (eds) *Rutter's Child and Adolescent Psychiatry*, 5th edn. Wiley-Blackwell, Chichester, pp. 565–586.

Further reading

Bowden-Jones H, Clark L. (2011) Pathological gambling: a neurobiological and clinical update. *British Journal of Psychiatry* **199**, 87–89.

Fuller E *et al.* (2008) *Drug Use, Smoking and Drinking among Young People in England in 2007*. The NHS Information Centre, Leeds. Available at: http://www.ic.nhs.uk.

Lynskey MT *et al.* (2010) Genetically informative research on adolescent substance use: Methods, findings, and challenges. *Journal of the American Academy of Child and Adolescent Psychiatry* **49**, 1202–1214.

NICE (2007) *Psychosocial Interventions for Substance Misuse*. National Clinical Practice Guideline Number 51. NICE, London.

Robbins M *et al.* (2011) Therapist adherence in brief strategic family therapy for adolescent drug abusers. *Journal of Consulting and Clinical Psychology* **79**, 43–53.

CHAPTER 27
Maltreatment

Maltreatment of children and adolescents became widely recognised in the USA in the 1960s and since then has been uncovered throughout the world wherever systematic enquiry has taken place. Most definitions incorporate two elements: (1) evidence of behaviour towards the child, which is likely to be damaging; and (2) evidence of harm to the child resulting from this. Note that intention is not part of the definition; some parents may feel they love their children dearly but nonetheless may harm them, albeit unwittingly. Sometimes maltreatment is easy to recognise, for example, a girl with scalded buttocks with a parent who confesses to dipping her in a boiling bath to teach her a lesson. At other times it is far harder, for example, a neglected boy who has conduct disorder and whose parents are of low intelligence. How much avoidable harm has been done, or would he have turned out this way even if well looked after? Information is far from precise on how much neglect is required to cause specific, measurable damage.

Abuse and neglect cases can be some of the most disturbing and heart-wrenching experiences in child and adolescent psychiatry, sometimes evoking horror and a wish to rescue the victim immediately. Therefore it is important to keep a sense of perspective on how good the evidence is that abuse is indeed happening, and to have a sympathetic team for emotional support to stop one becoming overwhelmed by, or cut off from, what is seen.

Types of maltreatment include:

- *Physical abuse* Non-accidental injury: head injuries, fractures, burns and scalds, bruises. Munchausen syndrome by proxy (factitious illness by proxy). Non-organic failure to thrive and psychosocial short stature.
- *Neglect* Lack of: physical and medical care, supervision, emotional closeness, stimulation.
- *Emotional abuse* Hostility, deprivation of attention, threats to abandon, inappropriate demands.
- *Sexual abuse* Penetrative, non-penetrative; intrafamilial, extrafamilial; of girls, of boys.

Child and Adolescent Psychiatry, Third Edition. Robert Goodman and Stephen Scott.
© 2012 Robert Goodman and Stephen Scott. Published 2012 by John Wiley & Sons, Ltd.

Epidemiology

Obviously, ascertainment methods and definitions will strongly influence reported rates. In England, about 3% of children under the age of 13 are brought each year to the attention of professional agencies for suspected abuse. A tenth of this figure, 3 per 1,000, are on the official Child Protection (Safeguarding) Register for the whole age range 0–18 years. This prevalence figure is more than doubled for the first year of life, but then settles down to around 3 per 1,000 for children aged 1–16, after which there is a considerable drop. Looked at another way, it is important to note that there is still serious abuse frequently coming to light in the 10–15-year adolescent age group. Fatal abuse occurs in about 1 in 10,000 of the population, with violence-induced intellectual disability being about as common in the first year.

In England and Wales, the most commonly registered predominant category of maltreatment is physical abuse, followed by sexual abuse, then neglect; emotional abuse is seldom registered. However, more common than all of these categories, accounting for about half of all registrations, is the non-specific 'grave concern', used where there is thought to be a serious risk of abuse, for example, because siblings are known to be abused, or because there is a convicted sex offender living at home.

The above figures refer to abuse reported to authority. A large epidemiological survey was carried out in the UK in 2,000 with nearly 3,000 respondents. Some 7% of children were rated as experiencing serious physical abuse in their families, 6% serious absence of physical care, 6% serious emotional maltreatment, and 5% serious absence of supervision.

In the USA, the Government has carried out National Incidence Surveys at regular intervals, and these indicate that the prevalence of abuse in children under 18 is 2.5–4%. The lower figure includes only demonstrated harm to the child, the higher includes danger of being harmed in the view of community professionals and child protection services. These figures are very similar to UK rates of ascertainment. However, unlike the UK, in the USA, emotional abuse is the commonest predominant form registered (1.2%), soon followed by physical abuse (1%, of which three-quarters are considered severe), neglect (0.9%), and sexual abuse (0.7%). There are over 2,000 deaths a year resulting from recognised abuse and neglect, in addition to over 6,000 homicides per year of children aged under 8, generally by family members.

These figures give the predominant type of maltreatment at the time of registration. However, more detailed studies show that there is a large degree of overlap, with multiple forms of abuse being the rule rather than the exception. Thus physical abuse severe enough to reach an official register seldom occurs in the absence of emotional abuse, and there is not infrequently a degree of neglect; intrafamilial sexual abuse tends to occur in an atmosphere of inadequate personal boundaries and emotional distortions; and so on.

Clinical picture

Physical abuse

The child is usually presented with some form of injury. The history from the family may include suggestive pointers:

1 Delay or failure to seek medical help.
2 The account of how the injury was sustained is vague, lacking specific detail, whereas the remainder of the circumstances are conveyed in convincing particularity.
3 The account varies in significant ways with retelling.
4 The account of the incident is not compatible with the injury sustained, for example, a child with sharp bruises and fractures is said to have rolled off a bed onto a well-carpeted floor.
5 The parental affect while giving the account is abnormal and does not appear to reflect the degree of concern and anxiety one would expect.
6 Parental behaviour during the enquiry is suspicious, with hostility, over-emphatic denial of any anger towards the child despite evidence of his behaving in a difficult way preceding the injury, and attempts to leave hospital early before medical investigations are complete.
7 Many abused children look sad, withdrawn and frightened, some show frozen watchfulness.
8 The child may say something strongly indicative of abuse.

Examination and investigation may show injuries that are strongly suggestive of non-accidental injury. It should be pointed out that no one pattern of physical injury is pathognomonic of abuse: rather each case needs to be taken individually in the light of all the evidence, especially the history. Some paediatricians have become oversold on physical signs alone. For example, there was a school of thought that believed anal dilatation was a sure sign of abuse. Subsequent studies have shown this not always to be the case, and led to some landmark court cases where 'expert' evidence was overturned.

The suggestive physical signs are well described in most paediatric text-books, and include suspicious patterns of fractures (including widespread fractures of differing ages revealed on skeletal survey), retinal and intra-cerebral bleeds from shaking, burns and scalds (including cigarette burns and scalds from forced immersion), and characteristic patterns of bruising (for example, due to gripping or throttling).

Other forms of physical abuse include deliberate suffocation and poisoning. Suffocation may be presented as an apnoeic attack or as near-miss or actual sudden infant death syndrome (SIDS). Some have suggested, not without controversy, that 10% of SIDS is due to suffocation; siblings of children on the child protection register have a far higher rate than controls. Poisoning may be presented as accidental when it is not, or simply as a mystery illness.

Munchausen syndrome by proxy, also known as factitious illness by proxy, refers to a child being presented to doctors by a parent (almost always the mother) who has induced the illness. The child is usually brought repeatedly by the mother to hospital for investigation, yet when she is away the symptoms and signs abate. The parents deny any knowledge of the cause of the illness. Other siblings have often been subject to fabricated illness too, and indeed one study found that 1 in 10 had died in mysterious circumstances. Forms of fabricated illness include, in descending order of reported frequency, respiratory arrests due to smothering, poisonings, seizures, apparent bleeding from a variety of orifices, skin rashes and other skin conditions, fevers and high blood pressure. As the mother spends more time on the ward it may become apparent that she enjoys medical attention; often mothers have nursing or other health-related training or experience. Other types of physical abuse such as non-accidental injury and non-organic failure to thrive often co-exist.

Failure to thrive refers simply to less-than-expected weight gain. It is a relatively common presentation in paediatric clinics. In the majority a medical condition is found, such as heart disease, lung disease, gut disease or hormonal problems. In a minority, however, no medical cause can be found. This group comprise non-organic failure to thrive (NOFT). A proportion of these will simply have undiagnosed medical conditions, but many arise in the context of deviant parent–child interaction patterns. The deviant interactions are especially common in this group at meal times, with the result that most cases of NOFT end up receiving insufficient nutrition (as do many cases of organic failure to thrive, where parent–child interaction is, by contrast, usually normal). To demonstrate that adverse upbringing is the cause, it is essential to document that the weight of the child catches up when they are placed in a benign environment (for example, a hospital ward, or with foster parents). Children with NOFT have been shown to be at far higher risk of later neglect and abuse than controls.

Neglect

This refers to an absence of appropriate care rather than positively inappropriate acts. However, the effects of neglect on children can be just as devastating as the effects of abuse, if not more so. Most areas of care may be involved:

1 *Lack of physical care*. This includes undernutrition and sometimes NOFT, recurrent infections, unkempt dirty appearance, housing dirty and disorganised.
2 *Lack of medical care*, with failure to bring the child for immunisations, failure to seek appropriate medical help for illnesses and accidents. This can result in avoidable complications of medical conditions, including defective vision from untreated squints, impaired hearing from untreated otitis, and occasionally death, for example, from hypothermia.
3 *Lack of enforced house routines, rules and supervision*. This leads to an increased rate of accidents at all ages, including domestic and road traffic. Younger children frequently wet and soil for no organic reason.

Older children are left to wander away from home and are exposed to a variety of risks, for example, playing on railway lines, associating with drug users, petty criminals, and sex abusers. There is a failure to learn to conform to social norms with resulting difficulties fitting in with other people and organisational arrangements, notably school rules. Disruptive behavioural disorders are common.

4 *Lack of emotional warmth and availability*. This often has profound effects on children's ability to enter into rewarding close relationships, as they have not experienced a normal reciprocal intimate relationship. Their social and emotional skills and feeling for how to develop friendships are usually impaired, and self-worth as a person is very low, sometimes leading into frank depression, but more often being seen as despondency and lack of social interest and responsiveness. Other emotional disorders such as anxiety and fears are not uncommon. Attachment patterns in younger children as measured on separation and reunion with parents are often abnormal, with a high frequency of the disorganised category being seen (see Chapter 32). Other neglected children are indiscriminately friendly, craving affection and physical contact, putting them at high risk of abuse. School-age children are unable to maintain significant friendships. Adults brought up in neglected and abusive environments frequently exhibit inadequate close relationships. This is reflected in abnormal features in the way they describe their relationships with their parents and other intimates, as elicited by the Adult Attachment Interview (see Chapter 32).

5 Lack of cognitive stimulation and encouragement in constructive pastimes. This leads to delayed language acquisition, short attention span with poor concentration, lower IQ, poor skill acquisition, poor attainments, lack of school and examination success, and a greatly diminished sense of competence and initiative.

Emotional abuse

Although emotional abuse is seldom the main cause for the recording of concern on official child protection registers in the UK, in many cases it is the predominant form of maltreatment going on in a family. Furthermore, it is almost invariably present in the other registered forms of maltreatment. However, because the immediate manifestations are less dramatic and a causal connection with child impairment is harder to prove, less is done about it. This is not because it is less harmful; research over the past two decades has increasingly shown the profound and enduring effects on children reared under these circumstances. Elements include:

1 *Extreme hostility and criticism*. Parents can come to see only the bad qualities in the child, and subject them to a withering fire of critical and demeaning comments, which the child is not equipped to deal with. Follow-up studies confirm that children and adolescents exposed to harsh emotional climates are themselves more likely to be cruel and bully others.

2 *Rejection and withdrawal of affection.* No warmth or cuddles are offered to the child, who is continually spurned when he or she makes overtures. This may lead to desperate emotional frustration and impaired close relationships, sometimes with deep distrust of intimacy and consequent withdrawal, or a desperate need for intimacy at any cost. Where a sibling is treated very differently, this exacerbates the feeling of rejection and differentially rejected children have a particularly poor prognosis.

3 *Deprivation of attention.* The child is ignored, especially when he is quiet or behaving constructively; when he seeks someone to play with or approval for an achievement, it is withheld. This leads to less socially acceptable behaviour, and to more antisocial behaviour and aggression.

4 *Inconsistency.* Behaviour that is accepted at one moment receives crushing criticism and heavy punishment the next; a parent who is warm and welcoming in the morning is cold and rejecting in the afternoon. This leads to confusion and inability to predict or trust.

5 *Threats of abandonment.* For what may be very minor acts of perceived misbehaviour, the child is threatened with expulsion from the home, and may have his suitcase packed, be driven to social services, and so on. The constant fear of abandonment precludes the development of a secure base for the building of relationships and often leads to anxious attachments.

6 *Inappropriate stresses and demands.* A child may see his depressed mother repeatedly being beaten by her partner, or taking an overdose. He may be told he is the reason his parents got divorced, and be used as a football in the ensuing acrimony, being asked to take sides, pass messages, act as peacemaker, and give comfort and protection.

Sexual abuse

One definition specifies sexual abuse as: 'the involvement of dependent, developmentally immature children and adolescents in sexual activities that they do not fully comprehend, and to which they are unable to give informed consent, and that violate the social taboos of family roles'. There is a range of severity of acts with a corresponding range of prevalence. Thus 'non-contact' abuse such as exhibitionism is reported to have occurred at some time in childhood by around half of all women. 'Contact' abuse including fondling is reported to have occurred in childhood by 15–20% of women, whereas penetrative acts with vaginal, anal or oral involvement are reported by around 2%. All of these figures are imprecise because of difficulties in ascertainment. Community surveys suggest that females are more often abused than males, with a ratio of 2 or 3:1, but in clinically referred samples the female preponderance is greater, at around 4 or 5:1. In clinical samples of sexually abused children there is a small excess of children from socio-economically deprived backgrounds, but this gradient is far less marked than for physical abuse and neglect, and is virtually absent in community surveys.

Sexual abuse can come to attention in many ways. The most common is the child or adolescent disclosing the abuse, usually to a friend, a parent or another trusted adult; telephone helplines are increasingly used too. Changes in behaviour are common. While precocious sexualised behaviour should clearly raise the suspicion of abuse, more non-specific changes occur frequently, such as sullenness and withdrawal, increased irritability and aggressiveness for no obvious reason, declining school performance and loss of friends. Older children and adolescents may take overdoses, run away from home, or abuse other children. There may be presentations directly related to penetrative acts: anal or vaginal bleeding or infections, urinary tract infections, enuresis or faecal soiling, venereal disease or pregnancy.

Risk factors for maltreatment

With physical and emotional abuse, there is no single risk factor that predisposes a carer to abuse a child, but rather a range of influences that make abuse more likely. Broadly, they can be divided into the following:

1 Poor parenting skills with deficient moment-to-moment interaction patterns; this is the final common pathway through which abuse is transmitted.
2 Stressful circumstances.
3 Child characteristics.
4 Weak parental attachment to the child.

These well-established risk factors are summarised in Table 27.1.

With sexual abuse, perpetrators are most commonly men, although around 10% of sexual abuse is committed by women, who may be co-abusers with men, sometimes acting under duress. The proportion where the perpetrator is a family member varies according to the study from around one-third to two-thirds. Within the home, fathers are the commonest perpetrators, accounting for around half of clinically seen cases. Stepfathers are disproportionately commonly involved, accounting for around a quarter of clinical cases. Girls living in a home with a stepfather are around six times more likely to be sexually abused than girls living with both biological parents. When sexual abuse does occur outside the home, the perpetrator is, nonetheless, still usually known to the child and has been trusted to be left alone with him or her, for example, a neighbour, friend of the family, friend of the child, teacher, babysitter, club leader, etc. Abuse by strangers is relatively uncommon, accounting for around 5–10% of all abuse. Sex rings are being increasingly recognised. The term refers to a group of adults who are abusing several children. Initially, they often bribe the children to become involved, but then go on to blackmail them and may use them to make pornographic videos or involve them in child prostitution. The prevalence is unknown, but one survey over two years, of an English city of three-quarters of a million inhabitants, uncovered 31 child sex rings involving 47 male perpetrators and 334 children ranging from 4–15 years old; 90% of victims were girls; two-thirds had been forced to perform oral intercourse, one-third anal or vaginal intercourse.

Table 27.1 Prediction of intervention success

Factor	Better outcome	Worse outcome
Parental	Acceptance of problems	Denial of problems
	Compliance with treatment	Refusal to cooperate
	Normal personality	Personality problems:
		• antisocial
		• sadistic
		• aggressive
		• abused in childhood
	Supportive partner	Abusive partner
	No psychiatric disorder	Alcohol abuse
		Substance abuse
		Psychosis
Characteristics of abuse	Less severe injuries	Severe injuries
		Burns and scalds
		Failure to thrive
		Mixed abuse
		Penetrative sexual abuse
		Longstanding sexual abuse
		Sadistic abuse
		Munchausen by proxy
Interaction with child	Normal attachment	Disordered attachment
	Able to show empathy	Unable to show empathy
	Responsive caregiving	Insensitive caregiving
	Puts child's needs first	Puts own needs first
Child	Healthy child	Special needs – physical or learning problems
	Resilient response to abuse	Extensive psychopathology
	One nurturing relationship	No positive influence
Circumstances	Good local childcare	No facilities
	Informal networks	Social isolation
Professional intervention	Well trained and resourced	Few resources or skills Lack of
	Therapeutic relationship	engagement

Source: Adapted from a scheme devised by Dr David Jones, to whom we are grateful for permission to use it.

Effects of maltreatment

To date, few specific outcomes have been linked with specific patterns of maltreatment. This is partly due to the wide overlap of types of maltreatment, so it is hard to study 'pure' abuse of one type. Even when 'pure' forms of abuse are studied, impairments are seen in a wide range of functions. It is plausible that many of these associated impairments are attributable to the maltreatment. This is a causal inference that is supported if the impairments improve or resolve once maltreatment ceases, for example, because the individual is taken into care. Without this improvement, it is important to consider additional explanations.

Thus, pre-existing or constitutional impairments may have predisposed the child to being abused. For example, an irritable temperament might be a cause rather than a consequence of abuse. Alternatively, the same genetic or psychosocial factors that predispose the child or adolescent to be abused may independently have predisposed the child to the additional impairments. For instance, the genetic and psychosocial factors that result in low parental IQ and thereby increase the risk of abuse also increase the likelihood of low IQ in the child, whether or not abuse has taken place.

Physical effects

These effects on growth can be marked in severe cases, with NOFT and psychosocial short stature described above.

Emotional regulation

More negative emotions are displayed, and emotional arousal to stressful circumstances happens more quickly and takes longer to calm down. Children may be hyperaroused and hypervigilant. More fear and hostility is shown in response to adult arguments. Four general patterns may be seen:

1 Emotional blunting and lack of social responsiveness.
2 Depressed affect with sad facial expressions, withdrawal and aimless play.
3 Emotional lability, with sudden shifts from engagement and pleasure to withdrawal and anger.
4 An angry emotional state with disorganised play and frequent outbursts in response to slight frustrations.

Recently, physiological studies have shown abnormal diurnal patterns of cortisol secretion in physically abused children that become more normal after a year of foster care. Likewise, other physiological indices of exacerbated reactions to stress are abnormal, such as adrenaline and noradrenaline responses to anxiety-provoking stimuli. Adults who were abused as children have raised levels of C-Reactive Protein, a general inflammation marker associated with higher subsequent risk of cardiovascular and other diseases.

Formation of attachments

Maltreated toddlers and infants show a preponderance of insecure attachment patterns in response to separation and reunion with their parents. Particularly common is the disorganised response, characterised by fear, disorientation, switches between approach and avoidance, odd expressions, freezing and other bizarre behaviours (see Chapter 32). The insecure attachment pattern tends to persist through childhood and into adulthood.

Development of self-concept

Maltreated children find it difficult to talk about themselves, and especially about their negative feelings, possibly because they have learned it leads to punishment at home. Measures of how they feel about themselves show low self-worth and low self-competence ratings.

Symbolic and social development

Play is reduced in quantity, and its quality is impoverished, with an increase in routine, stereotyped activity. Social play with other children is impaired. These deficits correlate well with the quality and sensitivity of mother–child interaction. Maltreated children show less sensitivity to the emotions of others, more negative expectations of people, less trust in them, and fewer ideas of how to initiate and maintain a social relationship. They are more prone to construe ambiguous stimuli as aggressive, and respond to this by becoming aggressive themselves. Observation of actual peer relationships shows lack of competence, inappropriate aggression in response to friendly overtures, and sometimes a mixed picture of aggression and withdrawal that leads to particularly strong rejection by the peer group. There is some evidence that this represents a disorganised 'fight or flight' response developed in the face of repeated overwhelmingly frightening experiences.

Cognitive development

Both language and non-verbal abilities are less well developed than in non-abused controls, and school attainments are even more reduced. This may be due to a number of mechanisms, including impaired cognitive development in a home environment lacking in rewarding reciprocal exchanges and stimulation; the inheritance of cognitive disabilities from similarly disabled parents, poor ability to concentrate on schoolwork and organise it; and apathy and lack of motivation.

Emotional and behavioural disorders

These are common in abused children. By adolescence this can result in extreme cases, both of violence with psychopathic personality, and of suicide and deliberate self-harm. An increased incidence of post-traumatic stress disorder is additionally reported in victims of severe physical abuse. Although these findings emerge from studies that compare maltreated children with controls from similar socio-economic groups and neighbourhoods, the families of the abused children often had disproportionately high levels of ongoing, chronic adversity and deprivation. It is therefore sometimes hard to disentangle the effect of the abuse from the chronic deprivation. Where there are multiple stressors of this kind, the rate of psychopathology may increase disproportionately.

Resilience

How common is it for abused children to be resilient, that is, to develop normally despite their adverse experiences? Even taking the relatively conservative criterion of absence of significant problems, few abused children are classified as resilient. If competencies are measured across a range of domains, the proportion of resilient children drops still further, to zero in many studies, although many develop normally in at least some domains.

Intergenerational transmission

The proportion of abused children who become abusive parents varies by study, averaging around 30%. While abusive upbringing clearly has a powerful influence, the worst outcomes are by no means inevitable. Even among girls brought up in children's homes because of grossly inadequate parenting, roughly half went on to provide adequate parenting for their own children.

Effects of sexual abuse

As with all types of abuse, it can often be difficult to know how much impairment has stemmed specifically from the sexual abuse, and how much from the generally disorganised and disordered family background. Although outcome studies on clinical samples are likely to miss individuals who were resilient to abusive experiences, they serve to highlight the damage done and typically show a variety of negative consequences that often last for many years.

Emotionally, victims often feel guilt and responsibility for the abuse, especially if they have come to enjoy the sexually arousing experiences. They may experience a sense of powerlessness in response to their inability to stop repeated invasions of their body. They may find it impossible to trust others, especially older people of the perpetrator's gender. The trauma of the abuse may lead to sleeplessness, nightmares, loss of appetite, other somatic complaints and self-destructive behaviour. Frank symptoms of post-traumatic stress disorder may be present, with intrusive thoughts relating to the actual abuse process and avoidance of any associated people and places. Self-esteem is often very low with feelings of disgust, contamination, dirtiness and worthlessness predominating. Helplessness and hopelessness are frequent, often with an element of anger. The incidence of depression is considerably raised.

Behaviourally, chronic disobedience, aggression, bullying and antisocial acts are seen in both sexes following sexual abuse, but especially in boys. Girls are more prone to self-cutting, burning themselves with cigarettes and anorectic responses. A proportion of children show inappropriate sexualised behaviour, including sexual contact or play with other adults or children and seductive behaviour towards relative strangers, for example, staff in residential establishments or in-patient units. There may be persistent overt masturbation in public. As they grow up, a number are drawn to prostitution. Boys who experienced homosexual abuse commonly show confusion and anxiety about their sexual identity. The proportion who go on to be sexually abusive of others is uncertain, but it is clear that a significant minority do.

Factors affecting the impact of sexual abuse include:

- How much coercion and violence were used.
- The duration of the abuse.
- The nature and severity of the abuse, including whether penetration occurred.
- The relationship with the perpetrator, with abuse by a trusted figure such as a father being particularly disturbing.
- Subsequent events, such as being taken away from the family home to a disruptive residential setting.

Another factor exacerbating the effect of sexual abuse is disbelief by the parent, typically the mother. Around a third of seriously abused girls are not supported by their own mothers, who may deny the abuse ever took place (despite clear evidence to the contrary) and elect to stay with the perpetrators, so rejecting their daughters. Studies of the impact of sexual abuse according to the age at which it occurs do not show any clear period when it is less damaging.

Assessment

The overriding principle in suspected child abuse is to get help. Notifying someone of concerns about children being abused is everyone's business – not just child professionals. In England there is a legal duty to do this, so that, for example, one cannot decide to ignore worrying suspicions of abuse if, say, one is a researcher who sees it happening in a family during a home visit. If suspected in clinical practice, a senior colleague should be informed as soon as possible, and the local social services department consulted. Physical abuse is often picked up initially by paediatricians, and managed in conjunction with social services. Child mental health professionals, however, may see injuries or detect other forms of abuse or neglect while seeing a child for a behavioural or emotional problem. If court proceedings are being contemplated, child mental health professionals may be asked whether significant harm has occurred to the child, what the prospects are for improvement in parenting style and whether the child should be removed from the family.

A thorough general assessment is very useful because less obvious aspects can be overlooked by an exclusive focus on the circumstances of abuse. It is especially important to see all members of a household, whether or not they are blood relatives, including step-parents, lodgers, etc. External reports are essential. GP and health visitor records provide information on regularity of attendance, previous injuries in the index child and other family members, and parental health and behaviour (having obtained parental permission). School reports are equally important. The assessment should cover all the factors depicted in Table 27.1, as well as an enquiry about the possible abusive practices, set within the context of overall parenting and family life. The child should be seen alone, and psychometric tests given if performance is failing significantly at school. Social services should be asked whether they know the family, and whether any of the children are on the Child Protection Register. If abuse seems likely, a child protection conference is likely to be held, to which a range of involved professionals will be invited. Nowadays, the parents are usually invited to attend some or all of the conference. Recommendations are made, which can include placing the child's name on the register and other protective steps.

Investigation of suspected sexual abuse can be carried out as a screening exercise if the level of concern is moderate, or as a full investigative process if suspicion is higher. There are extensive guidelines on how this should be done, and it is imperative to seek advice from a senior colleague with experience in this area. If the child is not overtly disturbed, social workers will often be the agreed party to conduct interviews, but if the child is showing evidence of marked disturbance, or there are special circumstances, such as intellectual disability or very young children, then a child and adolescent mental health professional may need to be involved.

Screening interviews must be carried out alone with the child, since if a family member committed the abuse, the child is unlikely to reveal this in their presence for fear of the consequences. For example, there may have been explicit physical threats, emotional blackmail, or a fear by the child that if they tell, the family will break up and they will lose a parent. After a general discussion of how things are at home and outside, what the rules and discipline are and who the child likes and does not like, it may be helpful to enquire about sleeping and bathing arrangements and how they look after their body. Questions may concern secrets, matters the child has not been able to tell anyone about, whom they would confide in if they had any worries, and whether anybody had done anything to them or touched them in a way they did not like. Asking such specific questions has been shown to increase the rate of disclosure of sexual abuse.

Full investigative interviews are a specialised skill, and are often carried out in conjunction with the police. They are usually videotaped as in the UK and a number of other countries they are admissible as evidence in court, instead of the child having to be a witness and be cross-examined. Anatomically correct dolls may be used, and often help prompt the child's memory. Some young children describe what happened to them and show this in vivid detail with the dolls in a way that is hard to disbelieve. Nevertheless, caution and judgement have to be applied to avoid over-interpreting the child's behaviour and being over-zealous in diagnosing abuse where there is doubt.

Physical examination of the anus and external genitalia is useful, but should only be carried out by paediatricians, gynaecologists or police surgeons trained for the purpose. Whilst tearing and bruising are strongly suggestive of abuse, weaker signs may be of uncertain significance, especially as norms are only just being established. Tests for the presence of semen, venereal disease and pregnancy should be considered. Because recovery from the physical sequelae can occur quickly, a negative physical examination does not rule out the occurrence of sexual abuse. In one series where the presence of penetrative abuse was well established, fewer than 40% of the children had physical signs.

Intervention

The management of established abuse is guided by three aims. The first is to prevent further abuse. The second is to mitigate the effects of what has already happened. The third is to meet the child's emotional, social and educational needs in the longer term, which may include deciding whether it is best for the child to live in their own family, making special educational provision and providing positive social experiences outside the home. A wide range of methods may be used, according to the particular circumstances of the case and resources of the agencies involved. For example, the interventions in one particular case might include:

- A court order forbidding access by the stepfather.
- Training in parenting skills for the mother to help her manage her child's conduct problems.
- Antidepressant therapy for the mother's low mood.
- Individual counselling sessions for the child.
- Extra educational provision for the child's learning problems.
- An anti-bullying programme at school.
- An application to rehouse the family in better conditions.

To achieve all this successfully requires good inter-agency liaison. Management of sexual abuse is guided by the same three aims:

1 There needs to be an assessment of the likelihood of re-abuse if the child is to remain in, or be returned to, the family where it happened.
2 Prevention of further abuse may require the removal of the offender or an enforceable system of protection.
3 The ability of the mother to accept what has happened and protect her child is important, as is the ability of the perpetrator to acknowledge his responsibility.

This is relevant for risk assessment, and to help the child begin to reverse guilt and self-blame; it may pave the way for the perpetrator's eventual reintegration into the family. However, court orders may need to be taken forbidding access if the child is believed to be at risk. Mitigation of the effects of abuse is likely to be helped by skilled therapy. Enabling the child to talk freely about sexual matters can allow them to go on to confront the awful experiences within a safe setting, and so begin to process them emotionally without dissociating and cutting off, or becoming paralysed with fear and anxiety. A variety of psychotherapeutic and cognitive-behavioural techniques may help in this task, and a number of controlled trials suggest they help reduce symptoms and distress. Groups may help children achieve cognitive understanding, put their experience in perspective, and receive support from others who have had similar experiences. Meeting the child's longer-term needs may include fostering a sense of self-worth and an ability to communicate about emotions and be assertive in threatening situations. An understanding of their own sexual responses and of the boundaries between appropriate and inappropriate sexual behaviour will need to be developed. Family work will need to address whether the mother has resolved the issue of split loyalties between the victim and the perpetrator. Severely affected children with profound mood disturbance, severe self-mutilation, anorexia or other symptoms may need an extensive programme of therapeutic work, often best undertaken in a therapeutic community or residential setting.

When maltreatment was first widely recognised, there was often strong pressure to remove the child from the family, frequently influenced by people's sense of outrage. Subsequent research showed that many of these children did badly, often because the substitute care was deficient. This was particularly the case in some children's homes, where there was a high turnover of poorly trained staff, and where the child was at risk of being abused by care workers or co-residents. Currently, the emphasis is on rehabilitating the child within the family wherever possible. Therefore, it is important to be able to predict when this will be successful. In clinical studies where treatment is given and children stay within their families of origin, the overall established rate of re-abuse is 20–70%. Factors predicting outcome are set out in Table 27.1. Parental acknowledgement that abuse has occurred, and a willingness on their part to stay in a treatment programme are two of the most important predictors of successful rehabilitation.

Where the chances of improvement are slight, the court may order that alternative care be provided for the child, such as foster or adoptive parents, or in the case of older children, placement in a residential home. In England and Wales, the Children Act (1989) states that:

> The primary justification for the State to initiate proceedings seeking compulsory powers is actual or likely harm to the child, where harm includes both ill-treatment (which includes sexual abuse and non-physical ill-treatment such as emotional abuse) and the impairment of health or development, health meaning physical or mental health, and development meaning physical, intellectual, emotional, social, or behavioural development.

The Act puts great emphasis on working with parents voluntarily to maintain the child within the family wherever possible.

Primary prevention of child abuse through intensive home visiting programmes for high risk mothers contacted antenatally has been shown to work, for example, in a programme called the Nurse–Family Partnership (named Family Nurse Partnership in England) but is not widely deployed.

Subject review

Gilbert R *et al.* (2009a) Child Maltreatment 1: Burden and consequences of child maltreatment in high-income countries. *Lancet* **373**, 68–81.

Gilbert R *et al.* (2009b) Child Maltreatment 2: Recognising and responding to child maltreatment. *Lancet* **373**, 167–180.

Glaser D. (2008) Child sexual abuse. *In*: Rutter M *et al.* (eds) *Rutter's Child and Adolescent Psychiatry*, 5th edn. Wiley-Blackwell, Chichester, pp. 440–458.

Jones DPH. (2008) Child maltreatment. *In*: Rutter M *et al.* (eds) *Rutter's Child and Adolescent Psychiatry*, 5th edn. Wiley-Blackwell, Chichester, pp. 421–439.

MacMillan H. (2009) Child Maltreatment 3: Interventions to prevent child maltreatment and associated impairment. *Lancet* **373**, 250–266.

Reading R *et al.* (2009) Child Maltreatment 4: Promotion of children's rights and prevention of child maltreatment. *Lancet* **373**, 332–343.

Further reading

Chaffin M *et al.* (2011) A combined motivation and parent–child interaction therapy package reduces child welfare recidivism in a randomized dismantling field trial. *Journal of Consulting and Clinical Psychology* **79**, 84–95.

Cicchetti D *et al.* (2011) The effects of child maltreatment and polymorphisms of the serotonin transporter and dopamine D4 receptor genes on infant attachment and intervention efficacy. *Development and Psychopathology* **23**, 357–372.

Fergusson D. (2008) Exposure to childhood sexual and physical abuse and adjustment in early adulthood. *Child Abuse & Neglect* **32**, 607–619.

Jones DPH. (2003) *Communicating with Vulnerable Children*. Gaskell, London. (An excellent little manual of good practice for the balanced and sympathetic interviewing of all children, including where sexual abuse is suspected.)

Swenson C. (2010) Multisystemic therapy for child abuse and neglect: A randomized effectiveness trial. *Journal of Family Psychology* **24**, 497–507.

PART 3
Risk Factors

CHAPTER 28
Intellectual Disability

Though both DSM-IV and ICD-10 use the term *mental retardation*, an increasing number of professionals and the general public dislike this term and avoid it. By contrast, the term *intellectual disability* is increasingly widely used, particularly in the USA. In the UK, the term *generalised learning disability* is still commonly used, but may lead to international misunderstanding, since *learning disability* in the USA often refers to individuals of normal intelligence who have specific reading or spelling difficulties. We have opted for the less ambiguous *intellectual disability*.

Definition

At its simplest, intellectual disability is defined solely by a general deficit in cognitive function that emerges during childhood. The threshold is generally operationalised as having an IQ level below 70 on a standardised IQ test where the population mean is 100 and the standard deviation is 15. Thus, an IQ below 70 is more than two standard deviations below average. Most definitions of intellectual disability also require impaired social functioning, involving reduced personal independence or a need for special care or protection. This double requirement for intellectual and social impairment is found in the ICD-10 and DSM-IV definitions of mental retardation. The same is generally true for legal and administrative definitions of intellectual disability, for example, for the definitions of mental impairment and severe mental impairment in English law. While most individuals with intellectual disability have educational as well as intellectual and social difficulties, these educational impairments are not central to the definition of intellectual disability.

Prevalence

1 *Mild intellectual disability*, as defined by IQ criteria of 50–69, affects about 2% of the general population, which is about what would be expected if IQ were normally distributed with a mean of 100 and a standard

Child and Adolescent Psychiatry, Third Edition. Robert Goodman and Stephen Scott.
© 2012 Robert Goodman and Stephen Scott. Published 2012 by John Wiley & Sons, Ltd.

deviation of 15. Many of these individuals are never identified by medical, educational or social services. Sometimes this is because their social functioning is adequate and they are coping well enough in mainstream schools, but in other instances they are drowning quietly without the extra input that might have helped them had their intellectual disability been recognised.

2 *Marked intellectual disability* is used in this chapter to refer to an IQ under 50, sometimes banded into three levels: moderate (IQ 35–49), severe (IQ 20–34) and profound IQ 0–20. Marked intellectual disability affects about 0.4% of the population, which is some ten times higher than would have been expected if IQ were normally distributed with a mean of 100 and a standard deviation of 15. In other words, there is a small extra 'hump' at the bottom of the normal IQ distribution. Individuals with marked intellectual disability are nearly always known to health, education or social services, either because of the severity of their educational difficulties or because of co-existing physical features such as cerebral palsy or epilepsy.

The two-population model

It is useful for some purposes to distinguish between two sorts of intellectual disability: *organic* and *normal variant* (sometimes described as 'subcultural'). The distinction can be clarified by an analogy. The genetic and environmental factors that account for the normal variation in adult height will inevitably result in some adults being at the lower end of the height distribution. In addition to these individuals with normal-variant short stature, there are other individuals with short stature due to organic conditions, for example, genetic syndromes such as achondroplasia. The organic group will tend to be shorter and to have more medical problems. The normal-variant group will have many relatives of below-average height (due to shared environment and polygenes), whereas most of the relatives of the organic group will be of around average height because they do not have the same organic syndrome. Using a specific height cut-off to determine short stature, it would be possible to define a very short stature group (which is mostly organic), as opposed to a moderately short stature group (which is mostly a normal variant), but no height cut-off would distinguish perfectly between organic and normal-variant groups.

For intellectual disability, the equivalent of a height cut-off is an IQ cut-off of around 50. As shown in Table 28.1, this approach does identify two relatively distinct populations. By comparison with mild intellectual disability, marked intellectual disability is more often associated with neurological disorder and less often associated with social disadvantage. Only mild intellectual disability is associated with a below-average IQ in relatives. Not surprisingly, an IQ cut-off of 50 cannot distinguish perfectly between organic and normal-variant cases. Though useful as a conceptual model, the two-population model of intellectual disability should not

Table 28.1 Characteristics of mild and marked intellectual disability

	Mild intellectual disability	Marked intellectual disability
Major CNS disorder	14%	72%
Prevalence in families of **low** socio-economic status	3.3%	0.8%
Prevalence in families of **high** socio-economic status	0.3%	0.4%
Male	46%	63%
Mean IQ of siblings	85	103

Source: Data from Broman *et al.* (1987).

be taken too literally: organic and normal-variant causes of intellectual disability may co-exist, with additive or synergistic effects.

Causes of intellectual disability

1 *Mild intellectual disability*. Most mild intellectual disability is assumed to be due to the same sorts of polygenic and environmental factors that determine IQ within the normal range. Just as the polygenic component is assumed to be due to many genes, each of which has a small but additive effect on IQ, so the psychosocial component seems to involve many factors, each of which has a small additive effect on IQ. Examples of adverse psychosocial factors include: lack of early stimulation; reduced access to books; and parental indifference to educational achievements. Adverse factors in the physical environment, such as exposure to low-level lead, may also add to the effects of genetic and psychosocial factors.

2 *Marked intellectual disability*. The organic causes that account for the majority of marked intellectual disability (and for some instances of mild intellectual disability) are conventionally subdivided according to their time of onset:

 (a) *Prenatal*: for example, chromosome abnormalities, single gene defects, congenital infections, fetal alcohol syndrome.

 (b) *Perinatal*: for example, intraventricular haemorrhage in premature neonates, severe neonatal jaundice. Though the role of obstetric complications was emphasised in old textbooks, it now seems unlikely that these are common causes of intellectual disability. If a child has a difficult delivery and subsequently turns out to have marked intellectual disability, was the delivery to blame? Not usually. More often, the obstetric complications were either irrelevant or a consequence of pre-existing abnormalities in the unborn child. Thus, children with chromosomal problems or prenatal brain damage are at greater risk of an abnormal delivery.

 (c) *Post-natal*: for example, encephalitis and meningitis, trauma due to child abuse and accidents, severe lead poisoning.

Several syndromes, including the fragile X syndrome and the fetal alcohol syndrome, have already been discussed in Chapter 1. Other relevant syndromes include:

- *Down syndrome*: affects up to 1 in 800 live births, with older mothers at much greater risk. This is the commonest single cause of marked intellectual disability, accounting for around a sixth of all cases: 95% are due to an extra chromosome 21 resulting from non-disjunction, something which more commonly affects older mothers; 4% are from translocations, which are familial; and 1% are mosaics. Physical features include: small head; round face; upslanting eyes; epicanthic folds; large fissured tongue; low-set simple ears; short stature; single palmar crease; incurved little fingers; and hypotonia. Cardiac and gastrointestinal malformations are common. There is an increased risk later in life of deafness, leukaemia and Alzheimer's disease.
- *Single gene disorders*: there are many rare genetic disorders that sometimes or always cause intellectual disability. As a rule of thumb, you can assume that these disorders are autosomal recessive unless you know otherwise. There are a few exceptions: the Lesch-Nyhan and Hunter (but not Hurler) syndromes are sex linked; and tuberous sclerosis and neurofibromatosis are autosomal dominant.
- *Sex chromosomal anomalies*: individuals with the common anomalies (XO, Turner syndrome, XXY, Kleinfelter syndrome, XXX and XYY) are usually of normal or low-normal intelligence, though there is some excess of mild and marked intellectual disability.

Diagnostic assessment of intellectual disability

Children with marked intellectual disability are usually referred to a paediatrician because of associated physical abnormalities or slow development, either noted by parents or picked up on developmental screening. Mild intellectual disability may not be noticed until learning difficulties become apparent in school. Parents and teachers are usually fairly accurate judges of a child's ability level. If asked, they are often able to give a good estimate of the mental age. Nevertheless, even experienced parents and teachers sometimes seriously misjudge intelligence. Thus, a child with autism and normal intelligence (as judged by non-verbal tests) may be thought to have a marked intellectual disability on the basis of his poor performance in verbal tests and his lack of commonsense. This kind of misjudgement may lead to an inappropriate placement in a school for marked intellectual disability. Even more commonly, children and adolescents with mild intellectual disability are believed by their teachers to be of near average ability, with poor academic performance being attributed to lack of effort, emotional problems, or social disadvantage. Once again, the misjudgement leads to inappropriate academic provision and pressure. Given this, it is often sensible to supplement parent and teacher reports with formal psychometric testing. Besides measuring IQ reliably, a detailed psychometric assessment generates a useful profile of the child's cognitive strengths and weaknesses. For children and adolescents of school age, the Wechsler Intelligence Scale for Children, fourth edition (WISC IV), or the British Ability Scale, third edition (BAS3) provide a suitably wide-ranging battery of verbal and visual spatial tests. The Vineland test of adaptive functioning is a useful index of social functioning, particularly since there are extensive population norms.

Diagnosis of the underlying cause of intellectual disability is based on:

1 a thorough history, with particular attention to family history, prenatal infections and prenatal alcohol exposure;
2 a careful physical examination, particularly for neurological signs, dysmorphic features and the skin signs of the neurocutaneous syndromes (see Chapter 1);
3 selected special investigations, particularly for the fragile X syndrome, chromosomal abnormalities and metabolic diseases.

Although very few treatable causes will be found, the search for a cause is valuable for genetic counselling and because many parents are relieved by a diagnostic label (partly because this opens the way to joining the relevant parent self-help group). In Britain, diagnosis and counselling are usually undertaken by paediatricians rather than psychiatrists.

Prevention of intellectual disability

Many approaches can reduce the prevalence of the organic syndromes that sometimes or always result in intellectual disability. Thus, widespread rubella vaccination can prevent congenital rubella. Neural tube defects can be reduced by folic acid supplementation given around the time of conception and in early pregnancy. Advice on alcohol consumption in pregnancy can prevent the fetal alcohol syndrome. Prenatal diagnosis of organic syndromes is increasingly possible on the basis of blood tests, ultrasound scans, chorionic villous sampling and amniocentesis. Specific treatments are rarely available, but parents may opt for termination of pregnancy. Continuing advances in obstetric and neonatal care may further reduce the rate of early brain damage, for example, by reducing the rate and complications of premature birth. Neonatal screening for phenylketonuria, galactosaemia and hypothyroidism permits early treatment before irreversible brain damage has occurred. Immunisation can protect children against diseases that cause meningitis (for example, Haemophilus influenzae type b) and encephalitis (for example, pertussis). Measures to reduce the rate of domestic accidents, road traffic accidents and physical abuse can reduce brain damage secondary to head injury.

Less progress has been made in reducing the rate of normal-variant intellectual disability. Some interventions have targeted the infants of mothers who themselves have an intellectual disability and live in socially deprived neighbourhoods. These programmes can result in significant increases in scholastic achievement and measured IQ, at least in the short term. Continuing input in the school years may help maintain these gains in the long term. Just as there is no one critical period after which environmental damage is irreversible, so there is no one therapeutic window after which environmental enrichment is no longer necessary. It is important, though, not to overestimate the likely effect of environmental interventions. One adoption study found that there was a 12-point IQ difference according to whether children were raised by adoptive parents from the highest and lowest socio-economic groups. A lasting effect of this size is well beyond anything that specific stimulation or educational intervention projects have yet achieved.

Provision of services for children with intellectual disability

Service provision is increasingly influenced by the desire for 'normalisation', that is, the promotion of as ordinary a life as possible in the community.

Social provision

Children and adolescents develop best if they grow up as part of a family. Nowadays, most children and adolescents with intellectual disability live with their biological family. This can be a very positive experience for parents and siblings, but there is often a substantial burden of care too, particularly with marked intellectual disability. However, this burden can be eased by extra assistance and support, for example, mobility allowances or respite care (usually arranged by social services). If the family's capacity to cope is overwhelmed even with maximum respite care, placement in an alternative family setting is highly desirable, either by adoption or long-term fostering. A specialist residential placement should only rarely be required.

Educational provision

The law in many countries insists that all children and adolescents are entitled to an appropriate education, no matter how severe their intellectual disability. No individual should be denied all schooling on the grounds that they are 'ineducable'. It is increasingly recognised that children and adolescents with mild intellectual disability can generally receive the extra help they need within mainstream schools. Those with marked intellectual disability are more likely to need to attend special schools, or special units within mainstream schools. Reports from doctors and other health professionals can help education authorities identify special needs and provide for them accordingly.

Medical provision

Appropriate medical care generally involves family doctors and paediatric teams. Contact with child and adolescent mental health services is not routinely necessary, but may be helpful for the high proportion of individuals with intellectual disability who have co-existent psychiatric problems.

Psychiatric disorders in children and adolescents with intellectual disability

In the multi-axial schemes of ICD-10 and DSM-IV, intellectual disability and psychiatric disorders are coded on separate axes (see Chapter 2). While intellectual disability is not itself a psychiatric disorder, it is a powerful risk factor for psychiatric disorders. Roughly a third of all children and adolescents with mild intellectual disability have psychiatric diagnoses, as do roughly half of those with marked intellectual disability. This compares with some 10–15% of children without intellectual disability when judged by the same criteria. The combination of intellectual disability and psychiatric disorder is particularly stressful for families, many of whom find it harder to live with the psychiatric problems than with the problems intrinsic to intellectual disability. Psychiatric problems are the commonest reason for family placements breaking down.

Type of psychiatric disorder

Among children and adolescents with mild intellectual disability, the mixture of psychiatric disorders is generally similar to that seen in children without intellectual disability, being dominated by ADHD, emotional and behavioural disorders. In marked intellectual disability, the mixture of psychiatric disorder is more distinctive. Thus, although ADHD, emotional and behavioural disorders are still common, so too are autistic spectrum disorders (see Chapter 4). Thus, a substantial minority of children with marked intellectual disability are socially aloof or relate to others in a bizarre way; their imaginative play is characteristically impoverished, and stereotypies can be prominent, and may be worsened by boredom, isolation, blindness or deafness. Severe ADHD features sometimes occur alone, and sometimes in association with simple stereotypies or features of autism.

Self-injury, such as eye-poking, head banging or hand biting, is another behavioural syndrome that is particularly common in marked intellectual disability. These behaviours have a functional component that can be shown to vary from individual to individual. Thus, in different individuals, self-injury may serve to reduce boredom, to attract attention, or to discourage unwanted attention. Difficulties with the acquisition of self-help skills (including feeding, toileting and dressing) are also common in marked intellectual disability, as are sleep problems. For a range of reasons including understandable frustration, poor impulse control, less good understanding of why changes are occurring, a substantial minority of children and adolescents with intellectual disability have fairly frequent temper outbursts, sometimes called 'challenging behaviour'; as the individual grows larger and stronger these may become increasingly hard to manage.

Specific behavioural patterns

Some organic causes of intellectual disability are particularly associated with specific patterns of psychiatric problems. The Lesch-Nyhan syndrome, for example, is much more likely to lead to severe self-injury than other organic disorders resulting in equally low IQs. When the organic syndrome is genetic or chromosomal, the common behavioural characteristics are referred to as the *behavioural phenotype* of the disorder. Other examples include the social anxiety and gaze avoidance associated with the fragile X syndrome; and the insatiable overeating associated with the Prader-Willi syndrome. Non-genetic syndromes can also have associated behavioural features, and these, too, are sometimes referred to as behavioural phenotypes. Thus congenital rubella is associated with features of autism, while the fetal alcohol syndrome is associated with ADHD.

Box 28.1 portrays four possible causal pathways that could account for the observed association between intellectual disability and psychiatric disorder. For some psychiatric disorders, the evidence supports possibility B, namely that the same biological factors that cause intellectual disability also, and independently, cause the psychiatric problems. Take autism, for example. A child with an IQ of 40 and tuberous sclerosis is at high risk of autism, whereas a child with an IQ of 40 and cerebral palsy is at much lower risk. Thus, IQ cannot account for this difference, which is almost certainly related to the different biological substrates of the two sets of disorders.

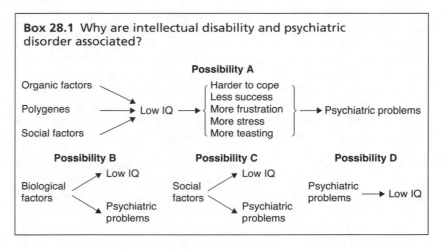

Box 28.1 Why are intellectual disability and psychiatric disorder associated?

For some other psychiatric disorders, however, the evidence favours possibility A, namely that low intelligence, whatever its cause, predisposes a child or adolescent to psychiatric problems. It is certainly plausible that low intelligence and poor academic attainments often undermine an individual's self-esteem and result in teasing by others. In addition, less intelligent individuals may find it harder to overcome everyday stresses, and may be more prone to 'act out' when under stress. For all these reasons, lower intelligence could well result in more anxiety, misery and anger. In the case of disruptive behavioural disorders, possibility A is supported by a fairly linear relationship with IQ. Within the normal IQ range, lower IQ is associated with more disruptive behavioural even when socio-economic background has been allowed for. The particularly high rate of disruptive behaviour among children with intellectual disability appears to be a continuation of this trend. It looks as though any cause of lower IQ, whether organic, polygenic or social, increases the risk of disruptive behavioural disorder.

There is little evidence supporting either of the other two possible explanations for the link between intellectual disability and psychiatric problems. The adverse social factors (such as lack of stimulation) that contribute to low IQ are different from the adverse social factors (such as harsh parenting) that increase psychiatric risk – arguing against possibility C. Finally, although psychiatric problems may interfere with school performance, they do not usually reduce measured IQ – arguing against possibility D.

Treatment

Treating the psychiatric disorders of children and adolescents with intellectual disability differs in emphasis but not in principle from treating similar disorders in children and adolescents of average intelligence. Behavioural treatment is particularly valuable in building up self-help skills and in reducing undesirable behaviours such as self-injury, stereotypies and frequent night waking. To be effective, behavioural therapy must be carefully tailored to the individual. For self-injurious behaviour, for example, advice to ignore a child during episodes of self-injury may be appropriate if the child uses the behaviour primarily to attract extra attention. However, it would only succeed in reinforcing the self-injurious behaviour if the child primarily used the behaviour to discourage unwanted attention. In addition to behavioural therapy, a wide range of other therapies can be deployed, including family therapy, cognitive therapy and supportive psychotherapy – depending on the nature of the problem and the age and cognitive level of the individual.

The role of medication in the treatment of psychiatric problems associated with intellectual disability remains controversial. In the short term, neuroleptics do reduce serious aggression and may therefore be useful in an emergency. However, the benefits usually wear off quite rapidly. It is then tempting to increase the dose to gain another temporary respite. Unless this temptation is resisted, the dose is likely to escalate progressively, leaving the individual on high-dose, long-term neuroleptic medication with all its attendant hazards (see Chapter 38). The pointlessness of this long-term medication is often only evident when the medication is finally withdrawn: aggression typically worsens for a while and then returns to its previous level. As a rule, challenging behaviour requires social and psychological management rather than pharmacological treatment. With this reservation, medication can be useful at times. Moderate doses of neuroleptics can sometimes reduce stereotypies, ADHD symptoms, self-injury and agitation, perhaps particularly in adolescents with intellectual disability and features of autism. Stimulants may sometimes improve the ADHD symptoms of children with IQs of around 40 or more, but rarely work for children with lower IQs. At any IQ, stimulants may exacerbate coexistent ritualistic and repetitive behaviours.

Subject review

Einfeld S, Emerson E. (2008) Intellectual disability. *In*: Rutter M *et al.* (eds) *Rutter's Child and Adolescent Psychiatry*, 5th edn. Wiley-Blackwell, Chichester, pp. 820–840.

Skuse DH, Seigal, A. (2008) Behavioral phenotypes and chromosomal disorders. *In*: Rutter M et al. (eds) *Rutter's Child and Adolescent Psychiatry*, 5th edn. Wiley-Blackwell, Chichester, pp. 359–376.

Further reading

Di Nuovo S, Buono S. (2011) Behavioral phenotypes of genetic syndromes with intellectual disability: Comparison of adaptive profiles. *Psychiatry Research* **189**, 440–445.

Moldavsky M. *et al.* (2001) Behavioral phenotypes of genetic syndromes: A reference guide for psychiatrists. *Journal of the American Academy of Child and Adolescent Psychiatry* **40**, 749–761.

CHAPTER 29
Brain Disorders

The preceding chapter considered the psychiatric complications associated with intellectual disability, with and without known brain disorders. This chapter is primarily concerned with the psychiatric effects of brain disorders on individuals who do not also have an intellectual disability.

A relatively rare risk factor

Unequivocal brain disorders are relatively rare in childhood, for example, about 0.5% of children have epilepsy and 0.2% have cerebral palsy. Current evidence suggests that these brain disorders are usually due not to perinatal complications, as used to be thought, but to genetic factors, prenatal insults and post-natal insults.

There is only very limited support for the notion of a 'continuum of reproductive casualty'. This theory suggests that severe obstetric and neonatal complications can result in death, cerebral palsy or intellectual disability, whereas mild obstetric complications more often result in ADHD, specific learning problems or clumsiness – a constellation sometimes referred to as 'minimal brain damage'. Since children from socially disadvantaged backgrounds are more likely to have experienced obstetric and neonatal complications, it is essential to adjust for social background when investigating the possible impact of these complications. Having done so, most studies suggest that obstetric and neonatal complications rarely, if ever, cause psychiatric problems in children who do not have overt brain disorders. One exception to this rule is an increase in concentration difficulties and perhaps social difficulties in neurologically intact children who were born weighing less than 1500g, usually as a result of marked prematurity. These very premature children are vulnerable to periventricular white matter damage that can lead to attentional problems in the absence of overt neurological difficulties – an effect that is probably only partly explained by a lowering of average IQ.

Child and Adolescent Psychiatry, Third Edition. Robert Goodman and Stephen Scott.
© 2012 Robert Goodman and Stephen Scott. Published 2012 by John Wiley & Sons, Ltd.

Table 29.1 Isle of Wight Neuropsychiatric Study

Children with	Percentage with at least one psychiatric disorder
No physical disorder	7
Physical disorder not affecting the brain	12
Idiopathic epilepsy	29
Cerebral palsy and allied disorders (IQ over 50)	44

Source: Rutter *et al.* (1970).

An extremely powerful risk factor

When present, overt brain disorders are powerful risk factors for child psychiatric problems, having an impact that is much greater than other physical disorders. This is well illustrated by epidemiological data from the Isle of Wight neuropsychiatric study (see Table 29.1). The particularly high rate of psychiatric problems associated with cerebral damage cannot be explained simply by the degree of disability or stigmatisation; there is convincing evidence of direct brain–behaviour links as well. It is striking, for example, that over half of a large epidemiological sample of children with hemiplegic cerebral palsy had psychiatric disorders, despite the fact that the physical disability was typically mild and that most children were of normal intelligence and attending mainstream schools. Another illustration of the importance of neurological factors is that in an epidemiological survey of British child and adolescent mental health (described in more detail in Box 3.1), individuals with neurodevelopmental problems made up just 3% of the general population, but accounted for 15% of psychiatric disorders.

At risk for which psychiatric disorders?

As a first approximation, the psychiatric problems of children and adolescents with brain disorders are similar to the psychiatric problems of children and adolescents without neurological problems: behavioural and emotional disorders are the commonest mental health problems in both groups. There is no single 'brain damage syndrome'. Moving beyond this first approximation, there are some differences in emphasis. Though all psychiatric disorders are more common in children and adolescents with neurological problems, autistic spectrum and ADHD disorders seem to be particularly over-represented. For example, in the Isle of Wight study, hyperkinesis (severe ADHD) accounted for 19% of psychiatric disorders among children with cerebral palsy, but only 1% of psychiatric disorders among neurologically intact children.

Parents and teachers frequently comment on the oppositionality and irritability of children and adolescents with brain disorders. Although these are often marked enough to warrant a diagnosis of oppositional-defiant disorder, it is relatively unusual for these individuals to develop the more seriously antisocial behaviours that are characteristic of severe conduct disorder. Anxiety as well as irritability may sometimes contribute to outbursts when individuals with brain disorders are faced with demands they have difficulty meeting. Episodic outbursts are far more likely to be behavioural than epileptic, although the latter possibility may need to be considered, particularly if the episodes are completely unprovoked or accompanied by other pointers to epilepsy, such as altered consciousness or a subsequent need to sleep.

Specific neurological disorders may be associated with especially high risks for particular psychiatric problems, for example, Sydenham chorea has been linked to an unexpectedly high rate of obsessive-compulsive disorder (see Chapter 14). Some of the behavioural consequences of child-hood brain disorders only become apparent in adulthood, for example, the high rate of adult-onset schizophrenia in individuals with developmental abnormalities of the temporal lobes. The current evidence suggests that there are few differences in the psychiatric consequences of left- and right-sided brain lesions. Studies of early-acquired head injuries have not revealed consistent effects of locus or timing of injury on rate or type of psychiatric problem.

Interaction with other risk factors

Having a brain disorder does not generally render children immune to the adverse effects of 'ordinary' psychiatric risk factors, such as exposure to marital friction. There is continuing controversy as to whether children with brain disorders are more vulnerable to ordinary risk factors or simply as vulnerable.

Mediating links

There are many possible mediating links between brain and behavioural disorders, though the relative importance of different links remains to be established. In some cases, the link may be relatively direct, for example, autistic impairments may simply reflect damage to the brain systems involved in communication and social interaction. In other cases, psy-chosocial factors, such as poor self-image, unrealistic family expectations, or peer rejection play an important part too. Specific learning problems and below-average IQ are common consequences of brain abnormalities. When present, these problems add to the stresses on the child, particularly if their special educational needs are unrecognised or unmet (as is all too often the case). Treatments for the physical disorder may also contribute to the psychiatric problems. Anti-epileptic medication can have adverse psychiatric consequences; regular physiotherapy can lead to considerable resentment because of lost play time; and repeated hospitalisations can disrupt family interactions.

Prognosis

Is the prognosis for any given psychiatric disorder worse if the child or adolescent also has a brain disorder? Clinicians and parents often suppose so, and this pessimism may be self-fulfilling if it leads to inappropriately low expectations or half-hearted therapy. The evidence is so limited at present that it is often preferable to work on the more optimistic assumption that the prognosis of the psychiatric disorder is independent of the presence or absence of coexistent neurological problems. Indeed, the families of children with brain disorders are often particularly receptive to professional advice, and may consequently be easier to help than the average family seen by child mental health services.

Treatment

In general, the psychiatric problems of children with brain disorders should be treated in just the same ways as the psychiatric problems of neurologically intact children. Biological treatments are neither more nor less useful than in ordinary psychiatric practice. However, since anti-epileptic medication may have behavioural effects, a change in dose or type can sometimes be helpful. Individual, family, and school-based treatments can all be useful. Parents are often helped by hearing that their child's problems are common consequences of neurological damage: the energy previously wasted on self-blame can then be diverted into more profitable channels. Equally, access to a parents' support group for children and adolescents with the same disorder can reduce the family's sense of isolation and powerlessness. Neuropsychological assessments of the individual's cognitive strengths and weaknesses can provide a helpful basis for advice to the school and education authority. Emotional and behavioural problems often improve dramatically when unrecognised learning problems are finally addressed, whether by provision of extra help in a mainstream school or by transfer to a special school.

Three specific points

1 A variety of rare dementing disorders – such as Sanfilippo syndrome (a lysosomal storage disease due to an autosomal recessive enzyme deficiency) and subacute sclerosing panencephalitis (a persisting infection of a resistant measles virus) – present in childhood with loss of established skills and a variety of additional emotional and behavioural abnormalities. Although the early symptoms of dementia can be mimicked by

purely psychosocial problems (such as sexual abuse), a dementing disorder should be considered in any child who presents with loss of skills. A full physical examination is mandatory, and special investigations may be indicated. The presence of psychosocial stressors does not rule out an organic disorder. For example, a child who has been sexually abused, or who has a drug-abusing mother, may also (and not coincidentally) have HIV encephalopathy.

2 Frontal lobe seizures are easily misdiagnosed as pseudoseizures: movements, postures and vocalisations may be bizarre; episodes may be brief; the termination may be abrupt with prompt return to responsiveness; and ordinary EEGs may be unhelpful. Combined video and EEG monitoring can be extremely useful.

3 It is not yet clear if mild head injuries (which are very common in childhood) have adverse psychiatric consequences. It is clear, however, that serious cognitive and psychiatric sequelae are common after severe head injuries, for example, after closed head injuries resulting in at least two weeks of post-traumatic amnesia. Roughly half of the survivors of severe head injuries develop psychiatric disorders, particularly if they had minor emotional or behavioural problems prior to the head injury, or if they are exposed to psychosocial adversities such as maternal depression or overcrowding. The risk of psychiatric disorder is not related to age, gender or locus of injury. Though the psychiatric disorders that follow severe head injury mostly involve the sorts of emotional and behavioural problems that dominate ordinary child psychiatric practice, severe closed head injury sometimes results in a distinctive syndrome of social disinhibition (resembling the adult 'frontal lobe syndrome').

Subject review

Harris J. (2008) Brain disorders and their effect on psychopathology. *In*: Rutter M *et al.* (eds) *Rutter's Child and Adolescent Psychiatry*, 5th edn. Wiley-Blackwell, Chichester, pp. 459–473.

Further reading

Goodman R, Yude C. (2000) Emotional, behavioural and social consequences. *In*: Neville B, Goodman R (eds) *Congenital Hemiplegia: Clinics in Developmental Medicine. No. 150*, Mac Keith Press, London, pp. 166–178.

Rutter M *et al.* (1970) *A Neuropsychiatric Study in Childhood: Clinics in Developmental Medicine. No. 35/36*. SIMP/Heinemann, London.

Rutter M *et al.* (1983) Head injury. In: Rutter M. (ed.) *Developmental Neuropsychiatry*. Guilford Press, New York, pp. 83–111.

CHAPTER 30
Language Disorders

Many specific language impairments are associated with increased rates of child psychiatric problems. This is not surprising, for three reasons. First, language impairments and psychiatric problems may sometimes share a common origin in brain abnormalities that interfere with 'higher functions'. Second, language dominates our lives: it is a powerful tool for thought and problem solving; it is our primary means for obtaining what we want from others; and it plays a key role in social cohesion, with human conversation functioning rather like mutual grooming among chimpanzees. Consequently, language impairments are likely to be frustrating and isolating. Finally, the same set of social communication difficulties may be construed as a language disorder by a speech-language therapist and as a psychiatric disorder by a mental health professional; the timber merchant, the botanist and the artist do not see the same tree.

Epidemiology

Specific language impairment (SLI) refers to language impairments that occur in the context of otherwise normal development and that are not part of a recognised syndrome; thus, a child would not be said to have SLI if he or she has an intellectual disability or Landau-Kleffner syndrome (see below). Estimates of the prevalence of SLI diverge widely, largely reflecting differences in the definition employed. At one extreme, severe and persistent disorders that result in substantial social impairment and occur in children of normal intelligence are quite rare, with a prevalence that is probably under 0.1%. At the opposite extreme, the prevalence of broadly defined language disorders may be as high as 15–25%, though many of these children have relatively minor delays or articulation problems that result in little or no social impairment and that resolve without treatment. Between the two extremes, significant language problems may be present in roughly 1–5% of schoolchildren. No matter which definition is used, there is a substantial male excess for all developmental language disorders.

Child and Adolescent Psychiatry, Third Edition. Robert Goodman and Stephen Scott.
© 2012 Robert Goodman and Stephen Scott. Published 2012 by John Wiley & Sons, Ltd.

Causation

Twin studies show that SLI is highly heritable. Studies of one large family with a dominantly inherited form of language disorder identified a mutation of the FOXP2 gene that affects the development of the brain (and other organs). However, mutations at this site have not turned out to be a common cause of SLI more broadly. Perhaps there are many rare mutants of strong effect, or perhaps there are common genetic variations that have small or moderate effects. It remains to be seen whether shared genes account for the co-occurrence of SLI with reading difficulties and autistic traits.

What about environmental risk factors for SLI? These have been harder to identify. At one stage, it was thought that otitis media with effusion ('glue ear') was a significant risk factor, but more recent studies suggest that any effect is relatively slight. Likewise, theories suggesting that growing up in a bilingual environment increases the risk of SLI, are not supported by the limited evidence.

Varieties of language disorders

Several different aspects of language can be affected by developmental language disorders (see Box 30.1). Language disorders include:

1 *Phonologic-syntactic language disorders* involve problems in the form but not the content of language. The child wants to communicate and says appropriate things, but there are problems with articulation or syntax, or both. Some children have *pure articulation problems* without any other language problems. Delay or deviance in speech-sound production makes these children harder to understand, and may lead to teasing. In cases of *expressive language disorder*, speech develops late and syntactic structures are several years behind age level. Articulation is often faulty too, but comprehension is within normal limits. *Receptive language*

Box 30.1 Different aspects of language

- *Phonology/articulation* refers to the production of speech sounds.
- *Prosody* refers to the expression and comprehension of those aspects of communication that are mediated by tone of voice and by variation in the way different syllables are stressed.
- *Syntax* refers to the production and comprehension of grammatically correct sentences.
- *Semantics* refers to the ability to encode meaning into words and decode meaning from words.
- *Pragmatics* refers to the ability to use and decipher language in a way that is appropriate to the wider social-interpersonal context, for example, drawing on knowledge of the context to grasp a message that is implicit but not explicit in the words themselves.

disorder is rarer, and nearly always involves a mixture of problems with language comprehension, language expression and articulation.

2 *Pragmatic language impairment* (formerly *semantic-pragmatic disorder*) refers to a set of problems concerning the use and content rather than the form of language. In a typical case, articulation and syntax are normal and the child scores well on formal tests of language, but there are problems with everyday conversation and comprehension that parents and teachers find hard to describe. Understanding is highly literal, and the child fails to use knowledge of the context to make sense of what is said. The child's own attempts to explain things or to tell a story do not make allowances for the listener's point of view, they miss out key details, or fail to organise the account into a coherent sequence. The child's speech may be dominated by rambling monologues or repetitive questioning. Prosodic impairments are common, for example, a monotonous tone of voice or abnormal pattern of stressing syllables. Many children with these pragmatic deficits meet all the criteria for childhood autism or Asperger syndrome in terms of associated social impairments, rigidity, and so on. Labelling such children as having both an autistic spectrum disorder and a pragmatic language impairment is not very helpful – it is not so much that these children have two separate disorders; more a case of different professional groups using different vocabularies. It may be more helpful to use 'social communication disorder' to refer to pragmatic language difficulties that affect social interaction, along with other mild or patchy features of autism that are too mild to warrant the diagnosis of an ASD. Some degree of pragmatic language impairment is common in children with severe phonologic-syntactic language disorders.

3 *Landau-Kleffner syndrome* (also known as *acquired epileptic aphasia*) is a rare disorder involving the loss of language skills after a period of normal development, usually starting between the age of 3 and 9. The loss is usually gradual, typically occurring over the course of months, though it can be more rapid. Receptive loss is noted first, with the child becoming increasingly unresponsive to spoken language. This may lead to deafness being suspected, though testing shows that hearing thresholds are normal. Loss of understanding is followed by loss of expressive language. The language changes are accompanied by EEG abnormalities, involving paroxysmal discharges that affect both hemispheres, often independently; these EEG changes are often most prominent during non-REM sleep. Seizures occur in roughly 50–70% of affected individuals, usually starting about the same time as the aphasia, and taking the form of generalised or simple partial seizures that are infrequent and mainly nocturnal. Perplexity, anxiety and temper tantrums are common at the time of onset, and may result in the child being referred to a child mental health professional, particularly when there are no evident seizures and the child's unresponsiveness is attributed to wilfulness. Affected children do not generally show autistic impairments in social interaction, but often show some degree of hyperactivity.

Differential diagnosis and assessment

Hearing impairment is the most important differential diagnosis since it is common, there are effective treatments and delaying these treatments can seriously disadvantage the affected individual. It is essential, therefore, that everyone with language delay should have their hearing properly assessed. Language delay can be part of an intellectual disability, and this possibility can only be ruled out by suitable tests of general mental ability, which obviously need to be judged by tests of non-verbal ability in the presence of severe language problems. Likewise, tests of general mental ability are helpful in distinguishing between the selective loss of language skills in Landau-Kleffner syndrome and the general loss of cognitive skills in progressive childhood dementias (see Chapter 24). A general psychiatric assessment is also important since autistic spectrum disorders (see Chapter 4) characteristically involve language delay or deviance, and may even begin with a developmental 'setback' in which established language skills are lost. Selective mutism (see Chapter 16) refers to a relatively rare group of children who are able to understand what other people say, but who restrict their own speech to a small group of very familiar people in specific circumstances; social anxiety is probably the key factor in most cases, but this anxiety may be aggravated by co-existent minor language problems. If a speech or language problem is likely to be present, referral to a speech and language specialist should be considered. There are many specific tests of articulation, expressive language and receptive language, with the Clinical Evaluation of Language Fundamentals (CELF) being widely used by speech-language therapists in the UK and the USA both for screening and for the diagnosis of specific language impairment.

Interventions for language disorders

There have been a few randomised controlled trials of speech and language therapy, which show:

- There is a significant effect of intervention when children have phonological or expressive language disorders.
- The results for children with receptive language difficulties are inconclusive, but the few studies that are available do not show a significant effect of therapy.
- For children with expressive language difficulties, treatment administered by parents under professional guidance seems as effective as treatment administered by clinicians.
- By contrast, treatment administered by clinicians may be more effective for children with phonological or receptive language difficulties.

Prognosis for language development

The prognosis for language development depends both on the type of language disorder and also on the presence of associated cognitive impairments. When a language disorder is associated with low IQ, the prognosis is generally worse. Within the phonologic-syntactic disorders, the chances of a complete recovery are highest for children with pure articulation problems and lowest for children with a receptive language disorder. A child with a receptive language disorder and a normal IQ is likely to make enough progress by adult life to communicate fairly well, but some noticeable language deficits usually persist. Studies of autistic spectrum disorders suggest that pragmatic deficits in language use and content can be very persistent. The prognosis in Landau-Kleffner syndrome is very variable, with severe persisting problems in some instances, particularly when the onset occurred before the age of 5 or 6.

Associated scholastic difficulties

Severe and persistent language disorders are associated with a substantial risk of academic difficulties, even if the child is of normal intelligence (as judged by non-verbal IQ). This risk is mainly for reading and spelling problems, though maths problems may also occur. Children whose language catches up completely do not seem to be at increased risk. Expressive and receptive language disorders carry a higher risk than articulation problems. Indeed, pure articulation problems may not result in any increased risk of academic problems.

Associated psychiatric and personality problems

Many studies have shown that children with language problems are at increased psychiatric risk. In some instances, the psychiatric risk may stem directly from the language disorder itself, for example, as a result of the teasing, frustration and social isolation engendered by communication difficulties. In other instances, however, the language and psychiatric problems may both stem from a single underlying cognitive or neurobiological disorder.

Children with language disorder are primarily at risk for anxiety disorders, ADHD and difficulties with social relationships. These problems are often more obvious in older children and adolescents than in younger children. There is little or no excess of disruptive behavioural problems. The rate of psychopathology is particularly high in individuals of low IQ, but the rate is also substantially increased in those of normal IQ. Psychiatric risk is primarily associated with expressive and receptive language problems, although children with pure articulation problems may be more liable to emotional problems.

Children with receptive language problems often show some degree of pragmatic language impairment. This may become more evident as the individual grows older. One follow-up study of children with receptive language problems and normal IQ found that over half had major problems with social relationships in adult life. In many instances, the failure to make friends or love relationships seemed to reflect a primary lack of social interest and skill; it was not simply a secondary consequence of the social restrictions imposed by communication difficulties.

These findings suggest some sort of continuum between classical autism and receptive language disorder. However, another follow-up finding points to differences rather than continuities between autism and receptive language disorder. Autistic spectrum disorders are rarely associated with subsequent psychosis, whereas receptive language disorder (with or without pragmatic language impairment and other mild features of autism) does seem to carry an increased risk of florid paranoid psychosis in adolescence.

Subject review

Bishop DVM, Norbury CF. (2008) Speech and language disorders. *In*: Rutter M *et al.* (eds) *Rutter's Child and Adolescent Psychiatry*, 5th edn. Wiley-Blackwell, Chichester, pp. 782–801.

Further reading

Bishop DVM, Adams C. (1989) Conversational characteristics of children with semantic-pragmatic disorder. II: What features lead to a judgement of inappropriacy? *British Journal of Disorders of Communications* **24**, 241–263. (This paper is full of examples of the sorts of language abnormalities found in semantic-pragmatic disorder.)

Law J, Garrett Z. (2004) Speech and language therapy: Its potential role in CAMHS. *Child and Adolescent Mental Health* **9**, 50–55.

Mantovani JF. (2000) Autistic regression and Landau-Kleffner syndrome: Progress or confusion? *Developmental Medicine and Child Neurology* **42**, 349–353.

Rutter M, Mawhood L. (1991) The long-term psychosocial sequelae of specific developmental disorders of speech and language. *In*: Rutter M., Casaer P (eds) *Biological Risk Factors for Psychosocial Disorders*. Cambridge University Press, Cambridge, pp. 233–259.

CHAPTER 31
Reading Difficulties

Reading difficulties affect up to 10% of children and adolescents and are of particular interest to psychiatrists because of the relatively strong links between reading difficulties and disruptive behavioural problems. Nearly all these reading difficulties are developmental in origin, though brain damage in childhood or adolescence can result in acquired reading disorders, and dementias lead to progressive deterioration in reading skills. Poor reading skills have a detrimental effect on children and adolescents' general academic trajectory and on their employment in adulthood. Children and adolescents who do poorly on reading tests are also more likely to perform poorly in other subjects, they have lower academic and reading self-concepts, and are more likely to leave school with no qualifications. Poor readers do not enjoy reading and they spend less time engaged in it, contributing to the continuation of poorer reading skills.

Background information about normal reading

When they start to read, children learn to recognise a small number of very familiar words (such as their own name) on the basis of visual clues from the overall shape of the word. At this early stage, they are generally unable to decipher new words. Subsequently, as they come to understand the principles of letter–sound correspondence, they acquire a phonological strategy for deciphering less familiar words. Eventually, as reading becomes fluent, most words are recognised as a single entity without the need for phonological decoding.

Though many linguistic and perceptual skills are involved in fluent reading, individual variation in reading ability is more closely related to linguistic than to perceptual abilities. In particular, preschool children's phonological awareness as indexed, for example, by their sensitivity to rhyme and alliteration, is a good predictor of how well they will subsequently learn to read (even when the effect of IQ is allowed for). Improving phonological awareness enhances subsequent reading skill.

Child and Adolescent Psychiatry, Third Edition. Robert Goodman and Stephen Scott.
© 2012 Robert Goodman and Stephen Scott. Published 2012 by John Wiley & Sons, Ltd.

Most twin studies suggest that genetic variation accounts for about 30–50% of individual differences in reading abilities. Environmental factors, including the amount of parental input and the quality of schooling, also have a major impact. Parent–child interaction centred on books contributes to children's success in reading. For young children who cannot yet read, parental storybook reading enhances children's language comprehension and expressive language skills which in turn helps learning to read later.

Specific reading difficulties (SRD)

Some children and adolescents have reading attainments that are substantially poorer than would be predicted from their age and IQ: these individuals are said to have SRD. Tests of reading attainment may assess reading accuracy or reading comprehension. Reading accuracy is typically tested by asking the individual to read words or passages of increasing difficulty. In English, it is relatively easy to tell when someone cannot read a particular word because he or she stumbles over it or mispronounces it. This is harder to judge in languages such as Spanish that have very predictable spelling – making it much easier to pronounce unknown words. Reading comprehension is tested by asking individuals questions about passages they have read, establishing how well they have taken in the meaning of the words. People with SRD often have less difficulty on tests of comprehension as opposed to accuracy since they can use clues from the general context to guess the overall meaning even when they have not been able to read some of the words. At the other extreme, people with hyperlexia do well on tests of reading accuracy, but do not necessarily understand what they have read.

The relationship at any given chronological age between reading age and IQ is shown schematically in Box 31.1. The correlation between reading age and IQ is fairly substantial (with a correlation coefficient of 0.6). Not surprisingly, brighter individuals are likely to be reading better. It is worth noting, however, that predicted reading age does not generally equal mental age – there is regression towards the mean. Thus, a 10-year-old with a mental age of 13 will not, on average, be reading up to 13-year-old level, while a 10-year-old with a mental age of 7 will, on average, be reading at better than 7-year-old level. Roughly 95% of children and adolescents fall within two standard deviations of their predicted reading age. SRD refers to those individuals, such as subjects B and C in Box 31.1 whose reading attainments are over two standard deviations (SDs) below their predicted reading level. This corresponds, at the age of 10, to being about $2\frac{1}{2}$ years behind the predicted level. Though most individuals with SRD are reading at well below the average for their chronological age (for example, subject B in Box 31.1), some very bright individuals with SRD do have average reading ability (for example, subject C in Box 28.1). Therefore because a child or adolescent has a normal reading age does not mean SRD is absent.

Conversely, being markedly behind in reading attainments (*reading back-wardness*) does not necessarily imply SRD because poor reading skills may be in line with the low intelligence (for example, subject A in Box 31.1).

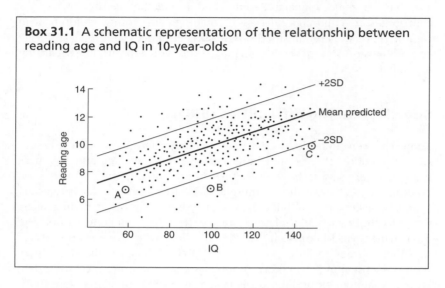

Box 31.1 A schematic representation of the relationship between reading age and IQ in 10-year-olds

Although it is somewhat arbitrary to define SRD in terms of reading attainments that are at least two SDs below the predicted level, this cut-off does identify a group who have a substantial and persistent disability. These individuals may represent an extra 'hump' at the bottom of the normal distribution curve of reading ability. Whether such individuals are qualitatively or just quantitatively different from individuals who are less far behind with their reading (for example, only 1 or $1\frac{1}{2}$ SDs behind) has not yet been resolved.

Epidemiology

SRD affects 3–10% of children and adolescents. Most studies show it to be two to three times more common in males than females. SRD is more common among the children of parents with manual rather than non-manual occupations. The prevalence of SRD at 10 years of age was 4% on the Isle of Wight and 10% in inner London; a difference that could be explained by social, school and family factors.

Associated features

1 Spelling is often more severely affected than reading itself, and problems with spelling may persist even if reading becomes reasonably fluent. Arithmetical skills are not typically as far behind as reading skills, though some delay is usual.
2 Spelling errors are often severe and bizarre. They are commonly non-phonetic (for example, 'umderlee' for umbrella) rather than phonetic (for example, 'mite' for might). Reading errors are often based on

attempts to guess the word from its shape rather than on faulty attempts to decipher the word phonologically. In both reading and writing, letters and words may be reversed, for example, 'p' for 'q', 'b' for 'd', 'saw' for 'was', a phenomenon sometimes labelled strephosymbolia.

3 Children with SRD are more likely than other children to have neurodevelopmental and neuropsychological impairments, including left–right confusion, poor coordination, poor constructional abilities, motor impersistence and language abnormalities. Whether these associated symptoms delineate a specific dyslexia syndrome is considered later. Children who have early delays in language, but who then catch up completely are not at greater subsequent risk of SRD.

4 Children with SRD span the IQ range from very bright to very dull. The mean IQ of children with SRD is average or slightly below average. Verbal IQ tends to be lower than performance IQ. This may reflect not only the centrality of language rather than visuospatial deficits in SRD, but also the fact that children who read little have less opportunity to build up the skills tapped by the verbal subtests.

5 Epidemiological studies have not supported clinical accounts that left-handedness or mixed dominance is over represented in SRD. One recent epidemiological study found an excess of both strong left-handers and strong right-handers among children with SRD.

6 SRD is more common among children from large families.

7 SRD is associated with a variety of psychiatric problems, as detailed at the end of this section.

SRD and reading backwardness: is this a distinction worth making?

Is there any point distinguishing SRD from poor reading that is in line with the individual's IQ, for example, distinguishing between subjects A and B in Box 31.1? The answer is controversial:

• Some experts, particularly those more closely linked to education, argue that there is little practical justification for the distinction. When an individual is struggling with reading, this is generally due to underlying phonological deficits – and what is required is extra help developing phonological awareness. Since this applies to those with reading backwardness as well as SRD, educators put less effort into assessing IQ in detail, investing the time instead in tests of language (including phonological awareness) along with briefer measures of non-verbal reasoning.

• Other experts, particularly those more closely linked to psychiatry, continue to favour 'disrepancy definitions' – obtaining detailed measures of IQ and reading attainments in order to identify significant discrepancies between actual and predicted reading ability, using the sort of regression analysis shown in Box 31.1. Their rationale for distinguishing between SRD and reading backwardness is that these two categories differ in prognosis and associated features (Box 31.2).

Box 31.2 Differences between specific reading disorder and reading backwardness

	More strongly associated with:	
	Specific reading disorder	Reading backwardness
Poor prognosis for reading	√	
Marked male excess	√	
History of relatively specific problems in speech and language development	√	
History of widespread developmental delays		√
Overt neurological disorder		√
Social disadvantage		√

SRD and developmental dyslexia

Is there a subgroup of children with SRD who warrant a diagnosis of *developmental dyslexia* on the basis that their reading problems are part of a wider neurodevelopmental syndrome that is clearly constitutional rather than environmental? Epidemiological evidence from the Isle of Wight study does not support the notion of a pure dyslexic subgroup. Although children with SRD were indeed more likely to have other neurodevelopmental and neuropsychological problems (poor coordination, constructional difficulties, left–right confusion, etc.), most of the children had only one or two of these additional problems and there was no evidence for two distinct groups of children: a dyslexic group with many associated problems and a non-dyslexic group with few or none. Furthermore, it made no difference whether a child with SRD had many or few associated neurodevelopmental problems as far as many important outcomes were concerned: prognosis, response to treatment, likelihood of associated psychiatric problems, or likelihood of having a positive family history of reading problems.

Thus there is currently little justification for distinguishing developmental dyslexia from SRD. Some educationalists and researchers avoid using the term 'dyslexia' at all, while others use the term to delineate a group of children with particularly marked deficit in phonological skills (even if some of these children have compensated for this deficit and read well). It is tempting to abandon such a controversial term. In the real world, however, a label of dyslexia is widely recognised, usually conveys the message that the child's reading problems are not the result of stupidity or laziness, and sometimes results in important practical benefits for the child (for example, extra time in examinations). Given this, there is no reason to deny any child or adolescent with SRD a label of dyslexia if this is to the individual's overall advantage (irrespective of whether or not additional neurodevelopmental symptoms are present).

Causation of SRD

SRD is not a uniform condition, though it is not clear if the heterogeneity is best conceptualised in dimensional or categorical terms. It seems likely that the aetiology and pathogenesis of SRD are also heterogeneous.

In most cases, phonological problems seem central. These make it much harder for affected individuals to increase their reading vocabulary by sounding out new words and thereby familiarising themselves with them. In a minority of cases, visual perceptual problems may be more important than language-related problems. Little is known about children who do well on tests of reading accuracy but poorly on tests of reading comprehension, except that they tend to have poor vocabulary and syntactic skills, and fail to use context clues.

SRD was initially investigated in English-speaking populations. Does the link between phonological problems and SRD primarily reflect the notorious unpredictability of English spelling? Surprisingly, phonological problems are also linked to SRD in phonologically predictable languages such as Italian and German. For children with SRD who speak these languages, sounding words out is not so difficult, but automatising this process is problematic.

Twin and family studies have demonstrated a substantial heritability, particularly among those with higher IQ. Linkage studies have implicated the short arm of chromosome 6 – a replicated finding that has led to the identification of two candidate genes (DCDC2, KIAA0319) whose mutations may disturb cortical neuronal migration. The psychosocial environment is also of great importance, as shown, for example, by the fact that SRD was more than twice as common in inner London than on the Isle of Wight.

Children and adolescents with neurological conditions such as cerebral palsy or epilepsy are at much greater risk of SRD than other children and adolescents with comparable IQs. In children with dyslexia in the absence of overt neurological disorders, it has been suggested that SRD arises from developmental anomalies in language-related areas of the left hemisphere. Neuroanatomical and neuroradiological studies have focused interest on the planum temporale, a region of the temporal lobe involved in phonological processing. In individuals who read normally, the planum temporale is typically larger on the left side of the brain than on the right side; this asymmetry often seems to be lost in individuals with SRD. The finding of an excess of strong left-handers and strong right-handers among children with SRD is intriguing. Annett's genetic model of handedness suggests that strong left- and right- handers are mainly homozygotes, whereas mild and moderate right-handers are mainly heterozygotes. Perhaps there is a heterozygote advantage for reading (analogous to the heterozygote advantage of the sickle cell trait).

Interventions for SRD

Children and adolescents with SRD are all too often thought of as lacking in intelligence or motivation by their parents or teachers. These views will tend to aggravate the poor self-image generated by repeated failures at academic tasks. Informing teachers, parents and the affected individual that the reading problems cannot be explained by low intelligence or inadequate effort can have a major impact for good, fostering attitudes that are both more realistic and more positive. Since some parents think that dyslexia is a sign of being particularly gifted, it is important to avoid the opposite error of fostering unrealistically high expectations, particularly if the individual is of average or below average intelligence. Listing famous people with dyslexia is not necessarily helpful.

It should be possible to provide most children and adolescents with SRD with adequate extra help for their reading and spelling within a mainstream school. In severe cases, and when the literacy difficulties are an insuperable block to academic progress in all other subjects, placement in a special unit or school may be helpful. Some schools specialise just in 'dyslexia' while others cater for a range of learning problems, including SRD.

Historically, most interventions to improve reading resulted in short-term benefits but no lasting gains. More recent interventions, combining reading instruction with intensive work on phonological awareness and motivation training, seem more promising. Increasing parental involvement in their children's reading can be beneficial.

Prognosis of SRD

It is unusual for children and adolescents with SRD to catch up entirely and many fall increasingly far behind, not because they are losing skills but because they make less progress each year than their normal peers. The prognosis for reading is improved by high IQ and an advantaged socio-economic background. Because their academic difficulties persist (with spelling problems often being even more persistent than reading problems), individuals with SRD typically end up with poor school qualifications even if they have no associated behavioural problems. As a result of their poorer qualifications and continuing problems with literacy skills, they are more likely than their peers to have manual jobs in adult life.

Psychiatric accompaniments of reading disorders

Many studies have shown that SRD is fairly strongly associated with ADHD, anxiety, depression, disruptive behavioural disorders and juvenile delinquency. Some of these links appear direct and others indirect. Thus, the link between SRD and anxiety seems direct – being expected to read when you have SRD is a stressful experience. By contrast, the link between SRD and behavioural problems seems indirect, being mediated by ADHD (or perhaps specifically by the inattentive rather than over-activity component of ADHD).

Even if the link is indirectly mediated via attention difficulties, the resultant comorbidity between SRD and behavioural disorders is considerable. Among 10-year-olds in the Isle of Wight study, for example, a third of children with SRD had disruptive behavioural disorders, and a third of children with disruptive behavioural disorders had SRD. Subsequent studies have shown that disruptive behaviour and poor pre-reading skills are already associated in preschool children. This is long before the child's disruptive behaviour could plausibly have interfered with schoolwork or led to criticism in the classroom – arguing against the notion that disruptive behaviour can usually be attributed to the frustration and marginalisation engendered by school failure. Equally, there is no convincing evidence that being disruptive in the classroom is what stops a child learning to read.

Follow-up studies suggest that those children with SRD who are free from additional psychiatric disorders in middle childhood are no more likely than their peers to develop psychiatric problems in their teens (with the possible exception of an increased risk of problems with temper control in adolescent girls with SRD).

When SRD is compounded by disruptive behaviour, the teenage prognosis is worse. These individuals are more likely to leave school at the first opportunity, obtain no qualifications, take up unskilled work, and have a poor work record.

Though SRD is associated with a relatively high risk of adverse psychiatric and psychosocial outcomes in childhood and adolescence, follow-up studies into adulthood suggest that the impact on adult adjustment is far less marked. Whereas school life centres on reading, adults have the freedom to adopt occupations and lifestyles that do not depend on reading skill. Perhaps this is why SRR in adult life does not lead to more psychiatric or social problems.

Subject review

Snowling MJ, Hulme C. (2008) Reading and other specific learning difficulties. *In*: Rutter M *et al.* (eds) *Rutter's Child and Adolescent Psychiatry*, 5th edn. Wiley-Blackwell, Chichester, pp. 802–819.

Further reading

Annett M *et al.* (1996) Types of dyslexia and the shift to dextrality. *Journal of Child Psychology and Psychiatry* **37**, 167–180. (This paper discusses Annett's genetic model of handedness and brain lateralisation and their possible relationship to reading difficulties.)

Carroll JM *et al.* (2005) Literacy difficulties and psychiatric disorders: Evidence for comorbidity. *Journal of Child Psychology and Psychiatry* **46**, 524–532.

Duff FJ, Clarke PJ. (2011) Reading disorders: What are the effective interventions and how should they be implemented and evaluated? *Journal of Child Psychology and Psychiatry* **52**, 3–12.

Schumacher J *et al*. (2007) Genetics of dyslexia: The evolving landscape, *Journal of Medical Genetics* **44**, 289–297.

Sylva K *et al*. (2008) Teaching parents to help their children read: A randomized controlled trial. *British Journal of Educational Psychology* **78**, 435–455 (This trial showed that parents can be taught specific techniques to increase children's reading age.)

CHAPTER 32
Insecure Attachment

This chapter discusses the development of attachment *patterns*, which is a process that should occur in all young mammals. There are a variety of common attachment patterns, some of which are referred to as insecure rather than secure. As described later in this chapter, at least some forms of insecure attachment are risk factors for psychopathology. Whereas insecure attachment is common and is not necessarily associated with psychopathology, full-blown attachment *disorders* are rare and necessarily involve psychopathology. Attachment disorders are considered separately in Chapter 17.

The nature of attachment

For over 25 years, clinical and scientific thinking about attachment has been strongly influenced by the theories and writings of John Bowlby (1907–1990), a British psychiatrist and psychoanalyst who moved well beyond the traditional limits of those disciplines, drawing heavily on ethology and cybernetics. Though many disciplines study behaviour, ethologists study animal behaviour (including human behaviour) from a perspective that emphasises ecological and evolutionary considerations. Ethologists consider the function and not just the form of a particular sort of behaviour, asking why that behaviour is adaptive in the ecological niche that the species has evolved to fill. In this context, attachment can best be understood as regulating the balance between security, on the one hand, and exploration and play, on the other. At one extreme, a young primate who always clung to a parent would be relatively secure from predators but would not learn vital independence skills. At the other extreme, an over-independent youngster might acquire many useful skills but meet a premature death. Key adults act as a 'secure base' – the child sets forth from this base to explore, and retreats back to this base when threatened and in need of protection.

According to Bowlby, a child's need to be attached to protective figures is as basic and as important as the child's need for food. This

Child and Adolescent Psychiatry, Third Edition. Robert Goodman and Stephen Scott.
© 2012 Robert Goodman and Stephen Scott. Published 2012 by John Wiley & Sons, Ltd.

contradicted earlier psychoanalytic theories that children became attached because they associated parents with food, the 'cupboard-love' theory of object relations. Bowlby's view was supported by Harlow's famous (and heart-breaking) experiments with infant monkeys. When separated from their mothers, the infant monkeys spent most of their time clinging to a cloth-covered model rather than the wire model that they got their milk from. The cupboard-love theory predicted the opposite, namely that infants would associate comfort with the wire model that provided them with food.

Bowlby's ideas on attachment were greatly influenced by cybernetics, which considers the ways in which a system can use information in order to attain its goals. Potential strategies can be illustrated by some of the different ways a heating system can be designed to maintain a relatively constant indoor temperature, which is the controlled variable. A thermostat inside the house provides feedback information on the controlled variable, boosting the heating when the indoor temperature is too low. The feedback completes a loop: the heating system influences the indoor temperature and, by means of the feedback, the indoor temperature influences the heating system. An alternative control strategy is to use information from predictor variables, sometimes referred to as feedforward. One instance is a heating system that is turned on in the autumn and off in the spring – a crude method favoured by many UK hospitals. A more sophisticated system could use an outdoor thermostat that turned the heating up when it was cold outside. The information from predictor variables is not part of a loop: although the season and the outdoor temperature influence the heating system, the reverse does not apply. In summary, feedback is from controlled variables whereas feedforward is from predictor variables.

In order to maintain an optimal security–exploration balance, attachment behaviour is regulated in part by feedforward from predictor variables. Thus, it makes good evolutionary sense for children to move closer to a protective adult when they are ill, or when strangers are around, or when it is dark. This feedforward control is supplemented by feedback from controlled variables. For example, if you watch young children exploring in the park, you will see that they usually behave as though they are attached to their caregiver by a long piece of elastic, venturing away on their own, but then moving back towards the caregiver again. The behavioural system that keeps the child from straying too far can be thought of as a feedback system in which the controlled variable is the distance between caregiver and child. Thus, too great a distance between child and caregiver activates the child's attachment behaviour and brings the child back to the optimum distance again, in much the same way that too low an indoor temperature activates a feedback-controlled heating system and brings the temperature up again.

A wide variety of attachment behaviours can serve the purpose of keeping the child close enough to a caregiver (just as a wide variety of heaters can serve the purpose of keeping a house warm enough). The child's ability to crawl or walk towards an adult is the most obvious sort of attachment behaviour, but calling out, smiling sweetly, or crying are also effective methods for bringing a caregiver closer. A child's anger at being separated from a caregiver can also serve a similar role: angry outbursts may motivate caregivers to maintain even closer contact in future to avoid further outbursts. Anger is rather a risky strategy, however, since it may make a reluctant caregiver even less likely to stay close to the child in future. A better strategy, when the caregiver is reluctant, is for the child to keep demands to the minimum since a reluctant caregiver is better than no caregiver at all.

Children generally develop clear attachments to a relatively small number of people, often described as attachment figures, in the second half of their first year of life. Many children have a hierarchy of attachment figures, for example, a child who is attached to both parents may usually turn to the mother rather than the father for comfort and security if both are present. While separation from familiar caregivers is relatively well tolerated in early infancy if the substitute care is good, separation from attachment figures at later ages is more stressful, particularly for children aged between about 6 months and 4 years. The impact of separation from, or loss of, an attachment figure is discussed in Chapter 33.

Attachment theory has been such a dominant theme in developmental psychology that other components of parent–child relationships have sometimes been underplayed, for example, play, teaching and limit-setting. The relative prominence of these different aspects of parent–child relationships varies between and within cultures.

Bringing together elements from cognitive psychology and psycho-analytic object relations theory, Bowlby proposed that young children internalise their experiences with attachment figures to generate internal working models of themselves, of other people, and of the relationship between themselves and others. Children who have experienced sensitive and responsive caregiving typically come to see others as caring and reliable, and themselves as loveable and worthy of care. Conversely, children who are rejected or ignored typically come to see others as uncaring and unreliable, and themselves as unlovable and unworthy. In later childhood and adulthood, the individual's behaviour to others will often create new relationships in line with prior expectations. For example, if you assume that other people are uncaring and then treat them accordingly, this will make it less likely that they will care for you – your expectations have been self-fulfilling. This is one factor that reinforces your expectations. Another factor is our tendency to selectively attend to and remember precisely those aspects of our experience that reinforce our internal working model, ignoring or forgetting contradictory experiences. The notion that *internal working models* of attachment figures play a key role in linking early attachment experiences to later social and psychological sequelae is appealing but confirmatory research is only beginning.

Secure and insecure attachment

Although nearly all children develop attachments, the quality of these attachments varies greatly. Much research on this subject has used the Strange Situation Procedure (SSP) devised by Mary Ainsworth to investigate the attachment of 12–18-month-old children. In this procedure, an infant is observed via a one-way screen or television camera while spending about 20 minutes in an unfamiliar room. One of the child's attachment figures and an unfamiliar adult enter and leave the room in a predetermined sequence (see Box 32.1). This highly artificial procedure is not supposed to be representative of the child's ordinary experiences. Just as cardiologists and endocrinologists use 'stress tests' to unmask pathology that may not show up in ordinary circumstances, so the SSP is a stress test designed to show how the child copes with the triple challenge of a strange setting, the presence of a stranger, and separation from the attachment figure. When the SSP was first introduced, a lot of emphasis was placed on how distressed the child became during the separations (phases 3 and 5 in Box 32.1). It has subsequently become clear, however, that the degree of distress about separation is primarily related to the child's temperament and not to the security of the child's attachment. Consequently, more attention is now paid to the child's response to the reunions (phases 4 and 7 in Box 32.1).

Box 32.1 The strange situation procedure

Seven phases are illustrated by the time lines below. Each phase usually lasts three minutes, though the separation phases are cut short if the child is really distressed. The sequence generates two separations and two reunions in about 20 minutes.

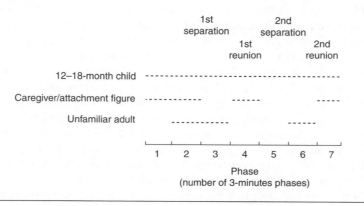

The original ABC classification used information from the SSP to classify children as securely or insecurely attached to that particular caregiver: type B is secure attachment, while insecure attachments are divided into type A (avoidant) and type C (resistant–ambivalent). (Mnemonic: Ay for

Ay-voidant.) More recently, an additional variety of insecure attachment has been recognised (type D = disorganised–disorientated); the children who are now included in this new category were previously scattered among the A, B and C categories. The characteristic child behaviours seen with each type of attachment are shown in Table 32.1. Table 32.1 also shows the approximate frequency of each type in normative American samples, as well as the most commonly associated care-giving styles, and the likely classification of the caregiver's own attachment type, as revealed by the Adult Attachment Interview (see below).

A secure attachment is obviously better than an insecure attachment – or is it? It is true, as discussed later, that a secure attachment is associated with modest increases in subsequent happiness and social success, at least in middle-class America. From an evolutionary point of view, though, it is important to remember that insecure attachments may well be adaptive responses to unfavourable circumstances, in much the same way that restricted growth (stunting) is an adaptive response to chronic malnutrition. If a caregiver is rejecting, an avoidant (type A) attachment may be the child's most adaptive strategy for getting some care without risking total abandonment. 'Half a loaf is better than no bread.' Conversely, if a caregiver is preoccupied and tends to ignore the child, exaggerated (type C) attachment behaviour may be the child's most adaptive strategy for getting his or her needs met. 'The squeaky hinge gets the oil.' Whether a disorganised (type D) attachment is ever adaptive is not yet clear.

The relative frequency of the ABCD attachment types as assessed by the SSP varies between and within cultures. To some extent, this may be an artefact of the assessment procedure. Thus, although a higher rate of resistant attachment has been described in Japan, this may be because young Japanese children are so rarely separated from their mothers that the SSP is far more stressful for them than for their American or European counterparts – and therefore far more likely to elicit marked and prolonged clinging. Such artefacts seem less likely to account for two other cross-cultural differences. In north Germany there is a higher rate of avoidant attachment, perhaps reflecting a cultural push towards early independence; and in Israel there is a higher rate of resistant attachment on kibbutzim, where young children sleep in a children's house, a setting where crying or distress may need to be intense and prolonged before a caregiver responds. Many American studies of infants who spend much of their week in non-maternal care also report an elevated rate of insecure attachment, perhaps reflecting the poor quality of some of this non-maternal care.

The rate of insecure attachment is increased by adverse family factors such as maternal depression, maternal alcoholism, or child abuse. This is most obvious for disorganised attachment, which is the sort of insecure attachment that best predicts future problems (see below). Thus, the rate of disorganised attachment varies from around 15% in two-parent middle-class samples to over 80% in maltreating families.

The ABCD classification generated by the SSP is specific to the child–caregiver pair that is assessed. A child who is shown to be securely

Table 32.1 The ABCD classification of attachment

Type	Characteristic child behaviour (SSP)*	Approximate % in non-clinical sample	Likely caregiving style	Caregiver's probable attachment type (AAI)**
A = Avoidant	Explores with little reference to caregiver. Minimally distressed by separation. Avoids or ignores caregiver on reunion.	15%	Actively rejecting of attachment behaviour or insensitively intrusive. Lack of tenderness. Suppressed parental anger.	Dismissing
B = Secure	Uses caregiver as a secure base to explore from. May be distressed by separation. On reunion greets caregiver positively, may seek comfort, then gets on with play/exploration again.	60%	Sensitive to child's signals. Responsive to child's needs. Prompt response to distress, buffering negative affect.	Autonomous
C = Resistant-ambivalent	Minimal exploration. Highly distressed by separation. Hard to settle on reunion, with ambivalent mixture of clinging and anger.	10%	Minimal or inconsistent responsiveness.	Preoccupied
D = Disorganised-disorientated	Lack of coherent pattern in exploratory or reunion behaviours. Fear or confusion in the caregiver's presence is suggested by disorganised and disorientated behaviours, for example, rocking, covering face, freezing, unexpected alternation of approach and avoidance.	15%	Parental behaviour is frightening or unpredictable. Not responding to infant's cues. Overrides infant's communications and goals. Sends infant double messages, for example, holds out arms and backs away.	Unresolved

Notes:
* SSP = Strange Situation Procedure.
** AAI = Adult Attachment Interview.

attached to one parent might, if reassessed with other caregivers, turn out to be insecurely attached to the other parent, to a nanny, or to a day care worker. Thus, while some young children are similarly attached to all their caregivers, others have a mixture of secure and insecure attachments. For this latter group with mixed attachment types, the current evidence suggests that subsequent development is particularly affected by the quality of attachment to the most important caregiver. Which caregiver is most important? The amount of contact seems relevant since several studies have shown that when infants spend most of their waking time in day care, their development is better predicted by the quality of their attachment to day care staff than by the quality of their attachment to parents. One important implication is that 'quality time' with parents may not entirely offset the ill effects on infants of prolonged low-quality day care. Behaviour genetic studies in twins suggest attachment patterns are predominantly environmentally determined, with no heritable component, suggesting that they are indeed formed by parenting behaviour.

Attachment throughout life

While the SSP tests the attachment security of children aged 12–18 months, newer assessments are emerging for older children. These newer assessments also generate ABCD categories on the basis of the child's response to reunion with a caregiver.

Thus, for example for children aged 4-8, doll-play tasks can be used. The child is asked to name dolls to match who is at home (for example, me, my mother and my brother) then a number of lively scenarios are commenced by an interviewer that are designed to trigger attachment behaviour (for example, an accident leading to a cut knee). At this juncture the child is asked to enact what happens next. If the 'me' person as enacted by the child gets well looked after by the mother, a secure designation is likely, whereas if the parent is indifferent or the child seeks no solace, one of the insecure categories is more likely to be assigned. Insecure patterns elicited by such 'story-stems' are predictive of psychopathology. In adolescence, a modification of the Adult Attachment Interview (see below) called the Child Attachment Interview has been devised for 8–15-year-olds, and again predicts psychopathology. Moreover, insecurity predicts symptoms over and above what is associated with poor parenting, suggesting that there is indeed value to the notion that an internal working model organises the child responses.

A child's attachment classification is moderately stable in childhood, age 5 year stability being of the order of 0.4 or 0.5. One explanation for this modest stability is that a child's internal working model of relationships is largely determined early in childhood and is then resistant to change. It should be borne in mind that assessment methods change as noted above, so some of the discontinuity may be due to different measurement methods. An alternative explanation, for which this increasing evidence, is that family circumstances are generally stable, for example, a mother who is sensitive and responsive to her infant is still likely to be sensitive and responsive to the same child several years later, thereby promoting secure attachment at each age. One way these alternative explanations can be distinguished is by studying what happens when family circumstances change markedly for the better or for the worse. For example, what happens if the caregivers of insecurely attached infants are taught to be more sensitive and responsive? Does this have no effect because early experience has already irreversibly moulded the children? Or do the children become securely attached because what counts is current rather than previous caregiving?

What limited evidence there is favours an intermediate answer. On the one hand, early attachment experiences typically do have lasting effects that cannot simply be attributed to the continuity of the environment. On the other hand, these effects are not totally irreversible and can be attenuated or even reversed by radically altered life circumstances. Thus for example in one study, over 90% of abused children taken into foster care had insecure attachment patters to their birth parents, but over half had developed secure patterns to their foster parents after being with them for at least 6 months, a rate similar to controls. This suggests that attachment patterns can indeed be altered by changes in parenting circumstances. Moreover there are now a number of well-validated interventions to increase attachment security in infancy. They all have a common element in increasing parental sensitivity to the child's signals so the child is better cared for in all interactions, but especially when distressed. To date, the most effective interventions use video feedback to show the parent the infant's signals and how best to respond.

There has recently been an explosion of interest in attachment in adult life. Close adult relationships commonly have an attachment component, providing security, comfort and a source of confidence. In adulthood, unlike childhood, the relationship is often a reciprocal bond between equals, with each adult being an attachment figure to the other, and commonly a sexual partner too. Research on attachment quality in adult life has drawn heavily on the Adult Attachment Interview (AAI), developed by Mary Main. This interview asks adults for descriptions and evaluations of their childhood attachment relationships, and also enquires about any separations or losses, and the effect these had on the respondent's development and personality. The respondent is asked to provide specific biographical episodes to substantiate global evaluations. The aim is not to reconstruct exactly what happened many years ago but to establish, through discourse analysis, the respondent's current state of mind with respect to attachment. Four categories have been identified, each of which has an association with one of the child ABCD categories (see Table 32.1).

1 *Dismissing*. The respondent can recall few affectively charged memories from childhood. Closeness and attachment are not valued. An idealised picture of parents is at odds with the specific details recalled. These

respondents resemble children with type A attachments – attachment behaviours and feelings are denied, restricted or repressed.

2 *Autonomous*. The respondent values attachment relationships and either gives a convincing history of emotionally supportive relationships in childhood or has come to terms with a childhood lacking them (called by some 'earned security'). Typically self-reliant, objective, and non-defensive, these respondents resemble children with type B attachments – attachment feelings and behaviours are expressed in open and balanced ways, with appropriate dependency and confidence in the attachment figure.

3 *Preoccupied*. The account of childhood relationships is confused, incoherent and unobjective. They are still caught up in childhood events and unable to move beyond them. Anger at parents is unresolved. These respondents resemble children with type C attachments – attachment feelings and behaviours are exaggerated and ambivalent.

4 *Unresolved-disorganised*. Discussions of potentially traumatic events are marked by striking lapses in the monitoring of reasoning or discourse, suggesting dissociated memory systems or abnormal absorption in unresolved traumatic memories. These respondents resemble children with type D attachments – disorganised.

Given the complexity and seeming subjectivity of this rating scheme, it is truly remarkable how well parent and infant attachment status correspond. When the parent's attachment type is classified using the AAI (whether before or after the child's birth), and when the infant's attachment to a parent is classified as A, B, C or D using the SSP, then roughly two-thirds of infants match their parents in attachment type. This concordance is all the more striking given the difference in assessment methods between analyses of transcripts of what adults say and analyses of videotapes of how infants behave.

Consequences of secure and insecure attachments

Many studies have compared the social and psychological development of securely and insecurely attached children. The picture that has consistently emerged is that securely attached children do better on average. However, not all securely attached children do well, and not all insecurely attached children do badly. It is still unclear whether this group difference arises because insecure attachment is itself the key risk factor; the alternative is that insecure attachment is simply a marker for wider-ranging family abnormalities that have the adverse long-term effects. Recent research suggests that children can do well despite being insecurely attached, so long as other things are favourable (good parenting overall, stable education, no unpleasant traumas, etc). Vice versa, children with secure attachment patterns who are brought up in poverty and fail to make good friendships, etc. typically do much less well. Thus, a lesson is that while attachment patterns are important, they are not wholly deterministic and clinicians should not forget to assess all the other factors that influence the life course. Over the longer term, if individuals are followed into their mid-twenties, attachment patterns are only modestly stable: infant classification typically correlates 0.2 with adult classification. This is partly explained by different life courses and experiences of the type indicated above.

Bearing these caveats in mind, a secure attachment nonetheless does increase the likelihood of the child subsequently forming harmonious relationships with adults and children. This is most evident for close relationships with family members and friends. Securely attached children are more cooperative and responsive with their mothers, more likely to comfort younger siblings, and more likely to have good friends. They are less likely to be non-compliant with parents, quarrelsome with siblings, or controlling with friends. The benefits of secure attachments are also evident with familiar but less intimate social partners. On average, securely attached children are less emotionally dependent on teachers and are better able to ask for a teacher's help when they face a challenge they cannot manage alone. Typically, they are also more popular with classmates and less often victimised, perhaps because they show more empathy for peers and engage in less conflict when playing. Attachment security has least influence on the quality of social interactions with unfamiliar adults or children. Such interactions are primarily influenced by the child's sociability, which is a moderately heritable temperamental trait. Conversely, genetic factors seem less important in determining the quality of close relationships.

Early studies, using the ABC classification of attachment, particularly emphasised the link between type A (avoidant) attachment and externalising problems such as aggression. It now seems likely that the more recently recognised type D (disorganised) attachment is the strongest predictor of externalising problems. For example, one study showed that disorganised attachment at 18 months predicted a six-fold increase in serious aggression towards peers in nursery school. Though the disorganised attachment often included avoidant elements, it was noteworthy that those children who had purely avoidant (and not disorganised) attachments were not subsequently more likely to be unusually aggressive towards peers. Perhaps severe family adversity launches children onto a developmental pathway characterised by disorganised attachment and dysphoria in infancy, oppositional defiant disorder in middle childhood, and more severe conduct disorder and juvenile delinquency in adolescence.

An increasing number of studies have used the AAI to investigate the attachment classification of adults with mental illnesses or personality disorders. In clinical samples, the likelihood of an autonomous (that is, secure) attachment is only about 10%, as compared with roughly 60% in low-risk samples. The remaining 90% of clinic patients are split fairly evenly between the three insecure attachment categories: dismissing, preoccupied and unresolved. So far, there are only hints of links between particular psychiatric diagnoses and specific types of insecurity, for example, between borderline personality disorder and preoccupied or unresolved attachment. Future research needs to integrate the insights gained from attachment theory with other findings from developmental psychopathology more broadly.

Subject review

DeKleyn M, Greenberg M. (2008) Attachment and psychopathology in childhood. *In*: Cassidy J, Shaver PR (eds) *Handbook of Attachment: Theory, Research, and Clinical Applications*, 2nd edn. Guilford, New York, pp. 637–665.

Further reading

Bakermans-Kraneburg MJ *et al*. (2003) Less is more: meta-analyses of sensitivity and attachment interventions in early childhood. *Psychological Bulletin* **129**, 195–215. (A classic review showing early interventions do not need to be prolonged in order to enhance parental interventions and promote secure attachments.)

Berlin *et al*. (2007) *Enhancing Early Attachments: Theory, Research, Intervention, and Policy*. Guilford, New York. (Has chapters on all the main interventions designed to improve attachment.)

Cassidy J, Shaver PR. (2008) *Handbook of Attachment: Theory, Research, and Clinical Applications*, 2nd edn. Guilford, New York. (Great overall review book covering scientific underpinnings and clinical applications.)

Futh A *et al*. (2008). Attachment narratives and behavioural and emotional symptoms in an ethnically diverse, at-risk sample. *Journal of the American Academy of Child & Adolescent Psychiatry* **47**, 709–718. (Shows that attachment insecurity as elicited by doll-play tasks predicts more psychopathology in 4–6- year-olds.)

Grossman K, Grossman K, Waters E. (2005) *Attachment from Infancy to Adulthood*. Guilford, New York (Has readable chapters on all the major longitudinal studies, which now go from infancy to adulthood.)

Scott S *et al*. (2011) Attachment in adolescence: Overlap with parenting and unique prediction of behavioural adjustment. *Journal of Child Psychology and Psychiatry* **52**, 1052–1062. (Shows that good parenting in adolescence is associated with attachment security, which, however, still has power to independently predict psychopathology.)

CHAPTER 33
Nature and Nurture

Until recently, many studies of children and adolescents' difficulties assumed that poor outcomes were due to the unsatisfactory conditions in which they were raised. In fact, the picture may be much more complex. Consider, for example, possible interpretations of the finding that children who are poor readers are more likely to come from homes where they do not spend much time reading to their parents. This finding would lead many to conclude that the children's lack of interest and ability in reading stemmed from a lack of parental attention and encouragement (one can almost hear the cries of 'that's only common sense'). However, there are many other plausible interpretations. One possibility is that although the parents love books and are good readers themselves, the child may have some constitutional reading difficulty ('dyslexia') which means that he finds being encouraged to read very unpleasant, as he cannot do it nearly as well as his younger sister. His parents will soon learn to back off to avoid the whining, resentment and misery they cause! Another possibility is that the parents and child all have genetically determined reading difficulties so that they all avoid anything to do with reading. A third possibility is that both parents and children could easily read if they had the opportunity, but they live in an environment where there are no books and the video is king. And of course more than one of these three explanations may be operating at the same time.

Sorting out what is cause and what is effect is no mere academic matter. If we are trying to improve people's lives, it is essential we get it right. At an individual level, there is no point, for example, in trying to teach a 'refrigerator mother' holding techniques to 'get through' to her autistic son if in fact he has a genetically determined inability to communicate which has consequently led his entirely normal mother to give up trying. At a policy level, there is little point in rebuilding a sordid estate in order to eradicate the high rate of child abuse and schizophrenia found there, if in fact the reason people with these difficulties have ended up living there is because of their multiple social handicaps, which they will take into any new situation, and which should be addressed in their own right. (It might be a good idea to rebuild the estate for lots of other reasons though.)

Child and Adolescent Psychiatry, Third Edition. Robert Goodman and Stephen Scott.
© 2012 Robert Goodman and Stephen Scott. Published 2012 by John Wiley & Sons, Ltd.

Before reviewing a number of commonly encountered family adversities (see Chapter 34), it is important to consider some general principles that help tease out causal relationships and disentangle nature from nurture.

Association is not the same as causation

Many family factors are associated with an increase in the rate of one or more child and adolescent psychiatric disorders. It is all too easy to fall into the trap of assuming that association implies causation. If a family characteristic (X) is associated with a child and adolescent psychiatric disorder (Y), it could be the case that X causes Y, but two alternative explanations also need to be considered: that Y is causing X, which is known as reverse causality; and that both X and Y are due to the operation of a third factor or confounder.

Reverse causality

It is plausible that a psychiatrically disturbed child or adolescent can influence family characteristics. For example, parental depression, anger, criticism, coldness, over-protection, punitiveness or disengagement could all be evoked by their child's symptoms. Some of the most powerful evidence for such effects comes from intervention studies. For example, one study showed that when stimulant medication reduced a child's ADHD, this usually led to less maternal criticism of the child, more maternal warmth towards the child, and an increase in the time that the mother spent with the child (see Chapter 5). Of course, it could still be the case that the parental negativity evoked by a child's ADHD is also damaging to that child's development. The evidence suggests that there is often a two-way effect: the children's characteristics do indeed influence parental behaviour, and the parental behaviour in turn has an independent effect on the children.

Third factors

If a mother and daughter are both particularly fearful of spiders, it seems natural to assume that the daughter has learned the anxiety from her mother. An equally plausible alternative is that the mother's fear and the daughter's fear have a common origin: perhaps mother and daughter share a genetic tendency to be fearful, or perhaps they have both watched the same horror film about spiders. Conceptually, adoption studies provide the most straightforward evidence for genetic third factors. If arachnophobia were completely genetic, then adopted children would resemble their biological parents but not their adoptive parents in this respect. Other approaches are needed to identify environmental third factors. For example, if having seen the same film accounts for parents and children both fearing spiders, then an epidemiological approach should be able to show that the association between parents' fears and children's fears disappears once allowance has been made for the effect of film viewing.

Children and adolescents inhabit three rather different social worlds: the family, the classroom and the peer group. Though distinct, the three worlds are related. Thus, children and adolescents who come from disadvantaged and disharmonious families are also more likely to be attending poor schools and spending time with disruptive peers. This can make it very hard to tell if an association is causal. For example, if individuals from disadvantaged families are more often truants, is this because a disadvantaged family environment directly fosters truancy, or is the family disadvantage simply a marker for poor neighbourhood schools that foster truancy? To complicate matters further, adverse factors cluster together within each of the individual's social worlds. At home, for example, overcrowding (one particular family-based risk factor) is linked to unemployment, poverty, parental mental illness and a host of other family-based risk factors. If overcrowding is associated with delinquency, is this a direct effect of overcrowding, or is overcrowding simply acting as a marker for other family-based risk factors? There are research designs and statistical techniques for trying to answer this sort of question.

Genes, shared environment and non-shared environment

Until the 1970s, it was widely believed that genes gave people their physical constitution, but that it was the way they were brought up that was responsible for their psychological characteristics. It subsequently became clear that both genes and environment were relevant to personality dimensions such as extroversion–introversion, to behavioural traits such as aggression, and to psychiatric symptoms such as depression. Much of this improved understanding of the role of genes and environment arose from conceptual and methodological advances in the analysis of twin and adoption studies. What follows is a brief introduction to *behavioural genetics*. The *variance* of a trait is a measure of how much that trait varies between people in the population being studied. *Heritability* refers to the proportion of the variance explained by genetic factors. Thus, a heritability of 25% for a particular trait means that genetic differences between people account for a quarter of that population's variability in the measured variable (under the conditions prevailing at the time of the measurement). The rest of the variance is conventionally divided between two environmental components:

1 *Shared or common environment* refers to environmental factors that make people living in the same family resemble one another (making allowances for resemblance due to genetic similarity). For example, poverty, damp housing or air pollution might lead anyone living in the family (mother father, son, lodger) to become more irritable. Or irrespective of your genetic heritage, if you are brought up in a French-speaking household, you speak French!

2 *Non-shared* or *unique environment* refers to environmental factors that are not shared by people living together, for example when only one

twin is knocked down by a bus (resulting in brain damage or PTSD) or only one twin has a best friend who is a drug addict. However, as discussed later in this chapter, the term 'non-shared environment' may be somewhat misleading since it may also incorporate measurement error and random factors in brain development.

The relative importance of genes, shared environment and non-shared environment is usually estimated from twin or adoption studies, though increasing use is now being made of comparisons of full-siblings, half-siblings and step-siblings growing up in reconstituted families. Box 33.1 summarises the twin and adoption findings for three traits: a trait that is entirely genetically determined, a trait that is entirely determined by shared environment, and a trait entirely determined by non-shared environment. In practice, most traits are mixtures of these.

Box 33.1 Twin and adoption findings

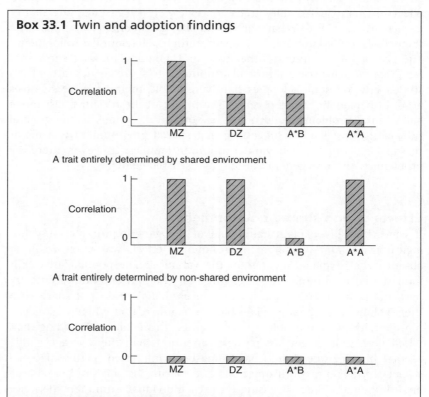

A trait entirely determined by shared environment

A trait entirely determined by non-shared environment

Notes: **MZ** = comparing **M**ono**Z**ygotic ('identical') twins
DZ = comparing **D**i**Z**ygotic ('non-identical' or 'fraternal') twins
A∗B = comparing early **A**dopted children with **B**iological parents or siblings
A∗A = comparing early **A**dopted children with **A**doptive parents or siblings

A *correlation* is a measure of similarity: a value of 1.0 means the two individuals are identical on the trait being measured, while a value of 0 means that the two individuals are no more alike than randomly chosen members of the population.

Genetic influence

Most psychological traits have been found to have a heritability of around 40–60%, that is, genetic differences between individuals account for roughly half of the observed variance in a given population. Disruptive behavioural problems are one likely exception to this rule, with most (but not all) studies showing a smaller genetic contribution to this sort of behaviour. At the opposite extreme, liability to autism may have a heritability of over 90%.

Effects of shared environment

In the 1980s, some behavioural geneticists made the dramatic claim, based mainly on twin studies, that shared family environment has little effect on many personality traits. A review in 1987 stated the matter particularly forcibly: 'What parents do that is experienced similarly by their children does not have an impact on their behavioural development.' The gist of the argument is that twin and adoption findings show that family resemblances are almost all attributable to shared genes rather than shared environment; adoptees hardly resemble their adoptive relatives at all in personality traits. Even at the height of these claims, disruptive behavioural problems stood out as important exceptions to the general rule, with most studies suggesting that shared environment is a major reason for disruptive behaviour running in families. However, there are problems with these generalisations, as discussed below.

Effects of non-shared environment

If genes typically explain about half of the variance for most psychological traits, and if shared environmental effects are often weak or absent, what explains the rest of the variance? The popular answer is 'non-shared environment', suggesting that children and adolescents are particularly influenced by the experiences that they do not share with their siblings. It is certainly plausible, for example, that when parents pay more attention to one sibling than another, this is more wounding than when both siblings get less parental attention than the 'average child'. Mental health professionals have long been interested in the effects of scapegoating and favouritism, which are specific instances of non-shared environmental effects. Focusing on each individual's unique experience of the family environment can be very helpful clinically. At the same time, it is unclear how powerful these non-shared environmental effects really are. It is wrong to suppose that if genes and shared environment only account for half of the variance on any given psychological trait, then the impact of non-shared experiences *must* account for the other half. As described below, non-genetic variance can have other explanations.

Precautions required when interpreting behavioural genetic studies

A number of problems can arise when behavioural genetic studies are interpreted without recognising the limitations of the methods used:

1 For many years, behavioural genetics studies were carried out by researchers who were more interested in genes than environments. Using twin and adoption studies, they were happy to estimate environmental effects indirectly without actually measuring the environment. In effect, the environment was assumed to be responsible for any variance that could not be explained by genetic effects. This assumption is a simplification since there are other potentially important sources of unexplained variance including measurement error, which is often greatly underestimated, and the role of chance in brain development. Fortunately, the best behavioural genetics studies nowadays include sophisticated environmental measures in genetically sensitive designs (for example, twin studies), generating direct measures of relevant shared and non-shared environments.

2 The average variation in environment across a given population may not be great, leading to an underestimate of its potential effects. For example, height in Western Europe is estimated to have had a heritability of over 90% in the seventeenth century, and has a similar heritability today. It would, however, be wrong to conclude that environmental factors such as nutrition have only a slight role to play in the determination of height – on the contrary, mean adult height has increased by about 15 cm over that time, and this cannot plausibly be attributed to a change in the gene pool. At first sight, it is puzzling to find that height can be so sensitive to nutrition despite a heritability of over 90%. The explanation lies in the restricted environmental variation at each time point. In the past, most Western Europeans resembled one another in being poorly nourished; nowadays they resemble one another in being well (or excessively) nourished. With relatively little variation in nutrition, most of the variance in height is genetic at any one moment. Nevertheless, the major change in average nutrition over three centuries had a major effect. What applies to nutrition applies to parenting too – for most of the population, there are not great differences in child-rearing style at any one time. This will make the effect of 'shared environment' seem small, but it does not mean that parenting cannot make a big difference, especially when it is outside the normal range. Sometimes the effects of extreme environments are evident from 'experiments of nature', where severe man-made or natural disasters affect lots of children or adolescents, almost at random. For example, severely deprived orphans, such as those studied from Romania in the late 1980s, all had very delayed development. For children in these circumstances, the shared environment does indeed matter. Randomised controlled trials that alter the environment can also be very informative since there should not be

pre-existing differences between the participants who were and were not exposed to the changed environment. While it is obviously not ethical to expose children at random to adverse environments, it may be ethical to randomise children to environmental improvements (for example, if there are insufficient funds to offer this to everyone). Such trials have shown, for example, that improving parenting leads to a large reduction in antisocial behaviour, and that early cognitive stimulation in deprived preschoolers leads to better adjustment and achievement in adulthood.

3 Twin studies may underestimate environmental effects if genotypes predispose individuals to environmental risks. For example, imagine a gene that made individuals more likely to become addicted to cigarettes. This would result in identical twins being more similar than non-identical twins in their smoking habits. In fact, it would be a genetic pathway to lung cancer – and yet it is the environmental risk (smoking) that is the final cause of the cancer. Simply reporting that lung cancer was highly heritability could easily result in the misleading view that there was little or no point in trying to use environmental interventions (such as taxing or banning cigarettes) to deal with what seems to be a very heritable problem. Similar issues arise in child and adolescent psychiatry. For instance, the combination of ADHD and a disruptive behavioural disorder has a high heritability, but this does not mean that environmental interventions are unimportant. That is because what is heritable is primarily the ADHD, but the symptoms of ADHD often evoke a style of hostile parenting that leads to the child or adolescent developing disruptive behaviour too. It would therefore be wrong to conclude that because heritability (as measured) is high, and shared environment influences (as calculated) are low or non-existent, that there are no treatments that might work by altering the environment. In fact trials show that improving the parenting of children who have both ADHD and disruptive behaviour can be very effective.

4 The distinction between shared and non-shared environments can lead to misunderstandings – even among experts! As noted above, non-shared environment is used to explain differences between family members after genetic influences have been allowed for. Sometimes this may indeed be due to non-shared influences. However, the difference can also be due to the same, shared environmental influences affecting individuals within the family differently, either directly or because they perceive it differently. Thus, living with a hostile parent might, for example, make one child anxious, another aggressive, leave a third indifferent, and the fourth may be made stronger. In this case it is the reaction to the environment that differs, not the environmental influence per se. This, then, is an interaction between a shared environmental influence and the child's susceptibility, but conventional behaviour genetics would badge it as non-shared environment. To take another example, the results of twin studies of schizophrenia show that 'non-shared' environmental influences are considerable and 'shared' environmental influences are insignificant. Again, this does

not necessarily mean that there is nothing in the shared environment bringing out schizophrenia in those genetically predisposed to it. For example, migration or discrimination may make one family member schizophrenic, while another may get depressed, or cope.

5 It is now well documented that some environments are genetically influenced, and this can lead to an overestimation of environmental effects. For example, cross-sectional studies show that in households where there are more books and where parents read more to their offspring, the children have considerably higher reading ages. It might be concluded that buying extra books and reading them to children will lead to big improvements in the children's reading ability, but it turns out that a third factor, parental IQ, mediates a good deal of the effect. While parents of higher IQ tend to read more to their children, their children tend to have higher IQ and are better readers anyway. This is not to say that increasing reading with children will not improve their ability, but that the effects may be more modest that anticipated.

Genes and environment interact

The notion that either genes or environments can act alone is over-simplistic: the two are always interacting. Through evolution, our genetic make-up is designed to be sensitive to the likely environment. We need to consider the mechanisms through which environments affect a given genotype, and what the mechanisms are through which genes influence the reaction to a given environment.

In the 1960s, longitudinal studies established that children's development was influenced by an interaction between temperament and upbringing, with temperamentally placid babies being less affected by insensitive parenting than temperamentally irritable babies. Subsequent adoption studies have shown how genetic sources of variation in temperament influence parenting, and interact with it. Observational studies show that the disciplinary practices of adoptive parents are more harsh and critical when their children have criminal birth parents, probably because the children are harder to cope with because they have inherited a tendency to more disruptive behaviour.

An influential Scandinavian adoption study examined which adoptees were convicted for criminal behaviour as adolescents. Each adoptee was classified according to both biological and psychosocial risk:

1 An adoptee was said to be at high *congenital* risk if the *birth parents* had criminal or alcoholic histories. Otherwise, congenital risk was said to be low. Any risk transmitted from birth parents was probably genetic, though the prenatal environment could also be relevant, for example, if high alcohol consumption by the biological mother during pregnancy influenced fetal brain development.

2 An adoptee was predicted to have received *worse rearing* if the *adoptive parents* had criminal or alcoholic histories. Otherwise, the adoptee was

classified as receiving better rearing. Any risk transmitted from adoptive parents was probably mediated by psychosocial factors.

Box 33.2 illustrates how high and low congenital risk interacted with better and worse rearing:

- Among adoptees experiencing better rearing, high congenital risk was linked to four times the rate of convictions, 12% versus 3%, suggesting a considerable biological effect.
- Among adoptees at low congenital risk, worse rearing more than doubling the rate of convictions from 3% to 7%, suggesting a substantial effect for psychosocial environment.
- The really striking finding was that when adoptees at high risk also experienced worse rearing, the conviction rate soared from 12% to 40%. This shows a strong interaction whereby increased biological risk leads to a far poorer outcome when combined with a less favourable environment. Or to put it another way, the effect of an adverse environmental influence is greater when combined with genetic (or other biological) susceptibility.

Paradoxically, the strong interaction between biological and environmental risk justifies some therapeutic optimism. This is because the adoptees with the double disadvantage of high congenital risk and worse rearing environment have the most to gain from intervention – potentially dropping their conviction rate in this instance from 40% to 12% if their adoptive parents can be helped to improve their child rearing. Far from being 'heartsink cases' for whom nothing can be done, they may be particularly dramatic responders.

In general, genetic liability can translate into poorer outcomes through several mechanisms. First, it may directly lead to psychopathology

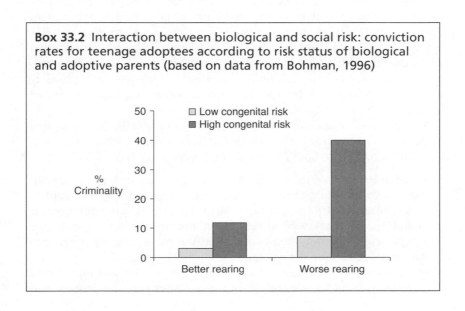

Box 33.2 Interaction between biological and social risk: conviction rates for teenage adoptees according to risk status of biological and adoptive parents (based on data from Bohman, 1996)

irrespective of usual variations in the environment, as appears to be the case for autism. Second, genetic liability may confer greater susceptibility to less favourable environments, for example, a child with a genetically irritable temperament may be more prone to have tantrums and develop behavioural symptoms in response to insensitive parenting. A recently documented example of this phenomenon is that children with one variant of the monoamine oxidase A gene are more prone to develop antisocial behaviour if their parents are relatively harsh, but not otherwise. Third, genetic liability may predispose an individual to seek out or end up in a context that has a higher exposure to known risk factors, for example, youths with conduct disorder are more likely to take drugs and alcohol.

Epigenetics and the environmental modulation of gene expression

Epigenetics refers to changes in gene expression that are *not* brought about by changes in the underlying DNA sequence. The crucial importance of epigenetic processes is evident from the combination of two facts. Firstly, nearly all of an individual's healthy cells have the same DNA (though there are exceptions such as the variation in B lymphocyte DNA brought about by the somatic hypermutation that increases antibody diversity). Secondly, our very existence as multi-cellular organisms made up of different types of cells depends on different profiles of gene activation in each cell type. Conjuring cellular diversity out of genetic identity involves epigenetic rather than genetic processes.

What epigenetic processes are involved? In some instances, changes in gene expression are brought about by adding methyl groups to the DNA itself, or by removing these again; these changes to do not alter the 'genetic code' that is stored in the sequence of base pairs along the DNA double helix. In other instances, epigenetic modification involves chemical changes to the histone proteins that are associated with DNA.

The epigenetic processes that bring about the differentiation of a single-celled zygote into many cell types have more to do with the embryo's internal logic than environmental influences. Nevertheless, fairly similar processes have been shown to be involved in the ways that the environment – including the social environment – can induce lasting changes in the brain, thereby affecting behaviour and physiology in a way that seems very relevant to child and adolescent psychiatry.

One particularly thoroughly researched example is the way early maternal care can have a lasting effect on rats' stress responses. Rat mothers vary in how much they lick and groom their pups, and 'high licked' pups grow up to respond less markedly to stress than do 'low licked' pups: when exposed to stress, low-licked pups show more fearfulness in their behaviour, and their hypothalamic–pituitary–adrenal response is more extreme. But, we hope you will ask, couldn't that be due to genetic effects or reverse causality? Good questions! In principle, it could be that there are one or more genes that promote pup-licking in the mother – with those same genes in the pups reducing stress response. The evidence against this comes from the lab equivalent of an adoption study. If newborn pups are brought up from birth by unrelated mothers, the pups have a modest stress response if fostered by high-licking mothers, just as the pups have an exaggerated stress response if fostered by low-licking mothers. But what about reverse causality? Maybe there is something about over-reactive pups that discourages mothers from licking or grooming them. The evidence against this is that a rat mother's tendency to lick and groom her pups seems more of a fixed trait than something that varies with each pup; for any given mother, the amount of licking and grooming is relatively constant from one litter to another, and from one pup to another. Thus the evidence does favour the straightforward interpretation that the level of pup licking alters the stress response. What is more, this seems to be a case of *early life programming* – the effect depends on what happens to the pup in its first week of life, and then generally lasts for its lifetime.

These findings are remarkable enough, but what is even more remarkable is that much is now known about the underlying epigenetic mechanisms. For example, when a pup receives a lot of licking and grooming in the first week of life, one key consequence is more serotonergic activity in the hippocampus. This triggers permanent changes to the pattern of methylation of a key promoter region in the gene for glucocorticoid receptors. The resultant increase of these receptors in the hippocampus amplifies the negative feedback effect of circulating cortisol, damping down excessive hypothalamic–pituitary–adrenal responses to stress.

In summary, the material summarised in this chapter shows that genes and environment constantly interact in complex ways. As more is discovered about these processes, it is to be hoped that more effective interventions can be devised.

Subject review

Thapar A, Rutter M. (2008) Genetics. *In*: Rutter M *et al.* (eds) *Rutter's Child and Adolescent Psychiatry*, 5th edn. Wiley-Blackwell, Chichester, pp. 337–358.

Further reading

Bagot RC, Meaney MJ. (2010) Epigenetics and the biological basis of gene x environment interactions. *Journal of the American Academy of Child and Adolescent Psychiatry* **49**, 752–771.
Bohman M. (1996) Predisposition to criminality: Swedish adoption studies in retrospect. In: Bock GR, Goode JA (eds) *Genetics of Criminal and Antisocial Behaviour*. Wiley, Chichester, pp. 99–114.

Dodge K, Rutter M. (eds) (2011) *Gene-Environment Iinteractions in Developmental Psychopathology*. Guilford Press, New York.

Fergusson, DM *et al*. (2011) MAOA, abuse exposure and antisocial behaviour: 30-year longitudinal study. *British Journal of Psychiatry* **198**, 457–463.

Plomin R, Daniels R. (1987) Why are children in the same family so different from one another? *Behavioral and Brain Sciences* **10**, 1–60.

Plomin R, Davis OSP. (2009) The future of genetics in psychology and psychiatry: Microarrays, genome-wide association, and non-coding RNA. *Journal of Child Psychology and Psychiatry* **50**, 63–71.

Stevens HE *et al*. (2009) Risk and resilience: early manipulation of macaque social experience and persistent behavioral and neurophysiological outcomes. *Journal of the American Academy of Child and Adolescent Psychiatry* **48**, 114–127.

CHAPTER 34

Coping with Adversity

Overcoming difficult circumstances is essential for survival. The success of the human species depends on our ability to respond to a whole range of problems intelligently and flexibly, to adapt adequately to a wide range of environments – or else to control the environment so it is within a 'comfort zone' and not damaging. Ideally, children and adolescent's upbringing ought to enable them to develop coping skills so they can deal with the challenges they will encounter in their society as adults. However, children and adolescents may not be in a position to overcome some fairly fundamental violations of their lives, which may then compromise the integrity of their development and undermine their ability to live a reasonably successful and satisfying life. This chapter starts by reviewing children and adolescents' reactions to a number of difficult and painful predicaments, and then goes on to discuss more generally how they may cope.

Common stressors

One way to categorise difficulties is into discrete major changes, sometimes called *life events*, and ongoing obviously difficult situations, sometimes called *chronic adversities*. Research on adults has shown that there is a third type of common stressor, sometimes called *daily hassles*. This term refers to everyday difficulties that can seem relatively insignificant in themselves, yet have proven to be important determinants of psychopathology. However, they are less well researched in children, so this account is mainly about life events and chronic adversities. As well as considering impact in terms of (1) psychiatric disorders, it is important to consider impact on (2) functioning, for example, in terms of ability to make good relationships and develop academic abilities and other competencies, and (3) subjective distress. All three will influence the general quality of life of the child, and their family too. Thus, if children are left without psychiatric symptoms, and are not upset, that is not to say all is well: they may have no friends and spend most of the day watching TV and not achieving

Child and Adolescent Psychiatry, Third Edition. Robert Goodman and Stephen Scott.
© 2012 Robert Goodman and Stephen Scott. Published 2012 by John Wiley & Sons, Ltd.

anything. Likewise, there may be no psychiatric symptoms, and children may be functioning fairly well in terms of school success and other achievements, but if they are frequently preoccupied by distressing recollections of how horribly they were abused, then this is not a good outcome.

Separation and loss

Attachment is a central theme in developmental psychology and psychiatry (see Chapter 32), and many studies have examined what happens to children when their attachment bonds are temporarily disrupted by separations, or permanently broken by losses. There is no doubt that children and adolescents often find separations and losses very upsetting, but it is less clear whether these unpleasant experiences on their own have serious long-term consequences for their functioning. Of course, it is highly desirable to prevent or reduce children and adolescents' short-term distress whether or not it has adverse long-term consequences. Nevertheless, the issue of long-term outcome is important.

Do traumatic separations or early losses predispose an individual to persisting psychiatric disturbance? In trying to answer this sort of question, it is crucial to allow for 'third factors' (see Chapter 33). For example, when studying the effects of divorce on children, it is important to ask how far any adverse effects are due to prior and continuing family discord rather than to separation from one of the parents. In this regard, it is striking that long-term psychiatric problems are more likely to follow the loss of a parent through divorce than through death. This suggests that the antecedents and consequences of loss are more important than the loss itself. Similarly, when children are taken into foster care, the poor quality of their previous care is more important as a predictor of future problems than the fact that they have been separated from their biological parents.

It is also important to remember that separations and losses may set in motion a series of adverse events that have lasting consequences of their own. For example, divorce may be followed by parental depression or less effective parental supervision, a change to a worse school, and less money for leisure activities that can promote self-confidence and friendships. These changes may have long-term effects on the child or adolescent's behaviour even if the divorce itself does not. Several lines of research confirm that the long-term impact of the death of a parent depends strongly on the quality of subsequent care.

Taking these various issues into account, most research findings suggest that although they are often extremely upsetting, separations and losses are not in themselves major risk factors for persistent psychiatric disturbance – but their antecedents or consequences often are. This is not to say that they may not be experienced as very painful and be a defining point in the individual's life, and perhaps strongly influence, for example, how the individual, in turn, decides to bring up his or her own children. Rather, the evidence suggests that in themselves, separations and losses do not lead to large and lasting increases in psychiatric disorders or worsening in psychosocial functioning.

Hospital admission

Since pain and illness activate a child's drive to stay close to an attachment figure, being admitted alone to hospital is a particularly stressful sort of separation experience. Over the course of several days or weeks, children admitted to hospital, who do not see their parents, go through sequential phases of protest, despair and detachment. These reactions to separation are observed most clearly when children are aged between 6 months and 4 years of age, and have been captured poignantly on the films made by James and Joyce Robertson. Though a single separation due to a hospital admission is not associated with an increased risk of subsequent psychiatric disorder, multiple admissions are associated with higher rates of later problems, mainly disruptive behaviour and delinquency. This increased risk is far more marked in discordant families, suggesting that many of the harmful long-term consequences of multiple hospital admissions may be mediated by an adverse impact on subsequent family relationships. Though separations are painful for the child, most families are able to buffer the child's distress during and after hospital admissions and thereby minimise the long-term consequences.

Studies carried out at a time when children's wards generally discouraged parental contact showed that the harmful effects of hospital admissions could be reduced by increased parental contact. Fortunately, as awareness of children's attachment needs has grown, hospital policies have shifted markedly so that parents are now usually encouraged to stay with their child for as long as they can, or even to 'room in' with them. For somewhat different reasons, the parents of premature babies on intensive care units are also encouraged to have frequent contact and interact with their children. Though the babies are too young to be specifically attached, increased contact promotes more sensitive and responsive parenting subsequently. Hopefully, by strengthening the parent's bond to the child, this will help counteract the raised risk of child abuse after premature birth.

Bereavement

The death of a parent is typically followed by a period of considerable distress that gradually diminishes over months. Distress may show itself through emotional symptoms, disruptive behaviour, or a mixture of the two. The severe depressive withdrawal seen in some adults is less marked in children. A year later, overt distress is generally much less evident, although other manifestations, such as lack of interest in school, may persist. There is certainly not a strong link with depression in subsequent adult life; whether there is a weak link remains controversial. Where there are adverse effects on psychosocial outcome in adult life, these are less associated with the bereavement itself, but arise more from indirect consequences such as becoming poorer, the surviving parent becoming depressed, or negative experiences with a step-parent. Traumatic death witnessed by the child, such as their mother dying during an attack by a partner, or during war, is associated with considerably higher morbidity.

Divorce

This often follows years of decline in the parental relationship, and this needs to be borne in mind when comparisons are made between children from divorced and intact families: the differences are in part due to pre-existing discord, poorer ability of the parents to relate, and so on. Parents tend to feel anxious, depressed, angry, rejected and incompetent during the first year after divorce, with these responses diminishing in the second. The divorced parents frequently remain ambivalent about their relationship with each other, often with resultant conflict; both the strong positive and negative feelings reduce if parents find another partner. Inconsistent parenting of children is frequent, especially of sons by mothers. Conversely, mothers may be greatly harassed by their sons, who may blame them for the loss of their fathers. Parents' lives are often dominated by practical issues such as not having enough money or difficulty getting all the household chores done.

Children are also affected. Both at home and at school, social interactions become markedly disrupted. There is much fantasy aggression, opposition and fearfulness, with a need to seek help from, and proximity to, adults; boys, especially, seek help from adult males. By comparison with other children, they are more negative and less positive to adults. Younger children usually hope desperately for a reconciliation even if pre-divorce life had been characterised by severe discord. There is great fear that the father might be replaced through remarriage. Prospective longitudinal studies show that for a year or two following divorce, children will, on average, experience a rise (of about a third of a standard deviation) in disruptive behaviour, anxiety and depressive symptoms. Later follow-up shows that though most of the children become well-functioning individuals, the divorce had a big effect on their lives. For example, they may be left with a lasting concern that their own intimate relationships will end in separation and divorce. If parents remarry, the children have to make further adjustments. While young children often show good relationships with their step-fathers, older children frequently do not. On average, boys are more distressed than girls by the divorce, while girls are more distressed than boys if their mothers remarry.

Family discord

There is a marked association between psychiatric disorder and being reared in a disharmonious home. Discord, angry arguments, hostility, and criticism are related to disruptive behavioural disorders in boys, and to emotional disorders in both sexes. Discord is a risk factor in itself, and not simply a marker for other risk factors such as poverty, lack of rules or poor supervision. For example, discord is a powerful predictor of psychiatric problems even in well-off households. The absence of warmth in family relationships is not as relevant as the presence of discord. Family discord is so often connected with poorly administered discipline that it has been hard to tease apart their respective impacts. However, when taking a history, one can ask about disciplinary consistency, and observe the number and tone of critical comments made by parents about their children, and about their partner. These have been shown to be a reliable risk factor.

In discordant households, there is good evidence that children and adolescents learn that aversive behaviours are an effective way of getting parental attention, so that parents inadvertently encourage tantrums and other undesirable behaviours, such as whining and disobedience. In young children, this effect may be relatively situational, with children behaving negatively when exposed to discord at home, but relating more normally to people outside the family. With time, however, the negative behavioural style becomes more set; the child appears to have internalised the parents' mode of interaction, repeating the same pattern in other relationships. Put another way, the children are being brought up to respond in a way that may help get their need for attention met at home, but that is maladaptive in the outside world. On a more positive note, scores of controlled trials have shown that parents can be taught better disciplinary methods and improved ways to relate to their children, which is accompanied by a reduction in discord and criticism. Such parenting programmes lead to marked reductions in disobedience and other antisocial behaviours, and an increase in social relationship skills.

Parental mental health problems

When parents have mental health problems, such as marked depression, drug misuse or a psychotic illness, their children are at increased risk of developing emotional and behavioural problems themselves, with a particularly marked increase in disruptive behavioural disorders. Sometimes, a parent and child will both have psychiatric problems because of shared genes, shared environment, or direct modelling. This may apply, for example, to some families where parents and children have anxiety or depressive disorders. More often, however, the adverse effects of parental mental health problems are mediated by the children's exposure to poor parenting, including parental hostility and marital discord. These factors increase the risk of emotional and behavioural problems in children in general. Parents with a personality disorder (whether antisocial or otherwise) are even more likely than parents with affective or psychotic disorders to have children who develop disruptive behavioural disorders. This link primarily reflects the greater tendency of parents with personality disorders to be inconsistent and hostile to their children. Child characteristics may also be relevant since, other things being equal, temperamentally difficult children are more likely to evoke parental hostility than temperamentally easy children.

Other adversities

Other adversities seen fairly frequently in clinical practice include maltreatment (see Chapter 27), victimisation (see Chapter 35), poverty, and the effects of war and subsequent migration.

Family size and birth order

Family size and birth order can be measured so easily and reliably that they are included as possible predictor variables in most studies of child and adolescent psychiatric problems. Researchers who find an association between psychiatric problems and family composition are likely to report that finding, whereas researchers who find no such association may concentrate on other positive findings and not even report the negative findings. The predictable result is a profusion of reported associations, most of which are not replicated by subsequent studies.

One of the few consistent findings to emerge from this muddled field is that children and adolescents from large families are at greater risk of disruptive behavioural problems and juvenile delinquency. Though this may partly reflect an association between large families and social disadvantage, family size probably has a direct effect too – with the number of brothers being a stronger predictor of externalising problems than the number of sisters.

Contrary to popular mythology, only children are not psychiatrically distinctive; children from small families are at relatively low psychiatric risk whether or not the family has one or two children. One important implication for our overcrowded planet is that parents who choose to have just one child need not feel that they are selfishly endangering their child's mental health.

Whereas most 'oldest' and 'youngest' children come from two-child families, 'middle' children must come from families with at least three children. Consequently, the link between larger family size and disruptive behaviour will inevitably make it seem as though middle children have more of these problems than oldest or youngest children if no account is taken of family size. It is not clear whether birth order has an effect on psychiatric problems once the effect of family size has been allowed for, although there may be a link between school refusal and being the youngest in the family.

Coping and resilience

Cumulative risk

Are some adverse experiences especially damaging, whereas others do little lasting harm? Several longitudinal studies now indicate that it is the dose rather than the type of stress or risk factor that is particularly relevant. Exposure to one or even two moderate stresses or risk factors only slightly raises the rate of psychiatric disorder, and may even have long-term advantages. Children who have encountered and coped with moderate stresses may be more resistant to stresses in later life than if they had been spared all stresses. (This is not a reason for deliberately stressing children, though it is a reason for encouraging them to take on challenges that they can successfully master.) Though exposure to one or two moderate stresses or risk factors may do little harm and perhaps some good, children are far more likely to be adversely affected when they experience multiple adversities. Once children face three or four stresses or risk factors, the rate of poor outcomes goes up three to five times compared with controls, and under these circumstances the majority of children suffer from psychiatric disorders. The main risk factors implicated are:

- biological risks (physical illness, especially brain injury; low birth weight);
- parental mental health, personality and intelligence (any psychiatric disorder, especially major psychoses, alcoholism and criminality; personality disorders are particularly important: each of these factors operates independently of upbringing style);
- family dysfunction (interparental discord, hostility and criticism, stressful life events);
- risky neighbourhood (high crime, violence, and drug availability; poor schooling, low social cohesion).

Resilience and protective factors

Though cumulative risks and major stresses usually have adverse effects, some children do considerably better than others, which has led to the concept of resilience under stress. The factors associated with better outcomes under stress are:

- personal attributes (for example, calm as opposed to irritable temperament, higher as opposed to lower IQ, stronger as opposed to weaker belief in own ability);
- family attributes (for example, warmth, closeness, cohesiveness);
- the use of outside support by the family and child, who has at least one strong positive, supportive relationship with an adult (who may be outside the immediate family, for example, a grandfather or aunt).

Most of these factors are associated with better outcomes, whether or not children are living in adverse circumstances. They therefore are not only 'protective' against stress but are 'promotive' of good functioning whatever conditions children are living under. This is what some researchers and clinicians mean by 'protective factors', while others prefer a narrower definition that excludes factors that are good for everyone. Narrowly defined protective factors help cancel out the effects of risk factors, but confer no added benefits to individuals who are not exposed to stress. An analogy drawn from physical health may make this clearer. Using a broad definition, a balanced diet is a protective factor since it promotes everyone's physical health, regardless of whether or not they have been exposed to infectious diseases or some other risk. By contrast, having a vaccination against rabies is a narrowly defined protective factor since it reduces the risk of getting ill if bitten by a rabid dog, but does not make people healthier if they are not exposed to rabies. In the field of mental health, many more factors have been identified as protective in the broad sense than in the narrow sense (but see Box 37.2 on p. 314 for an example of protective factors operating in the narrow sense).

Mechanisms

A rather diverse list of adversities has been given above. It is now worth considering what they have in common, and how they may disrupt normal development. The environments that damage children tend to be:

- disorganised, inconsistent and unpredictable;
- harsh and punitive;
- dangerous, frightening and anxiety-provoking;
- lacking in stimulation;
- lacking in individuals who respond sensitively to the child's need.

These adverse features can be present in the immediate environment of the family, and/or in the wider social community in which the child lives. Their impact on the child is likely to be due not only to the number of adverse risk factors, but also the extent to which they are constant and widespread as opposed to intermittent and limited in scope.

The experiences may exert their harmful effects by hindering the development of healthy responsiveness and social development, which depend on:

1 well-modulated emotional regulation;
2 secure attachment relationships;
3 competent social perception and skills.

Evidence is accumulating that each of these is damaged by chronic adversity.

Emotional regulation can be measured: behaviourally in the ability to exert self-control when frustrated, in contrast to explosive outbursts with little provocation; physiologically in terms of arousal (for example, heart and respiration rate, blood pressure, skin conductance), and; biochemically in terms of levels of hormones affected by stress, such as adrenaline and noradrenaline, and cortisol. Animal, and now human, studies are finding that in the abused young, these systems are far more prone to show large reactions to relatively small stimuli, and to take far longer to down-regulate. Thus, for example, the diurnal cortisol rhythm of children taken into foster care because of abusive parenting is abnormal. Encouragingly, it becomes more normal after a year in stable foster care.

Secure attachment relationships are compromised by adverse parenting, which is associated with increased rates of all types of insecurity. A dismissive parenting style is associated with an avoidant attachment pattern, an ambivalent parenting style by a resistant pattern, and an unpredictable, abusive parenting style by a disorganised pattern. Insecure attachment is in turn associated with more psychopathology and worse functioning. On the more positive side, there have now been over 70 controlled studies confirming that interventions that increase parental sensitivity and quality lead to more secure attachment patterns (see Chapter 32).

The social understanding and skills of abused children are usually altered. Their perception and interpretation of social cues make them more likely to infer hostile intent, and they are more likely to believe that an aggressive response by themselves will achieve their goal. They are poorer at generating solutions to hypothetical social problems, and in real-life social encounters display fewer prosocial skills and less ability to deploy constructive, positive behaviours and strategies. They are especially poor at negotiating interpersonal differences and conflict of wishes. Many of these perceptions and response styles are entirely understandable in the light of the children's experiences, and indeed may have been necessary to survive. However, they do not lead to success in new relationships and tasks.

In summary, ongoing adversities are not just distressing; they often damage the growing child's social, cognitive and emotional capacities. Children who are relatively immune to these stresses usually have protective factors present that enable them to develop adequate emotional regulation, secure attachments and appropriate social skills.

Clinical implications

Assessment of children with psychological problems should include appraisal of protective factors as well as characterising the nature and intensity of adversities. The formulation should describe explicitly the child's strengths and capabilities. Wherever possible, steps should be taken to ameliorate adverse circumstances. In any case, and especially when adversities cannot all be corrected, helping the child develop competencies is likely to mitigate the impact of psychiatric disorders and improve confidence and self-esteem. Thus, for example, in a conduct-disordered boy who is reasonably good at football, encouraging the parents to take him to an afterschool training club may be beneficial; in a depressed girl with dancing ability, helping this develop through classes may likewise improve confidence and sometimes symptoms. For some children, particularly where both home and school experiences are unpleasant, such activities may be the main or only positive experience in the week.

More formally, there are social skills and problem-solving interventions that teach children how to develop these general abilities. For particular circumstances, such as living with chronic medical conditions, there is a range of psychological interventions. They are proven to work in clinical trials, but unfortunately are often not easily available.

Subject review

Jenkins J. (2008) Psychosocial adversity and resilience. *In*: Rutter M *et al.* (eds) *Rutter's Child and Adolescent Psychiatry*, 5th edn. Wiley-Blackwell, Chichester, pp. 377–391.

Luthar S. (2006). Resilience in development: A synthesis of research across five decades. In: Cicchetti D, Cohen D (eds) *Developmental Psychopathology*, 2nd edn, Vol. 3: *Risk, Disorder, and Adaptation*. John Wiley & Sons, Inc., Hoboken, NJ, pp. 739–795.

Sandberg S, Rutter M. (2008) Acute life stresses. *In*: Rutter M *et al.* (eds) *Rutter's Child and Adolescent Psychiatry*, 5th edn. Wiley-Blackwell, Chichester, pp. 392–406.

Stein A *et al.* (2008) Impact of parental psychiatric disorder and physical illness. *In*: Rutter M *et al.* (eds) *Rutter's Child and Adolescent Psychiatry*, 5th edn. Wiley-Blackwell, Chichester, pp. 407–420.

Further reading and viewing

Belsky J, Pluess M. (2011). Beyond adversity, vulnerability, and resilience: Individual differences in developmental plasticity. *In*: Cicchetti D, Roisman G. (eds) *The Origins and Organization of Adaptation and Maladaptation*. pp. 379–422. John Wiley & Sons, Inc., Hoboken, NJ. (A thoughtful essay combining theory of adverse events, attachment, and new genetic findings on differential susceptibility; the book has many good chapters on resilience.)

Coleman J, Hagell A (2007) *Adolescence, Risk and Resilience: Against the Odds*. John Wiley & Sons, Ltd, Chichester (An easy-to-read book that focuses on adolescence and the evidence of what interventions help young people survive difficult predicaments.)

Cummings EM, Davies PT. (2010) *Marital Conflict and Children: An Emotional Security Perspective*. Guilford Press, New York.

Hetherington E.M, Kelly J. (2002) *For Better or for Worse: Divorce Reconsidered*. Norton, New York. (This book is a lively account for the general reader, of the largest and perhaps best study of divorce, in the USA. It includes the impact on children six years later, as well as the different styles of coping by mothers and fathers.)

Kim J, Cicchetti D. (2010) Longitudinal pathways linking child maltreatment, emotion regulation, peer relations, and psychopathology. *Journal of Child Psychology and Psychiatry* **51**, 706–716. (A nice longitudinal study showing how one thing leads to another: abuse leads to poor regulation of emotions which in turn leads to aggression and few friends.)

Robertson J, Robertson J. (1959) *A Two-year-old Goes to Hospital*. Concord films, Ipswich. (This is a very moving documentary of a child's reaction to separation from his parents. Highly recommended viewing.)

McNeal C, Amato PR. (1998) Parents' marital violence: Long-term consequences for children. *Journal of Family Issues* **19**, 123–139. (Representative longitudinal study of 400 families showing that marital discord early in children's lives was associated later with less closeness to parents, lower self-esteem and happiness, and more distress and violence in their relationships as adolescents.)

Shure MB. (1996) *Raising a Thinking Child*. Pocket Books, New York. (This is a classic manual for parents, showing them how to teach their child problem-solving skills applicable to everyday social conflicts.)

CHAPTER 35

School and Peer Factors

Though family life undoubtedly has a powerful influence on many aspects of development, it is important to remember that most children and adolescents inhabit more than one social world. Even in the toddler years, experiences in day care can be very different from experiences at home. From the preschool years onwards, peer relationships become increasingly important. Close friendships can buffer children and adolescents from the impact of other adversities, while peer rejection, victimisation or involvement in a deviant peer group can all contribute to the onset of psychiatric problems. The peer group and the family are two different social worlds; the classroom is a third social world, and it, too, can influence emotional and behavioural problems for better or for worse. A supportive teacher and success in some area of the school curriculum can promote self-esteem and resilience, while a hostile teacher and school failure can have the opposite effect. A chaotic classroom, like a chaotic family environment, can train children and adolescents to become coercive and disruptive by rewarding these behaviours through greater attention and fewer demands. It is important to consider classroom and peer factors in any assessment, and not just when the individual's emotional or behavioural problems are mainly restricted to the classroom or playground. Stresses in one setting sometimes present with psychiatric problems in a different setting; stresses at home (such as sexual abuse) may lead to behavioural problems that are most prominent at school, while stresses at school (such as bullying) may lead to distress or disturbance that is more evident to parents than to teachers.

Bully-victim problems

Bullying refers to repeated and deliberate use of physical or psychological means to hurt someone, without adequate provocation and in the knowledge that the victim is unlikely to be able to retaliate effectively. Most bullying occurs in school rather than on the way to or from school. Bullies and victims are commonly in the same school year. Although pupils

---

are supposed to be supervised at school, most bullying goes unrecognised by teachers, and the victims commonly feel unable to report the bullying either to teachers or parents. Roughly 2–8% of pupils are bullied at least once a week, and 2–4% engage in bullying at least once a week. Less severe levels of victimisation and bullying are substantially commoner. English studies have found similar rates of bullying in childhood and adolescence, though studies elsewhere have reported that bullying declines with age. Most bullies are boys, and there may be a small excess of boys among victims too. Physical aggression is most characteristic of boys' bullying; girls' bullying is more likely to involve social exclusion or whispering campaigns.

Bullies are more likely to have witnessed domestic violence. They, in turn, are typically aggressive not only to their peers but also to their siblings, parents and teachers. They have a positive attitude towards violence and little empathy for victims. At least among boys, bullies are likely to be physically stronger than their peers. The development of aggressive personality patterns may reflect both temperament and parenting (with the parents of bullies being more prone to use power-assertive child-rearing methods, and failing to provide adequate warmth, control and supervision). Most bullies are not especially prone to anxiety, insecurity, or poor self-esteem (though there may be a minority of anxious bullies who dominate their victims in order to bolster a fragile sense of self-worth). Bullies are not generally unhappy or unpopular at the time. In the longer term, bullies are at an increased risk of criminality and alcohol abuse in adulthood.

Some pupils are both bullies and victims, often referred to as *bully-victims*. These individuals may be described as *provocative* (or high-aggressive) victims. Provocative victims show a high level of aggression and disruptive behaviour: picking fights, taunting others, getting people into trouble and being easily angered. Clinical experience suggests that individuals with ADHD are particularly likely to become provocative bully-victims.

By contrast, *passive* (or low-aggressive) victims are anxious, insecure, quiet individuals who withdraw when attacked and may cry. They typically lack friends and have very poor self-esteem. Among boys at least, passive victims are likely to be physically weaker than their peers. A cautious and sensitive personality probably predates the victimisation, but many of the other characteristics of victims are as likely to be consequences as causes of victim status. Victimisation may be more likely in larger schools. It is uncertain how far victimisation is influenced by physical appearance, physical disabilities, or minority group status. While there is no doubt that victims often experience considerable distress at the time, the long-term consequences are less clear. Possible consequences include lasting problems with self-esteem, peer relationships, and intimate friendships. One study showed that frequent victimisation at age 8 increased the rate of attempted and completed suicide by age 25, but the nature of the link varied with gender. In males, the link disappeared after controlling for behavioural and depressive symptoms; whereas in females early victimisation did predict later suicidal behaviour even after allowing for behavioural and depressive symptoms.

Systematic interventions can reduce the rate of victimisation in schools (by about 50% in one carefully planned intervention in Norway). The unacceptability of victimisation has to be made clear to all pupils, and the policy must be backed up by adequate supervision, and by firm but non-hostile sanctions. Victims need to know that they will get the backing of the school, their parents and their class if they report bullying.

Peer popularity and unpopularity

The most common technique for assessing peer relationships is 'sociom-etry', which commonly includes asking each pupil in a class in private which three classmates they would most want to play with ('positive nom-inations') and which three they would least want to play with ('negative nominations'). They may also be asked about other characteristics, for example, which three of their classmates fight most.

At one stage, popularity and unpopularity were viewed as the opposite end of a single dimension, as if a low number of positive nominations and a high number of negative nominations had the same meaning. Nowadays, it is more common to view popularity and unpopularity as different dimensions, generating a wider range of associated categories, shown in Box 35.1.

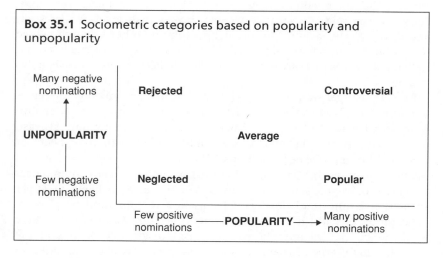

Box 35.1 Sociometric categories based on popularity and unpopularity

In the past, studies of 'unpopular' pupils typically lumped together rejected and neglected children even though these two groups differ in several important respects. The peer problems of rejected children and adolescents are more persistent, and more often associated with aggressive and disruptive behaviours, loneliness, misery and academic difficulties. In the longer term, rejected children and adolescents are more likely to drop out of school, engage in delinquent behaviour and have mental health problems (though it is still unclear whether peer rejection contributes directly to these later problems, or simply acts as a marker for a life-long maladaptive behavioural style). Rejection is probably related mainly to the individual's social behaviour, though physical appearance, academic and athletic limitations, and minority group status may all be relevant (and some social groups may need a scapegoat or outcast). An aggressive and disruptive style is the most common identifiable reason for peer rejection. Marked self-isolation, particularly if combined with socially inept or eccentric behaviour, is also liable to result in rejection. Lesser degrees of shyness and withdrawal are more typical of neglected individuals, and probably do not have serious long-term consequences. Controversial individuals are typically characterised by a mixed social style, incorporating both aversive and prosocial elements.

Institutional factors

Rates of child and adolescent psychiatric problems, absenteeism and delinquency vary markedly and consistently from school to school, often paralleling differences in examination results. Much of this can be explained by differences in catchment area and intake. Even when intake characteristics are allowed for, however, schools continue to differ in their impact on pupils' behaviour and academic attainments. Some of these differences can be explained by school ethos and organisation. Pupils are less likely to develop disruptive behaviour problems when they attend a school where they are frequently praised and given responsibilities, where the teachers provide models of good behaviour, and where standards are high, lessons are well organised, and working conditions are pleasant. These factors seem obvious enough, but it is important to remember that the following equally 'obvious' factors have not been shown to have a marked impact on school effectiveness: size of school, age or layout of buildings, continuity of teaching staff, or type of pastoral care. Variations in class size within the 25–35 range seem to have little effect on school effectiveness, though much smaller classes (8–15) may have benefits if teachers take the opportunity to adopt a more individualised style of teaching – with these benefits being more marked for children who are younger, have special needs, or come from disadvantaged backgrounds.

Oldest/youngest in class

In most classes, the oldest pupils are roughly a year older than the youngest pupils. Many studies have shown that the youngest pupils tend to be educationally disadvantaged. They also appear to be slightly disadvantaged in terms of their mental health. Thus, one large study showed that the average rate of emotional and behavioural difficulties is greatest in the youngest third of the class and lowest in the oldest third – an effect evident in 11–15-year-olds as well as 5–10-year-olds. This effect of 'relative age' is not strong at the individual level, but even moderate effects that apply to many individuals can be important from a public health perspective. Abolishing the effect of relative age could potentially eliminate about 8% of child and adolescent psychiatric disorders.

One possible explanation for the vulnerability of the youngest pupils in a class is that their emotional and intellectual immaturity makes it harder for them to hold their own socially and academically in their peer group. Smaller size and lesser strength may also be risk factors for bullying and marginalisation, particularly among boys. In addition, teachers commonly forget to make appropriate allowances for relative age, which may lead to younger pupils being unfairly regarded as failing when they are performing adequately for their age – something that may well be stressful. Taking the class register in birth order rather than alphabetical order is one easy way to raise teachers' awareness of relative age. Though being one of the oldest in a class is generally beneficial, it may carry its own risks, such as being bored, or being trained to be coercive (since aggressive interactions are more likely to be rewarded when the perpetrator is bigger and stronger by virtue of being older).

Interventions

For children and adolescents who do not have friends, social skills programmes that specifically target building friendships have been proven effective in controlled trials. More indirectly, the power of peer relationships can be harnessed to help psychological problems. This is useful, when a child's behaviour has been improved at home but peer pressure seems to lead him to be oppositional in class. Teachers can set up a scheme whereby, for example, the class is divided into three groups, and the group that behaves best during the morning gets a reward at lunchtime, perhaps ten minutes extra break or first choice on the lunch menu. If a child misbehaves, his peers are responsible for stopping the misbehaviour (and they usually do this with alacrity). Such an approach has also been proven effective in trials, and can have enduring effects on future mental health.

Subject review

Hay DF *et al.* (2004) Peer relations in childhood. *Journal of Child Psychology and Psychiatry* **45**, 84–108.

Rutter M, Maughan B. (2002) School effectiveness findings 1979–2002. *Journal of School Psychology* **40**, 451–475.

Smith P. (2004) Bullying: recent developments. *Child and Adolescent Mental Health* **9**, 98–103.

Further reading

Bowes L *et al.* (2009) School, neighborhood, and family factors are associated with children's bullying involvement: A nationally representative longitudinal study. *Journal of the American Academy of Child and Adolescent Psychiatry* **48**, 545–553.

Deater-Deckard K. (2001) Recent research examining the role of peer relationships in the development of psychopathology. *Journal of Child Psychology and Psychiatry* **42**, 565–579.

Frankel F. (2010) *Friends Forever: How Parents Can Help Their Kids Make and Keep Good Friends.* Wiley, New York.

Goodman R *et al.* (2003) Child psychiatric disorder and relative age within school year: Cross-sectional survey of large population sample. *BMJ* **327**, 472–475.

Kellam S *et al.* (2008) Effects of a universal classroom behavior management program in first and second grades on young adult behavioral, psychiatric, and social outcomes. *Drug and Alcohol Dependence* **95**, S5–S28.

Klomek, AB *et al.* (2009) Childhood bullying behaviors as a risk for suicide attempts and completed suicides: A population-based birth cohort study. *Journal of the American Academy of Child and Adolescent Psychiatry* **48**, 254–261.

Viding E *et al.* (2010) The contribution of callous-unemotional traits and conduct problems to bullying in early adolescence. *Journal of Child Psychology and Psychiatry* **50**, 471–481.

PART 4

Treatment and Services

CHAPTER 36

Intervention: First Principles

Parents, children and adolescents come to mental health services for a variety of reasons. They bring with them a number of beliefs and fears about the nature of the problem and what needs to be done. They will be carrying out an assessment of the service they receive from the moment they come through the door.

Engaging the family

If the family feel poorly handled and not understood, they are unlikely to come back again. If this happens, then no matter how thorough and accurate the clinical evaluation has been, the opportunity to do useful therapeutic work will have been lost, and the family may also have been put off seeking help at some later date. Discovering the family's beliefs and fears, and responding to them sensitively is vital to the whole process of engagement. If they feel they are understood, and treated as respected individuals, then the chances of their taking part in treatment will be far greater. This calls for considerable flexibility in response rather than one fixed 'right' way of doing things.

When are labels useful?

It can take considerable courage to walk through a door where the service is for 'mental' problems, and some parents are fearful that either they or their children are going to be labelled mad, bad, abnormal, or sick in the head. They may be fed up with being made to feel useless by a range of people in authority who tell them that what they are doing is wrong. Under these circumstances being told, for example, that their son has a serious condition labelled 'conduct disorder', and that they need a course of instruction to learn the 'right' way to handle their child may play into their sense of inadequacy and despair. For such a family it might have been

Child and Adolescent Psychiatry, Third Edition. Robert Goodman and Stephen Scott.
© 2012 Robert Goodman and Stephen Scott. Published 2012 by John Wiley & Sons, Ltd.

more constructive to have said that their child is indeed strong-willed and can behave in an antisocial way at times, but he or she has many strong points that have become obscured by his or her reaction to the stress of school difficulties. The parents clearly are doing their best for their child by bringing him or her to be seen. If they receive support to do more of the useful things they are already doing, there is hope for improvement.

In other families the reverse may be true, and an approach which gives a diagnostic label can take the strain off family relationships and help all involved parties to focus on the child's needs. This can work for a number of reasons:

1 An official 'label' is, for some families, the single most important thing they take away from their contact with child mental health profession-als. Particularly with 'out of the ordinary' disorders, such as childhood autism or Tourette syndrome, it can be an enormous relief to know that the problem has been recognised. It is no coincidence that demons in fairy stories often lose at least some of their power once they have been named. A child and family's sense of isolation is usually lessened once they know that other children and families have similar problems. Professionals should inform families of relevant voluntary groups. There are local and national parents' organisations for some child psychiatric disorders. By joining these groups, families are able to meet other people in similar situations, and may also gain access to newsletters, pamphlets and talks.

2 A diagnosis may also be the 'passport' children and families need to be allowed access to special educational help, extra allowances, special holidays, and so on.

3 A diagnosis often comes with a prognosis. When the prognosis for natural remission is good, the family may be happy to leave well alone and let time do the work. Indeed, defusing anxiety about the future may hasten spontaneous recovery.

4 Explaining the implications of a diagnosis is also an opportunity for conveying important information on the nature and origin of symptoms. This, too, may have therapeutic value, as illustrated by the follow-ing three examples. Knowing that childhood autism is not caused by parental unresponsiveness may help parents and others move beyond guilt and blame. Teachers and parents may find it easier to deal constructively with a hyperactive child once they know that he or she is not just being naughty. Knowing that Tourette syndrome is a neurobiological disorder may help dispel ideas of 'possession'.

5 A label can be used in therapeutic work to stop a child being scape-goated. For example, rather than blaming a child's propensity to jump up and down during dinner and fidget constantly on his wickedness and unswerving desire to wind up his mother, the parents may be helped to 'externalise the problem' and see that it is his hyperactivity that's making him fidget. Then both the boy and his parents can be on the same side in trying to beat the difficulty.

Symptoms and social impairments both need to be addressed

Treatment is unlikely to be effective if the problem has not been characterised accurately. The most skilled therapist will not get very far if an important contributory factor has been overlooked and is preventing progress. Therefore, an accurate assessment and formulation is essential before embarking on a management and treatment plan. It is often a mistake to focus exclusively on psychiatric symptoms. As described in Chapter 1, a psychiatric disorder should usually only be diagnosed if two conditions are met: (1) the child has a recognised constellation of symptoms; and (2) these symptoms have a significant impact. This adverse impact often takes the form of social impairment affecting home life, schoolwork, friendships or leisure activities. Both symptoms and social impairment may need to be targeted by the intervention plan. Thus, with a depressed adolescent, treating the low mood and sleeping problems may not be enough. It may also be essential to decide how to tackle the issue of lapsed friendships, and work out a plan for catching up with missed schoolwork and even where symptoms may be hard to tackle directly, much good may be done through promoting skills and self-esteem, for example, by getting children to develop their interest in sport by joining a club where they are encouraged to develop their ability and are appreciated by their peers.

Complex problems may need complex solutions

The sorts of problems that present to child mental health specialists are rarely simple. Take, for example, a boy who presents with conduct problems. A careful assessment may suggest that all of the following are relevant:

- an inherited tendency to hyperactivity;
- dietary intolerance to citrus fruits and additives;
- specific reading difficulties;
- a tendency to see other people as hostile when they are not;
- a family environment that has trained him to act coercively to get attention and avoid demands;
- inadequate parental supervision;
- membership of a deviant peer group.

Perhaps tackling just one of these factors can help; the resultant improvements in one area may break a vicious cycle and allow the child to recover. More often, however, clinical experience suggests that it is necessary to target several problem areas at once. Interventions for child mental health problems may target:

- *the child's physiological function*, for example, diet, medication;
- *the family's knowledge of a condition*, for example, explanatory leaflets;

- *the external contingencies around the child's behaviour*, for example, parent training programmes, behavioural therapy for specific symptoms;
- *the internal world of the child*, for example, cognitive therapy, interpersonal therapy;
- *family relationships and beliefs*, for example, reduction in negative expressed emotion, family therapy;
- *peer relationships*, for example, social skills training, group therapy;
- *school activities*, for example, extra help with reading, anti-bullying programme;
- *the family's economic and social environment*, for example, change of housing, befriending programmes for isolated families;
- *alternatives to care in the family*, for example, fostering, admission to a residential community.

These are not mutually exclusive and several may be combined.

Working with other agencies

Many of the children and families seen by mental health services also need special input from other agencies, most notably education and social services. It is essential that each agency defines its role clearly and works in partnership with the other agencies, not at cross-purposes. Liaison meetings should be a means to an end rather than an end in themselves!

Treatment need not mirror aetiology

A disorder caused by physical factors may need psychological treatment, and vice versa. It is not always necessary to fight fire with fire; it is sometimes appropriate to fight fire with water! Thus, a child's hysterical paralysis may respond better to physiotherapy than psychotherapy. Medication may help a child's hyperactivity even if that hyperactivity is due to being raised in a grossly inadequate orphanage. Equally, a child with genetically caused learning disability may benefit from special education. An adolescent with biologically determined schizophrenia may benefit from reduction of parental negative expressed emotion.

Selecting treatment approaches

There is increasing emphasis on evidence-based provision, with moves in this direction generally being further advanced for health provision than for educational or social work provision. An evidence base is vital because clinical wisdom and commonsense are surprisingly fallible. 'Self-evidently' beneficial interventions may turn out to be worse than nothing. For example, one careful randomised trial of an intuitively appealing package of social and psychological interventions for children at high risk of delinquency showed that the intervention significantly worsened their long-term outcome. Other plausible interventions have also been shown to have little or no effect. Thus, conventional tricyclic antidepressants seem ineffective for depressed children and adolescents. There is also controversy about the effectiveness of the newer selective serotonin reuptake inhibitors (SSRIs), though on balance it does seem likely that at least one, fluoexetine, does work with adolescents (see Chapter 10). Similarly, many of the psychological treatments for children administered in everyday clinical settings are ineffective, or almost so.

On the positive side, treatment trials, and meta-analyses based on these trials, have shown that an increasing range of specific treatments for child psychiatric disorders are effective (see Box 36.1 for examples). But how effective are they? It is not enough to know that a particular treatment makes a statistically significant difference; it is also essential to know whether the size of this difference is large enough to be clinically significant. A tiny effect that is of no clinical relevance could still be statistically

---

Box 36.1 Examples of effective and ineffective treatments

There is extensive and sound evidence for the effectiveness of:

- Stimulant medication for ADHD.
- Parent training for disruptive behavioural disorders.
- Behavioural methods for soiling and enuresis.
- Family therapy for anorexia.
- Cognitive behavioural therapy for a number of anxiety disorders and post-traumatic stress disorder.
- Behaviourally-based video feedback for infants with insecure attachment patterns.

There is reasonably sound evidence for:

- Fluoxetine medication, cognitive behavioural therapy and interpersonal therapy for adolescent depression.
- Cognitive behavioural therapy and clomipramine medication for obsessive compulsive disorder.
- Behavioural approaches for school refusal.
- Home visiting schemes for physical maltreatment.
- Teacher classroom management techniques for child antisocial behaviour in school.

There is evidence that the following have little or no effect, or are harmful:

- Unfocused family work for disruptive behavioural disorders.
- Anger management for disruptive behavioural disorders.
- Medication for disruptive behavioural disorders (in the absence of hyperactivity).
- Social skills therapy given in clinic settings for peer relationship problems.
- Social work and general support for delinquency.
- Tricyclic medication for adolescent depression.
- Intensive behavioural approaches for the core symptoms of autism.
- Intensive treatments based on 'breaking through defences' or 'rebirthing' for children with attachment disorders.

significant given a large enough trial or meta-analysis. There are several ways of measuring how effective a treatment is. The commonest one is effect size, which expresses change in 'standard deviation' units. For example, if untreated hyperkinetic children are an average of 2.5 standard deviations above the population mean on a measure of hyperactivity, and if treatment with stimulant medication brings them down to an average of 1.4 standard deviations above the population mean, the effect size is said to be 1.1 (i.e. 2.5 minus 1.4). A great advantage of this measure is that it allows direct comparisons of diverse treatment modalities, such as medication and psychological therapies, and of diverse outcomes, such as different measures of depression or measures of symptoms and social impairment.

Successful psychological therapies typically have effect sizes of around 0.6 to 0.8 when administered in research settings. In ordinary clinic settings, however, the average effect size of psychological therapy may be less or even zero. What is this disparity due to? The exclusion of hard-to-treat children and families from research trials is likely to explain part of the difference. There are many other plausible explanations too, though only some are supported by the empirical evidence (see Box 36.2). The overall message for mental health professionals is both sobering and optimistic. It is sobering because if psychological therapies as currently used in everyday settings sometimes have little or no effect, then it seems difficult to justify the cost involved; but optimistic because three changes in emphasis could boost effectiveness in future. These changes are: a shift in emphasis towards behavioural and cognitive approaches; the use of specific, focused

---

Box 36.2 Why is psychological therapy much less effective in routine clinical practice than in research trials (following Weisz, 2006)?

Probably relevant
- Clinics make less use of behavioural and cognitive approaches.
- Clinics rely less on specific, focused therapy methods.
- Clinics are less likely to structure therapy (for example, through treatment manuals) or monitor therapy to ensure that the therapist adheres to the treatment plans.
- Clinics treat cases with high degrees of comorbidity and families who attend irregularly – both criteria for exclusion from many research trials.

Probably irrelevant
- Research studies are more recent than clinic studies.
- Some research trials use subjects who are recruited volunteers rather than referred patients.
- Clinic settings are less conducive to success.
- Clinicians are less effective than research therapists.
- Research therapists have had special training in the methods just prior to the intervention.
- Clinics have to provide for a range of children, and a range of problems.
- Clinics are less likely to provide brief interventions.

treatment methods rather than vague, diffuse or mixed approaches; and the use of structured therapy methods (for example, through treatment manuals), with sufficient monitoring to ensure that therapists consistently adhere to treatment plans. Good training programmes and ongoing expert supervision help therapists to deliver evidence-based treatments with fidelity to the intended approach. Conversely, there is increasing evidence that lower levels of therapist skill lead to less good outcomes.

It obviously makes good sense to use treatment approaches that have been shown to work. In practice, though, it is not possible to rely just on published trials and protocols. For example, formal trials are usually on children who meet the full diagnostic criteria for operationalised syndromes, whereas many clinic cases have diffuse or partial syndromes that do not meet these criteria. How should they be treated? Comorbidity is also an important issue: the presence of more than one condition in the same person is the rule in clinical practice rather than the exception. So if a child has three comorbid diagnoses, should the child be given three manualised treatments in succession or simultaneously? There is almost no evidence on the best approach for comorbid disorders. In addition, a child or family's circumstances and preferences may make standard protocols unworkable. There is clearly still a key role for clinical judgement and improvisation – extrapolating from published evidence on what works, but not following it slavishly. Finally, for less severe cases who are well motivated, there is a growing evidence base that encouraging families to work though a suitable self-help book or website can be effective, especially if backed up by modest support, for example, fortnightly phone calls.

Modify treatment according to outcome

Having decided on a course of treatment, it is not enough just to give the treatment; it is also important to monitor the outcome. The treatment goals should have been recorded at the outset. Have these been attained? This can be judged clinically, though it is often helpful to seek independent corroboration, for example, by administering short questionnaires to the child or adolescent being treated, to parents or to teachers. If the goals have not been attained, it is often sensible to reassess the individual and review the formulation before giving up or pressing on with more of the same. Perhaps the individual has been resistant to treatment because the initial diagnosis was wrong: a revised formulation may suggest a revised treatment. Even if the original formulation still seems correct, it may be appropriate to switch to a different treatment. Even when trials have shown that treatment X usually works better than treatment Y, a minority of patients may respond better to Y than to X. If the individual and family are keen, a second-choice treatment can be tried when the first-choice treatment fails.

There is an increasing trend in services to undertake routine monitoring of outcomes. As the service develops, the progression may go from (1) measures at initial assessment only to (2) assessment initially and at termination or after, say, six months, to (3) repeating the measures after each session. Each has its benefits: (1) helps make sure you are not missing anything major, (2) makes you honest about whether you are doing any good (and also provides your bosses and commissioners with evidence on how effective you are), and (3) enables you to modify treatment as you go along, for the reasons suggested above. There may be resistance among clinicians to doing such monitoring but in our view it is essential as a means of developing better outcomes for children and weeding out ineffective therapies. If it is not undertaken, there is a risk that the self-interest of therapist will win out over the children's interests – rather than give what works best for children, clinicians might ignore this in favour of what they feel most comfortable with, were trained in twenty years ago, know how to do, get most money for, find quickest, or are told by their organisation to do.

To be practicable, measures need to be short, easy to enter onto a database, and fed back to the team at regular intervals. They probably should include, at initial assessment and termination, a broad overall screen (for example, the SDQ) an index of impairment or function (for example, the CGAS), and a scale for the severity of the main condition; the last can be used for session by session monitoring. While it is good to have the clinician's view, there is a risk that this alone may not be accurate as they may wish to make their results look better than they are, so the young person (if old enough) and family need to complete measures too. Details of such a system can be obtained by visiting the website of the Clinical Outcomes Research Consortium (http://www.corc.uk.net), which also allows services to see how they compare with others.

Subject review

Weisz J, Bearman SK. (2008) Psychological treatments: overview and critical issues for the field. *In*: Rutter M *et al.* (eds) *Rutter's Child and Adolescent Psychiatry*, 5th edn. Wiley-Blackwell, Chichester, pp. 251–268.

Further reading

Carr A. (2009) *What Works with Children, Adolescents and Adults? A Review of the Effectiveness of Psychotherapy*. Routledge, London.
Fonagy P *et al.* (2005) *What Works for Whom? A Critical Review of Treatments for Children and Adolescents*. Guilford Press, London.
Henggeler SW *et al.* (1997) Multisystemic therapy with violent and chronic juvenile offenders and their families: The role of treatment fidelity in successful dissemination. *Journal of Consulting and Clinical Psychology* **65**, 821–833.
McCord J. (1992) The Cambridge-Somerville study: A pioneering longitudinal-experimental study of delinquency prevention. *In*: McCord J, Tremblay RE (eds.) *Preventing Antisocial Behavior: Interventions from Birth*

through Adolescence. Guilford Press, New York. pp. 196–206. (This careful, classic study puts an end to any notion that commonsense interventions are bound to do more good than harm: the young people getting the relatively intensive intervention did notably worse.)

Nock M, Kazdin A (2005) Randomized controlled trial of a brief intervention for increasing participation in parent management training. *Journal of Consulting and Clinical Psychology* **73**, 872–879. (Shows that talking to families for 5–15 minutes during the first, fifth, and seventh sessions about the barriers to implementing treatment and how they might overcome them led to greater adherence and attendance.)

Shirk S, Karver M. (2003) Prediction of treatment outcome from relationship variables in child and adolescent therapy: A meta-analytic review. *Journal of Consulting and Clinical Psychology* **71**, 452–464. (Shows that the quality of the therapist-family alliance predicts on average 20% of the treatment gain.)

Weisz JR *et al*. (2006) Evidence-based youth psychotherapies versus usual clinical care: a meta-analysis of direct comparisons. *American Psychologist* **61**, 671–689.

Weisz J, Kazdin A. (2010) *Evidence-based Psychotherapies for Children and Adolescents*, 2nd edn. Guilford Press, London. (Nice summaries of the most effective therapies plus useful overviews of general issues.)

CHAPTER 37

Prevention

The adage 'prevention is better than cure' encapsulates an attractive idea. The pain and suffering of established disorders will be avoided, as will the considerable expense of treating them. Medicine provides some excellent examples: stopping smoking prevents needless lung cancer and heart attacks, as well as asthma in children exposed to the smoke; folic acid in pregnancy prevents babies' risk of being born with spina bifida; immunisation with polio vaccine prevents paralysis from poliomyelitis. Since in all countries in the world the majority of children and adolescents with psychiatric disorders are not treated by specialists at all, and even the best resourced countries have insufficient services to do so, prevention may be especially relevant. But can prevention be applied in practice to child and adolescent psychiatric disorders? And will it be cost effective? There are downsides to over-enthusiastic implementation of prevention programmes. Given finite resources to spend on mental health, there is a risk that treatment services for established conditions will be cut back. This will be unwise for two reasons. Firstly, even cheap and effective prevention programmes are never going to eliminate the development of substantial numbers of cases (and indeed may increase the demand for the treatment of established conditions by detecting more of them). Secondly, more expensive, less effective prevention programmes may not be better than effective, curative treatment. This chapter aims to explore the conditions that are necessary for prevention to be effective in improving child mental health, and give some examples of where it has been attempted in practice.

Types of prevention

Primary prevention stops the occurrence of the disorder in the first place; *secondary prevention* stops the development of complications of the disorder. In child and adolescent mental health, we may want to aim for more

---

Child and Adolescent Psychiatry, Third Edition. Robert Goodman and Stephen Scott.
© 2012 Robert Goodman and Stephen Scott. Published 2012 by John Wiley & Sons, Ltd.

than preventing one or more disorders. We may also aim to prevent symptoms or problems that would never quite have been severe enough to be a disorder; or prevent distress; or prevent the development of poor psychosocial functioning. Each of these additional goals can be pursued with or without the others.

Prevention programmes may be:

1 *Universal*, covering the whole population. Potential advantages include the opportunity to make the intervention generally acceptable and part of the usual culture, so avoiding stigma; it may be easier to deliver interventions universally too, as in putting fluoride in the water or teaching all schoolchildren about the risks of taking drugs. Disadvantages are the cost and resources required to implement universal cover, especially if the intervention has no effect on most of the population. In the child mental health domain, a potential example of a universal approach would be a series of television programmes influencing parents to spend more time reading with their children and interacting with them warmly while setting firm limits; there is good evidence that this style of parenting improves attainment and reduces conduct problems, especially in less advantaged populations.

2 *Targeted/Selective*, covering that part of the population at elevated risk of developing a condition. Potential advantages include efficient use of resources, thus avoiding unnecessary expense directed to individuals who do not need it. Disadvantages include the need to have a screening procedure that is acceptable, sensitive and specific, so that it picks up those likely to have developed the condition, but not those who wouldn't have. Also, the screening procedure and the intervention may be perceived as stigmatising, which may hinder uptake. For example, a parent may not appreciate being invited to a group run by the social services department for those believed to be at risk of abusing their children. Another disadvantage is that although the targeted population may be at considerably higher risk, most cases will occur in the rest of the population. Thus, in the UK in the poorest tenth of the population, the prevalence of conduct disorder is around 18%, compared with around 5% in the rest of the population. Implementing a prevention programme that was totally effective in eradicating conduct disorder in those at risk because of poverty would still miss nearly three-quarters of cases.

3 *Indicated*, covering those children who already show early signs of the condition. An advantage of this approach is that it is most effective in terms of only being used where necessary. Disadvantages include the fact that considerable damage may already have occurred by the time intervention is given, making the intervention more complex, costly, and less effective than earlier prevention would have been. However, intervening at this stage is still likely to be easier than when the full-blown condition and its consequences for school work, friendships and family relationships have been long established.

Box 37.1 shows some of the terms used when using screening tests.

Box 37.1 Screening test terminology

		True diagnosis	
		Case	Non-Case
	Positive	a	b
Screening test result	*Negative*	c	d

True positive	a	Correctly identified case
True negative	d	Correctly identified non-case
False positive	b	A non-case misleadingly identified as positive by the screen
False negative	c	A case misleadingly identified as negative by the screen
Sensitivity	a/a+c	the proportion of cases correctly identified
Specificity	d/b+d	the proportion of non-cases correctly identified
Positive predictive value	a/a+b	the proportion of screen positive predictions that are cases
Negative predictive value	d/c+d	the proportion of screen negative predictions that are non-cases

---

Conditions that make prevention feasible

1 For targeted prevention programmes, there needs to be an effective screening or identification test or procedure. This needs to be sensitive, that is, it should not miss many cases (low false negative rate), and specific, so that cases that would not get the disorder are not identified unnecessarily (low false positive rate). However, since most psychiatric conditions are dimensional, some false positive cases may not be a bad thing, since the children an adolescents in question may have substantial problems that could befit from intervention even if they don't quite have a full set of symptoms warranting a diagnosis. There are now good psychometric data across large and diverse populations on easily administered screening instruments such as the Strengths and Difficulties Questionnaire (SDQ) that show the power to predict emotional and behavioural disorders with acceptable sensitivity and specificity.

2 There needs to be an effective preventive intervention that is taken up by a substantial proportion of the population to whom it is offered. For example, as shown below, there are effective programmes for conduct disorder.

3 There are serious, long-standing consequences if the full-blown condition develops. The case for prevention is particularly strong if the

condition requires expensive services. Thus, prevention of depression would lead to greater reduction of suffering and cost savings than the prevention of spider phobia. Worldwide, depression is reckoned to be the most expensive of all adult mental disorders due to its high prevalence and impact.

4 Prevention is especially indicated if there is no effective, available and relatively inexpensive treatment for the full-blown condition. For example, autism prevention might reasonably be prioritised over the prevention of specific phobias since there are cheap, rapid and effective treatments for the latter.

Targeting risk and protective factors

Much is known about what predisposes children and adolescents to psychiatric disorders, as described in Chapter 34 and much of the rest of this book. Some risk factors are relatively specific, such as having a strong genetic loading for schizophrenia. Other risk factors are more non-specific, predisposing individuals to a range of disorders, and usually to poorer psychosocial functioning too. Examples of relatively non-specific risk factors include low IQ and academic attainments, neurodevelopmental problems, poor parenting, lack of at least one trusting relationship, disrupted care, lack of a source of self-esteem, antisocial friends and a badly organised school. Poverty is associated with a plethora of difficulties, although the fact that it indexes them well (and so can be used as a marker for a targeted intervention) does not necessarily mean it is causal. Therefore, abolishing poverty may not reduce the prevalence of disorders to a great extent (which is not to say that it is not desirable for other reasons). Since the impact of risk factors is usually cumulative (see Chapter 34), the best prevention strategy may be to target several risk factors simultaneously.

Many of the risk factors for child psychiatric disorders fall outside the clinical remit of child mental health professionals. This, of course, does not stop them from joining with other professionals and members of the general public in promoting measures that reduce these risk factors. For example, although there are many good reasons for promoting improvements in education, child mental health professionals can provide evidence from their clinical work and research that one of the knock-on benefits will be improvements in emotional and behavioural adjustment during the school years, and later in life too. Similarly, there are many good reasons for controlling traffic and reducing accidents, but child mental health professionals can add their evidence that this will reduce chronic and incapacitating psychological consequences, such as childhood PTSD or the neuropsychiatric consequences of severe childhood head injuries.

Even where symptoms or a disorder cannot be directly prevented, psychosocial functioning and quality of life may be improved by boosting protective factors. These are especially important where there are a number of risk factors operating. Box 37.2 illustrates this point with data from a study of 7,000 18-year-olds. A risky lifestyle was defined on a scale of 0–8 risks, involving being in the worst 10–20% of the population for (i) drinking alcohol; (ii) drug use; (iii) being known to social services; (iv) having special education needs; (v) truanting; (vi) having conduct problems at school; and (vii) running away from home. The presence of protective factors was counted up to maximum of 5 from (i) good physical health; (ii) higher IQ; (iii) emotional control; (iv) social skills and maturity; and (v) energy levels. In the absence of risk indices, having protective factors in childhood made little difference to crime rates. But in their presence, the protective factors conferred very substantial benefits, greatly reducing the crime rates. The implication is that to maximise the effectiveness of prevention programmes in child mental health, these programmes should promote skills and resilience as well as targeting the symptoms of disorder.

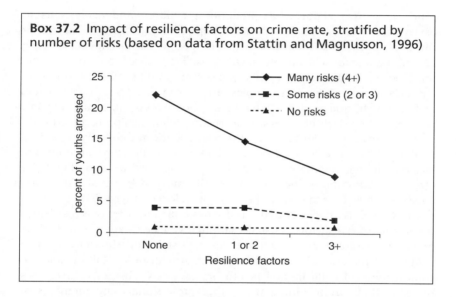

Box 37.2 Impact of resilience factors on crime rate, stratified by number of risks (based on data from Stattin and Magnusson, 1996)

An exciting prospect for preventive programmes in childhood is their potential for large effects, if they prevent disorders and improve functioning over the lifespan. Yet so far, few have been widely adopted, despite accumulating evidence of effectiveness. This is perhaps surprising where medical preventions of much more dubious benefit are endorsed by the state, for example, in the UK medication that shortens the course of influenza by only one or two days. One reason for the lack of implementation of child psychiatric preventions is the paucity, at present, of good evidence of the burden of disorders. There are few 'cost of illness' studies for most child psychiatric disorders, and no generally accepted Quality of Life (QoL) measures that allow comparison with the impact of physical disorders. Medical illness QoL measures cover dimensions such as pain, mobility, ability to communicate, and ability to care for oneself. These do not correspond closely with the ways in which mental disorders typically lead to impairment. For example, this may be by interfering with the ability to *be productive* (indexed, for example, by successful school work, successfully taking part in constructive pastimes and sporting activities, the capacity to take part appropriately and helpfully in everyday household activities, such as shared mealtimes, trips out of the house, and so on). Secondly, mental disorders may impair the ability to *maintain good relationships* with parents, siblings, peers and other adults such as teachers (indexed, for example, by successfully doing joint activities, good communication and emotional support). There are well validated measures of psychosocial functioning, but they are not generally recognised to be equivalent to quality of life measures.

The example of conduct disorder

Conduct disorder illustrates what might be achieved in preventive child psychiatry. It meets the four criteria for feasibility:

1 It is relatively easy to screen for risk, for example, short questionnaires of antisocial behaviour symptoms can be filled in by teachers and parents. A high score predicts future conduct disorder well, especially if combined with other factors such as hyperactivity and poor peer relationships, which are also covered by some screening questionnaires.
2 There are effective interventions (see discussion below).
3 There are serious and expensive consequences if the condition develops. Early-onset conduct disorder has lifelong consequences, including a markedly increased risk for frequent offending, drug addiction, low scholastic attainment, unemployment, disrupted relationships, violent injury and premature death. One community-based 'cost of illness' study found that by age 28, individuals who had had conduct disorder in childhood cost society ten times as much as controls.
4 Treatment for established disorders is expensive and typically only partly successful. While in adolescence comprehensive treatment programmes such as multisystemic therapy have been shown to reduce offending by 20–50% in demonstration projects in the USA, it is very expensive to deliver (around £20,000–£30,000 per case), and in most countries, including the UK, there is little capacity to deliver it.

Literally hundreds of randomised controlled trials have shown the effectiveness of parent training, with *clinically referred* children with conduct symptoms. Recently, a number of large randomised controlled trials have examined the effectiveness of targeted prevention programmes based on improving multiple factors in *at risk* children drawn from the general population. The Families and Schools Together project (FASTrack) took 1,000 5-year-olds who were above the 90th percentile for antisocial behaviour. Over a whole school year, half were randomised to receive the following input:(1) a weekly group on child management for their parents, including live coaching in the presence of their child; (2) individual academic tutoring for two hours a week; (3) teachers were instructed in classroom management skills; (4) twice a week all children had emotional literacy classes that stressed understanding of their own feelings including anger and frustration; and (5) each week, the index children had to spend an hour with a well-adjusted classmate, to promote friendships with prosocial, not anti-social peers. Despite the admirable theoretical grounding of this enormous prevention project, effects were modest, typically improving antisocial behaviour by only around 0.2 standard deviations, and longer-term follow-up is showing diminution of these gains, with at best some small effects on the most severe cases. However, since a total population was involved (with over 75% of the at risk families attending), the health gain is perhaps worthwhile, albeit at considerable cost.

Better results have been obtained in terms of absolute effectiveness and cost effectiveness by delivering only the parent training element, but using it to target multiple risk factors. One recent UK trial taught parents child management skills and how to read with their children, based on modern understanding of the acquisition of literacy. Antisocial behaviour, hyperactivity and reading all improved by around 0.4 standard deviations. A feature of this trial was the strong emphasis on high quality implementation, leading to high *treatment fidelity*. Evidence is emerging that treatment fidelity has a strong influence on outcomes, with effectiveness depending crucially on high quality training followed by high quality ongoing supervision with videotaping of therapist activity.

Prevention of other disorders

Programmes exist for anxiety and depressive symptoms, and these have been shown to be reasonably effective in trials. Some involve parents, and some see the child or adolescent directly. One advantage of seeing the individual directly is that typically, a substantial proportion of parents do not turn up for prevention programmes. As might be expected, they tend to come from the families at greatest risk, for example, from disadvantaged, poor single-parent families. If the child or adolescent can be seen alone at school, parental involvement in the intervention may not be necessary (although consent should be sought, and it is usually best to let them know what is going on). Drug use prevention programmes abound in the USA, usually targeting teenagers. Unfortunately only about a third of families at risk take part, and results are modest.

Prevention of risky predicaments

A number of trials of parenting programmes have shown reductions in abusive parenting and acts of child abuse. However, widespread implementation of parenting programmes in high risk groups is lacking, since agencies who might lead in offering them, such as social services departments, are often too busy trying to cope with severe child protection cases. Some shifts are occurring, but there is a long way to go. Interventions to mitigate the effects of divorce have been proven to reduce emotional and behavioural symptoms.

The future

Widespread implementation of prevention programmes will depend partly on further research to delineate the advantages and cost effectiveness of prevention programmes, and partly on persuading governments that worthwhile gains are realistic. For substantial change to occur, a shift in the beliefs of the whole population will be necessary, which will almost certainly require considerable use of broadcast media such as television. Particularly in developing countries, maternal education has been shown to be an important key to reducing family size and hence improved nutrition and material circumstances for children, which in turn promotes healthier and more rewarding lives. In the UK and the USA a number of reports have come out for professional bodies and politicians commending prevention of mental health problems and promotion of child well-being, but whether they will be acted upon to any degree is another matter.

Further reading

Allen G. (2011) *Early Intervention: Smart Investment, Massive Savings: The Second Independent Report to Her Majesty's Government*. London: Cabinet Office (An example of a politician reviewing the evidence and urging that early intervention through evidence-based programmes will save society money.)

Carr, A. (2002) *Prevention: What Works with Children and Adolescents*? Brunner-Routledge, Hove.

Conduct Problems Prevention Research Group. (2007) Fast Track randomized controlled trial to prevent externalizing psychiatric disorders: Findings from grades 3 to 9. *Journal of American Academy of Child and Adolescent Psychiatry*, **46**, 1250–1262.

Durlak J. *et al.* (2011) The impact of enhancing students' social and emotional learning: A meta-analysis of school-based universal interventions. *Child Development*, **82**, 405–432.

O'Connell, M *et al.* (2009) *Preventing Mental, Emotional, and Behavioral Disorders Among Young People: Progress and Possibilities. Reports of the US National Academy of Sciences*. Washington, DC: National Academies Press. Availabl at: http://www.nap.edu/catalog/12480.html.

Stattin, H. and Magnusson, D. (1996) Antisocial development: a holistic approach. *Development and Psychopathology*, **8**, 617–645.

Vitaro V, Tremblay RE. (2008) Clarifying and maximizing the usefulness of targeted preventive interventions. *In*: Rutter M *et al.* (eds) *Rutter's Child and Adolescent Psychiatry*, 5th edn. Wiley-Blackwell, Chichester, pp. 989–1008.

CHAPTER 38

Medication and Diet

Medication: general principles

Parents often feel uneasy about using medication to alter their children's behaviour or emotions; teachers and mental health professionals may feel the same. These concerns are understandable and partly justified. For example, children and adolescents with an intellectual disability may be given high doses of neuroleptics for long periods in a futile attempt to suppress their challenging behaviour. But even though it is true that psychotropic medication can be used unwisely, it is important to remember that suitable doses of the right medication used for an appropriate indication can be of great benefit. The continuing use of terms such as 'chemical cosh' or 'chemical straitjacket' by some journalists when describing the use of evidence-based treatments is inaccurate and unhelpful.

Prescribing for children and adolescents is not simply a matter of scaling adult doses down in proportion to body weight. Because of age-related changes in pharmacokinetics and pharmacodynamics, paediatric psychopharmacology is both quantitatively and qualitatively different from adult psychopharmacology.

Pharmacokinetics

The relationship between the dose administered and the effective concentration in the brain depends on several pharmacokinetic factors (see Box 38.1). Developmental considerations are relevant to each of these factors – these will be described first for children. Compliance may depend more on the motivation of parents and teachers than on that of the child. Absorption can be influenced by the fact that stomach acidity is generally lower in children. This reduces the rate of absorption of acidic drugs such as tricyclics (since less of the drug is in the lipid-soluble un-ionised form). Children have particularly active livers, so clearance is fast for drugs metabolised by the liver. This results in an exaggeration of the normal 'first pass' effect, that is, a particularly high fraction of the medication absorbed by the gut is cleared by the liver from the portal circulation

Child and Adolescent Psychiatry, Third Edition. Robert Goodman and Stephen Scott.
© 2012 Robert Goodman and Stephen Scott. Published 2012 by John Wiley & Sons, Ltd.

before it even reaches the systemic circulation. Distribution is affected by the relatively high proportion of extracellular fluid in young children; the greater diversion of medication to the extracellular fluid tends to reduce the amount in blood and brain. The blood-brain barrier is more permeable in children than adults so drugs can get through more easily, but this easier access to the brain may be partly offset by a higher concentration of drug-binding proteins in the cerebrospinal fluid.

Box 38.1 Relationship between the dose administered and the effective concentration in the brain

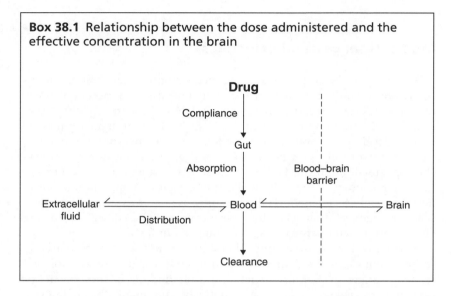

The various pharmacokinetic differences between children and adults pull in opposite directions, with bioavailability being reduced in children by faster clearance, slower absorption and a greater volume of distribution, but increased by greater blood-brain permeability. The effect of rapid hepatic clearance often dominates. As a consequence, weight-for-weight doses for psychotropic drugs are often 50–100% higher for children than adults.

The need for relatively high doses decreases as children get older, dropping fairly sharply around puberty. By mid to late adolescence, drug dosage follows adult norms.

Blood levels are useful for adjusting the dosage of some drugs, such as tricyclics and lithium, but are unhelpful with other drugs, for example, stimulants. Children and adolescents are very variable in their response to medication and the dosage prescribed needs to be titrated primarily against clinical response, seeing recommended drug dosages (and recommended blood levels) as helpful guidelines rather than rigid limits. Because the appropriate dosage is hard to predict in advance, it is sensible to start with a low dose and work up slowly. Once-a-day doses improve compliance but divided doses may be needed to reduce peak and trough effects.

Pharmacodynamics

Once a drug has reached the brain, its effect depends on its interactions with drug receptors. There are major developmental changes in the number and relative proportion of different types of receptors. Since a single drug may activate multiple receptor types, and since these various receptor types may have markedly different effects, developmental changes in the balance of receptor types can result in the same drug having very different effects on children and adults. Perhaps this is why stimulants can produce euphoria in adults but not in children, tending, if anything, to make children dysphoric. Psychotropic drugs that work in adults do not necessarily work in children, and vice versa. Furthermore, drugs familiar to adult psychiatrists for one set of disorders may be used by child and adolescent psychiatrists for a rather different set of disorders. For example, tricyclics work well for adult depression but not for childhood or adolescent depression, yet relatively low doses of tricyclics can be used to treat childhood enuresis or ADHD.

Medication: specific groups of drugs

Stimulants

Either methylphenidate or dexamfetamine is usually the drug of choice for the treatment of ADHD (including the subgroup of ADHD that meets the ICD-10 criteria for 'hyperkinesis'). They have mixed dopaminergic and noradrenergic actions. Indications and side effects are discussed in detail in Chapter 5. They have a powerful effect, usually reducing ADHD by around one standard deviation. Since most of those treated with stimulants are two or three standard deviations above the average, stimulants typically reduce rather than abolish ADHD symptoms – emphasising the need for educational and behavioural help too. When ADHD is associated with disruptive behavioural problems, stimulant treatment often improves these behavioural problems as well as the ADHD symptoms.

The fact that stimulants have a short half-life and duration of action can be an advantage: doses in the morning and at midday improve attention for schoolwork and homework, but unwanted suppression of appetite and sleep wear off by evening, allowing the individual to catch up on food intake and then get to sleep. Disadvantages of the short half-life include fluctuating effectiveness during the day and rebound worsening of symptoms in the late afternoon or early evening. If these are troublesome, slow-release preparations are available.

ADHD in children with autistic spectrum problems or an intellectual disability may also be helped by stimulants, but sometimes at the cost of a worsening in repetitive behaviours (see Chapters 4 and 28).

Given mixed evidence as to whether stimulants usually precipitate or aggravate tics, some clinicians avoid using stimulants for treating ADHD when the child or adolescent has a tic disorder or a strong family history of tic disorders, employing alternatives such as guanfacine or imipramine instead. Other clinicians still choose stimulants as their first-line treatment for ADHD in those with tics, using low to moderate doses if possible, and watching carefully to see whether tics worsen.

Atomoxetine

This is an alternative to the stimulants. It is an inhibitor of the noradrenaline transporter, thereby raising synaptic levels of noradrenaline – but also indirectly increasing dopamine levels in the frontal cortex. It has a smaller average effect size than the stimulants (around 0.6 standard deviations) and it takes longer to become effective (2-6 weeks). It is often used as a second-line treatment when stimulants have not worked or have had unacceptable adverse effects. Atomoxetine can have adverse effects of its own, including nausea and sedation.

Alpha-2 agonists

Clonidine and guanfacine are specific alpha-2 agonists that can reduce the symptoms of ADHD and tics, and may sometimes be the treatment of choice for the combination of tics and ADHD. While clonidine has been around for longer, guanfacine is often preferred nowadays because it causes less sedation and does not result in rebound hypertension after withdrawal. Alpha-2 agonists generally have a smaller effect size than stimulants for ADHD and a smaller effect size than neuroleptics for tics, but they may nevertheless be useful for either ADHD or tics when other medications have failed or resulted in unacceptable adverse effects. Particularly in the treatment of tics, affected individuals and their families may prefer a lesser reduction in symptoms from guanfacine to a greater reduction from neuroleptics – making this choice in order to avoid serious neuroleptics adverse effects such as dyskinesias (from typical neuroleptics) or weight gain and metabolic disturbance (from atypical neuroleptics).

Tricyclic antidepressants (TCAs)

Nocturnal enuresis can be treated with low to moderate doses of TCAs (for example, 25–75 mg of imipramine nocte), though it is almost always preferable to use a behavioural approach or desmopressin instead (see Chapter 17). ADHD can also be treated with low doses of TCAs if stimulants have failed or are contraindicated (see Chapters 5 and 13). In full dosage, clomipramine (a TCA that acts primarily on serotonin reuptake) has been shown to be helpful for obsessive-compulsive disorder (see Chapter 14). Judging largely from adult evidence, TCAs may also be useful in panic disorder. Meta-analyses do not support the use of TCAs in the treatment of depressed children and adolescents.

   In the low doses used in the treatment of enuresis and hyperactivity, TCAs have relatively few side effects. With high doses, however, common side effects include dry mouth, headache, sedation and malaise. There is also a risk of cardiac arrhythmias and sudden death, especially with desimipramine. To reduce this risk, an ECG should be carried out before embarking on anything more than low-dose treatment, in order to check that there are no pre-existing arrhythmias or cardiac conduction problems. Further ECGs should be obtained as the dose is progressively increased, to monitor for the warning signs of prolonged P-R and Q-T intervals.

Selective serotonin reuptake inhibitors (SSRIs)

These are of proven value in the treatment of obsessive-compulsive disorder in children and adolescents (see Chapter 14). Fluoxetine is the only antidepressant approved by the US Food and Drug Administration (FDA) for the treatment of depression in children and adolescents, reflecting trial evidence that is stronger for fluoxetine than other SSRIs. The superiority of fluoxetine over placebo is clearest for severe depression – the benefits are less certain for mild and moderate depression. It is currently uncertain whether fluoxetine has a greater effect when combined with cognitive-behavioural therapy (see Chapter 10). There are concerns that SSRIs increase the risk of self-harm or suicide. In the light of reported levels of adverse effects with different SSRIs, the British Government guidelines do not support the use of SSRIs other than fluoxetine for depressed children or adolescents (see Chapter 10). There is limited evidence that SSRIs may be helpful for some anxiety disorders and selective mutism (see Chapters 9 and 16). Common side effects include nausea, vomiting, agitation, insomnia and headaches.

Monoamine oxidase inhibitors (MAOIs)

The availability of a selective and reversible MAOI, moclobemide, has made this class of drugs easier and safer to prescribe, since adverse interactions with a normal diet are now very unlikely. Nonetheless, the use of MAOIs for ADHD, social phobia and resistant depression should be regarded as experimental approaches for specialist centres only.

Neuroleptics (antipsychotics)

These are particularly useful in the treatment of children and adolescents with psychotic disorders, tic disorders and mania (see Chapters 11, 15 and 23). They may sometimes be useful for children and adolescents with autistic spectrum disorders or an intellectual disability (see Chapters 4 and 28). There is limited evidence that low doses of neuroleptics (particularly atypical neuroleptics) can add to the benefits of stimulant treatment for ADHD. Given the uncertainty and the risk of side effects, this combination should probably only be tried by specialist clinics. Neuroleptics are not appropriate long-term treatments for the aggressive behaviour of children with an intellectual disability (see Chapter 28).

Neuroleptics should always be used with considerable caution because of their potentially serious side effects. Sedation can interfere with learning. In the first few weeks of treatment, neuroleptics commonly cause extrapyramidal side effects such as acute dystonic reactions or Parkinsonism – a risk that is lower with atypical neuroleptics. When using typical neuroleptics, such as haloperidol, there is a case for giving antimuscarinic drugs, such as benzhexol, prophylactically to prevent extrapyramidal reactions. The antimuscarinic can be withdrawn after about six weeks because it is rarely needed beyond that time and often does more long-term harm than good. Clozapine is an atypical neuroleptic that can be very useful in the treatment of resistant schizophrenia, but that is not much used otherwise because it can cause blood dyscrasias, especially in children.

The Neuroleptic Malignant Syndrome is an uncommon but potentially fatal hazard. The four cardinal features of the full syndrome are pyrexia, muscular rigidity, mental changes, such as mild confusion, and evidence of autonomic dysfunction, for example, pallor, sweating or shivering. Blood tests may show raised creatinine phosphokinase and a high white count. Since the early symptoms can progress in less than 48 hours to hyperpyrexia, rigidity, circulatory collapse and multiple organ failure, it is obviously essential to monitor carefully any child or adolescent who develops suspicious symptoms while on neuroleptics, discontinuing the medication immediately if suspicions seem to be confirmed. The full syndrome requires intensive care and muscle relaxants.

Long-term treatment with neuroleptics can lead to the eventual emergence of dyskinesias, which may be irreversible even if medication is stopped. The risk of these tardive dyskinesias is related to the lifetime dose, and may be further increased if antimuscarinics have also been administered for long periods. There is little evidence for the frequent assertion that neurological damage also increases the risk of tardive dyskinesias.

Lithium

This is widely used for the treatment and prophylaxis of bipolar affective disorder in adults, and may be of similar value in children and adolescents, though the evidence is suggestive rather than conclusive. Lithium may possibly also have a role in the treatment of severe outbursts of aggression that are triggered by minimal provocation and that have been resistant to appropriate psychological management. Lithium dosage is adjusted to obtain a plasma level of around 0.7–1.0 mmol/litre on samples obtained 12 hours after the most recent dose. Common side effects include nausea, fine tremor, thirst, polyuria and enuresis. Since there is a risk of hypothyroidism, thyroid function tests should be carried out before and during treatment. Routine monitoring of renal function is probably unnecessary. Excessive dosage leads to potentially fatal toxicity. The common early signs are coarse tremor, worsening gastrointestinal disturbance and mild confusion. Since these warning signs of toxicity may be less prominent in those with intellectual disability, lithium needs to be used with particular caution in this group.

Antiepileptic medications as psychotropics

Carbamazepine, valproate or lamotrigine can be used instead of lithium to prevent recurrences of bipolar affective disorder, though the evidence is weak and there is a risk of serious adverse effects, for example, hepatic failure and pancreatitis with valproate and toxic epidermal necrolysis with lamotrigine. Beyond this possible indication, there is no good evidence that antiepileptic medications improve emotional or behavioural problems in children and adolescents who do not have epilepsy (even if they do have minor EEG abnormalities). However, newer medications such as pregabalin have trial evidence of effectiveness among adults for the treatment of anxiety disorders and have been prescribed for adolescents by specialists with experience of the condition and the medication. For those children and adolescents who do have definite seizures, antiepileptic medications can have both positive and negative effects on psychopathology: reducing seizures sometimes improves mental health, but antiepileptic medication can also result in sedation, irritability or hyperactivity.

Benzodiazepines, antihistamines and other minor tranquillizers

Although these are among the most commonly prescribed psychotropic drugs for children and adolescents, they are also, arguably, the least justified. Long-term problems with sleep or anxiety problems are much more likely to respond to psychological approaches. Benzodiazepines may sometimes be useful in the treatment of intense acute anxiety, for example, before a medical procedure (though it is better still to desensitise individuals in advance if they are going to encounter feared procedures or situations repeatedly).

Diet

Doctors have been prescribing diets for millennia, and diets are still an important treatment for a wide range of physical problems, including eczema, migraine, phenylketonuria and intractable epilepsy. Specific foods may need to be avoided, because they trigger off allergic reactions, or because they have other sorts of adverse effects. As one example of a non-allergic effect, fava beans contain oxidising agents that interact with an inherited enzyme deficiency to precipitate haemolytic crises in individuals with favism. When it is unclear how a particular dietary ingredient has an adverse effect, it is better to speak of dietary *intolerance* rather than dietary *allergy*.

Does dietary intolerance trigger child psychiatric problems? Food colours in the diet do appear to make things worse in some children with ADHD, though the effect size is not large. There is stronger evidence for the clinical utility of an approach based on the 'few foods' diet. Individuals with ADHD are initially started out on a very restricted diet that excludes not only artificial additives but also many natural foods, including dairy and wheat products and most fruits. If there is no improvement after two or three weeks, the diet is abandoned. The few foods approach only works for some people with ADHD.

If behaviour does improve on the few foods diet, the excluded foods are re-introduced one at a time to identify which of them trigger behaviour problems. In some instances, it is possible to carry out double-blind challenges to establish whether a particular food really does make a difference. Controlled evaluations do suggest that this approach can identify foods that worsen behaviour. There is no one culprit – different individuals are intolerant to different foods, and many are intolerant to several foods. Artificial additives are common culprits, but so, too, are dairy products, chocolate, wheat, oranges, tomatoes and eggs. It is unusual for an individual to react only to additives; most of those who are sensitive to additives are also sensitive to one or more natural foods as well. Although diet is often thought of as a treatment for ADHD, the individuals who respond to the 'few foods' approach typically become less irritable and disruptive as well as less hyperactive and inattentive. Whether the same approach would help individuals who were irritable and oppositional but not hyperactive is unclear.

The few foods approach is very hard work for all concerned and not all families can see it through to completion. Cooking a special diet for weeks on end is more than some busy parents can manage and buying special foods can also be very expensive. Furthermore, there is little point embarking on this approach if the child or adolescent is likely to cheat frequently by stealing from the fridge, buying forbidden foods, or eating other children's school lunches! Is it possible to predict in advance who is likely to respond to diet? Unfortunately, it is not possible to predict from blood or skin tests (not to mention more dubious tests involving hair analysis or dowsing). Two clinical pointers to a good response are, first, that parents have previously noted reactions to food and, second, that the child or adolescent has cravings for particular foods (which may turn out to be the foods that trigger behavioural problems). Parental observations and the child or adolescent's cravings can be used to design a tailor-made exclusion diet; if behaviour is improved, the excluded foods are reintroduced one by one to identify the culprits. How this 'short cut' compares with the few foods approach has yet to be formally evaluated.

Other physical treatments

- *Electroconvulsive therapy* (ECT) is rarely used for children and adolescents and has not been adequately evaluated. It may be considered when adequate trials of medication have not relieved severe depression or catatonia.
- *Surgery*. Psychosurgery is not indicated for children or adolescents, but it is worth noting that successful epilepsy surgery may cure children or adolescents not only of their seizures but also of associated behavioural problems. For example, hemispherectomy for hemiplegic children and adolescents with intractable seizures often relieves not only seizures but hyperactivity and irritability too. It is unclear whether this behavioural improvement stems from the abolition of seizures, the withdrawal of antiepileptic medications, or the removal of dysfunctional brain tissue.

Subject review

Riddle MA *et al.* (2001) Paediatric psychopharmacology. *Journal of Child Psychology and Psychiatry* **42**, 73–90.

Volkow N, Swanson J. (2008) Basic neuropharmacology. *In*: Rutter M *et al.* (eds) *Rutter's Child and Adolescent Psychiatry*, 5th edn. Wiley-Blackwell, Chichester, pp. 212–233.

Further reading

Committee on Toxicity of Food (2000) *Adverse Reactions to Food and Food Ingredients*. Department of Health, London.

Daughton JM, Kratochvil CJ. (2009) Review of ADHD pharmacotherapies: Advantages, disadvantages, and clinical pearls. *Journal of the American Academy of Child and Adolescent Psychiatry* **48**, 240–248.

CHAPTER 39

Behaviourally-based Treatments

Behavioural methods used to be based on the notion that all behaviours are learned, and so can be unlearned. However, a less extreme form of behaviourism that is perhaps more acceptable states that the expression of most behaviour is influenced by antecedent events and consequent responses. Altering these may change the frequency of the behaviour.

Classical conditioning involves stimulus-contingent effects, as described by Pavlov in 1927. A previously neutral stimulus becomes associated with one that triggers the physiological response, and in time the new stimulus alone (now called *conditioned*) leads to a similar response. Treatments based on this model condition new physiological responses, such as relaxation to the stimulus. Examples that work well with children and adolescents include systematic desensitisation for post-traumatic stress disorder and phobias.

Operant conditioning involves response-contingent effects, as described by Skinner in 1938. Responses to stimuli, or indeed behaviours of any kind, become more frequent or stronger if they lead to rewarding consequences (*positive reinforcement*), or to escape from unpleasant consequences (*negative reinforcement*). Behaviours become less frequent if previously rewarding consequences are taken away (*extinction*), or if they lead to unpleasant consequences (*punishment*). Treatments based on this model consistently change the contingencies that follow a behaviour. This may be to increase desired behaviour through rewards (a star chart for clean underpants without soiling), or to reduce undesired behaviour through punishment (being made to clean the floor after throwing dinner on it). This approach also includes ensuring that undesirable symptoms or behaviours are not unintentionally rewarded, for example, ensuring that a child is not rewarded for psychogenic abdominal pain by being allowed to miss school and stay at home.

Social learning theory, developed by Bandura in the 1960s, led to a general widening of the behavioural model to recognise the primacy of human relationships in influencing learning. In children and adolescents, Patterson confirmed the central role of parental attention in providing rewards, and showed that in families where there is little positive interaction, children

---

Child and Adolescent Psychiatry, Third Edition. Robert Goodman and Stephen Scott.
© 2012 Robert Goodman and Stephen Scott. Published 2012 by John Wiley & Sons, Ltd.

may behave antisocially to get attention, even though this may be of a negative kind. Treatments based on this model increase the attention paid by carers to children when they behave desirably (for example, by speaking warmly to a child who is playing quietly) and withdraw attention when the child is behaving undesirably (for example, by turning away and stopping talking to a child who is screaming). An example of this approach working well is the use of parent training to reduce a child's antisocial behaviour.

Behavioural methods in practice

Assessment

Rather than initially ascribing meaning to a behaviour, a functional analysis is performed. The **A**ntecedents, **B**ehaviour itself, and **C**onsequences (ABC) are carefully characterised in great detail (see Box 39.1). Examples of antecedents: before a tantrum in a 4-year-old: mother's nagging demand at bedtime, or, sibling takes toy; before a panic attack in a 15-year-old: outdoors on a big playing field, or, in a crowded marketplace; before psychogenic abdominal pain in a 10-year-old: a row between parents, or, due to hand in difficult homework. Sometimes changing the antecedents alone ('stimulus control') is sufficient to alleviate the problem.

Box 39.1 An ABC analysis

Antecedent events (the setting)	Experiences for child just prior to behaviour People present Places Times of day Situations
Behaviour	Nature: detailed description of what actually happened Onset date Frequency Severity Duration of episodes
Consequences	Changes in demands and expectations of child by others Changes in attention and social set-up Attainment of child's immediate goals and wants Impact on siblings and parents

---

Methods for gathering information include: detailed behavioural descriptions from parents, charts, diaries, visits to home or school to observe behaviour in context, or videos of this.

Behavioural analyses thus concentrate on the here and now of what actually happens. The meaning to the parents of the behaviour ('he's becoming a criminal like his uncle'), and their explanations for it ('it's the crisps, doctor') may usefully be explored, but are not part of a strict behaviourist approach.

Negotiation of goals with parents and young person

1 Specify the target behaviours as precisely as possible. Many parents find this difficult, having diffuse concerns: 'he's disobedient', 'he's a Jekyll and Hyde', 'she's sad', etc. The work is to help the parent work out specifically what is worrying.

2 Assess the impact of the behaviours on the child's or adolescent's life, and on that of the siblings and parents, considering the following domains:

   (a) emotional/personal impact
   (b) social
   (c) developmental
   (d) learning/competence
   (e) self-esteem.

   Going through this list often helps the parents review the overall impact from their child's point of view, rather than just their own. For example, they may have arrived concerned by the smell and inconvenience to themselves of a boy who soils. Assessing the impact may make them aware of the social impact on friendships and emotions. This is often helpful in reducing negativity, and in engaging sympathy and motivation to implement the treatment programme. Parents also become fully aware of the long-term disadvantages of the current situation, rather than just the immediate inconvenience, which may further add to the gains they can visualise from engaging in therapy.

3 Agree the desired outcome in behavioural terms. Again, this will not be a generality ('he should become nice to me') but specific ('he will dress himself after being asked only once in the morning, without shouting at me; he will be in bed by 8.30 at night'). If a child has frequent major tantrums lasting over five minutes involving kicking and throwing, an appropriate target may be to reduce this to once a week. Total abolition is unrealistic and unnecessary.

4 Formulate the positive behaviours desired. This may not come easily to parents, who are more inclined to think in terms of stopping negative behaviours such as fighting, running, shouting, wetting the bed, etc. The desired behaviours in each case might be: play nicely with your brother, walk calmly, speak quietly and use the toilet properly. The major part of behavioural work is not the elimination of unwanted behaviour (a child who is only aware of what not to do has no help in finding his or her direction, and if totally obedient would stay rooted to the spot), but the promotion of desired behaviour in its place, so the unwanted behaviour simply fades away. Once the desired behaviours have been formulated, it is possible to start planning an intervention plan, with emphasis on

how to make it clear to the child or adolescent what is desired, how to introduce it into the individual's repertoire and practise it, and how to reward it once it starts occurring.

5 Explain in a way that can be understood by everyone in the family:

   (a) why the child or adolescent is currently behaving the way they are, framing the explanation in terms of learned habits and the circumstances maintaining them, rather than in terms of fixed character traits or inner conflicts.

   (b) that this way of looking at things shows that there is a possibility for change, but this will require some change from everyone.

Techniques

To increase desired behaviours:

- *Positive reinforcement*: reward desired behaviour through praise and rewards.
- *Negative reinforcement*: remove aversive stimulus after desired behaviour has occurred (for example, stop nagging when child goes to bed).
- *Explain underlying theory to parents, and child*: this includes helping them formulate the treatment in a way that makes sense to them and is attractive.
- *Train skills* with rehearsal, and role-play.
- *Remove interfering conditions*.

To reduce undesired behaviours:

- *Stimulus change*: remove or change controlling antecedent stimuli.
- *Extinction*. This should follow removal of previous reward identified with reinforcement of the behaviour, for example, no longer giving attention to child who is naughty. Parents need to be warned that for a period, the child will work even harder to get back to the previous status quo and behaviour may worsen, the 'extinction burst'. Ignoring may mean involving more than just parents, for example, preventing an aggressive youth getting admiration from his peers.
- *Differential reinforcement* of incompatible behaviour. As noted above, this principle is central to much behavioural work. The desired or prosocial behaviour that should be occurring is identified and rewarded, such as sitting nicely during mealtimes instead of running around, playing cooperatively instead of fighting, spending the night in the bedroom rather than wandering downstairs, etc.
- *Punishment*. This can involve the application of mildly noxious stimuli following inappropriate behaviour. In everyday childrearing this is frequently a telling off or verbal criticism. Mild occasional physical punishment, such as a light smack once a week, has not been shown to be deleterious to children, whereas prolonged heavy painful punishment in an atmosphere of cold, hostile rejection is certainly deleterious. Physical punishment is often popular with parents as it may temporarily suppress behaviour, and so be very rewarding for the parent, but often

the behaviour re-emerges later and has not been truly extinguished. It may have a role in immediate suppression of damaging behaviour, such as putting fingers into power sockets, or running across the road, but needs to be followed by explanation and plentiful reinforcement of actions incompatible with those being punished. This is very different from the destructive cycles that can occur when desperate parents use harsh physical punishment in extreme, inconsistent, retaliatory ways, without accompanying choices or encouragement for more acceptable alternative behaviours. For all these reasons and because of instances of abuse, application of aversive stimuli is seldom a part of therapeutic programmes, which tend to use other methods, seeing reduced parental use of physical punishments as an index of successful substitution of more appropriate methods. Even mild physical punishment is against the law in some countries, providing all parents with a clear message that they need to rely entirely on non-physical approaches to discipline.

- *Time out*. This is shorthand for 'time out from positive reinforcement'. Usually it involves taking a child aged around 3–8 away from the context where the behaviour occurred, to a dull quiet place for a few minutes. This differs from extinction since the child is removed from all the usual general social stimulation and reinforcement, not just from a specific identified reinforcer. It has the advantage of being a high-impact procedure that is not noxious (although it may well be perceived by the child as a punishment). There are a number of practicalities to setting up a time out programme. These include the following: the rules must be clear, and it should be given for fairly major infractions; a warning and an alternative behaviour should be given to the child before applying it ('please stop hitting and sit down or you'll go to time out'); the child should be taken there in a calm way, using physical force if necessary but not hurting the child; the space or room must be cleared of entertaining items; the parent or teacher must keep an eye on the child but not engage in conversation or recrimination (this would unwittingly be giving attention); and the child must be calm for a minute before coming out.
- *Response cost*. Here specified amounts of reinforcers are withdrawn from the child when he or she displays the unwanted behaviour. This requires that a previous reward system is in place, involving money, points, privileges, etc.; there has to be something positive to withdraw.
- *Over-correction*. The child is required not only to put right what he or she did wrong, but do more by way of restitution. A variant gets the child to over-learn a response physically incompatible with the original misbehaviour, for example, repeatedly taking shoes off on entering a house having trailed mud in previously.
- *Desensitisation*. The repeated exposure to an aversive stimulus in a situation where the child is relaxed and reassured. For example, going up through a hierarchy of phobic stimuli while the child is practising relaxation techniques with the mother present. This method is notably successful in treating PTSD and specific phobias.

A note on rewards

- Every child is different. Help parents decide what is motivating, and always check with the child or adolescent and ask for their suggestions.
- Rewards may be intangible, such as time with parents, etc. Tangible rewards do not have to be expensive; they can be sitting in a parent's place at dinner, wearing special clothes, extra TV etc. There are many other alternatives to money and presents.
- They need to be given as soon as possible after the behaviour has occurred (not a bike for Christmas).
- Check what unintended rewards a child or adolescent is getting for undesired behaviour (for example, peer approval). Be aware of when desired behaviour is occurring and monitor if it is being rewarded (is the child actually being ignored when she is playing quietly?).
- Check that rewards are being consistently applied.
- Switch rewards every few days. Many parents will say 'I tried that, it worked for a few days then didn't work.' But how many adults would find the same chocolates just as exciting after getting them for ten days in a row?
- When stuck for a reward, consider the Premack principle, which is to use as a reward what a person chooses to spend most of their free time doing. This could be playing on the computer, lying in bed, or whatever is acceptable. For an autistic child, it could include twirling their hands in front of their eyes.
- With older children and adolescents (and parents!), cultivate self-rewarding. Like rewards given by others, these may be intangible (for example, praising oneself for good behaviour), or tangible (for example, a treat).

Implementation

To learn a new behaviour, a individual must know *what* to do, *how* to do it and *when* to do it. If parents are to change their child's behaviour, they, too, must be equally clear. For the change to occur will require competence, or being able to do it, and *performance* repeatedly, which requires the will to do it.

The intervention will only rarely consist of the mechanical implementation of standardised techniques for altering the frequency of behaviours. Rather, most contemporary behavioural therapy draws upon these behavioural principles but adapts them into a wider context. General measures employed include:

- *Planning ahead,* for example, reducing school pressures on a phobic girl, avoiding taking a hyperactive boy to the supermarket, taking fight-prone siblings out *to the park rather than keeping them indoors.*
- *Negotiating with the child or adolescent.* Many parents make what seem to them to be reasonable demands, only to find them disobeyed, which leads to a major confrontation. Getting parents to negotiate basic situations (for example, bedtime routines, or what the family does on

Saturdays) pays big dividends. However, this requires parents to stop and listen to their children and find a compromise that achieves the goal. In return, children and adolescents get to realise their views have been taken into account.

- *Addressing beliefs and mood states of family members*. Early behavioural programmes were successful, but only in that proportion of cases where the parents carried out the instructions, which was often only half or less of those enrolled. Most practitioners now would spend a considerable amount of time addressing parents' fears and worries ('If I leave him to scream I feel a bad mother', 'I can't bear to ignore crying out at night since it reminds me of being left as a child').

- Adapting the programme according to progress. This is central to behavioural approaches, where success is carefully measured, and if it is not occurring then this is examined in detail and the plan revised, or a new strategy tried, or a course of action more acceptable to the parent found. Rather like a game of chess, particular moves do not produce victory in themselves, but have to be repeatedly adapted as part of an overall strategy to succeed.

Evaluation of behaviourally-based therapies

Criticisms

Behaviour therapy is soulless and ignores the world of the mind, treating people like dogs or pigeons. Motivation, dreams, fears and beliefs about ways of doing things are ignored. By concentrating on the presented symptom, a behaviour therapist may entirely miss the broader meaning of the difficulty for the individual and the worries and stresses that led to the difficulty arising in the first place. By thinking in a 'scientific, logical, linear' manner, the behaviour therapist may miss the network of relationships and systems in the background that are maintaining the symptom behaviour. A child's tantrums may be the result of a disturbed attachment relationship with the mother and require far more than a few star charts to put right. No place is given for the intangible but essential parts of the therapeutic relationship. Some problems, such as a disability or a bereavement, cannot be taken away. Yet families and children often gain a great deal from being helped to come to terms with these predicaments and can move forward with sympathetic counselling. It is chiefly effective only for circumscribed complaints, and cannot tackle general relationship difficulties as may occur following sexual abuse or neglectful parenting.

Rejoinders

While early behaviourism in the 1950s and 1960s may have been somewhat mechanical, nowadays it is an approach that is flexible, and practitioners take the individual's meanings, beliefs and relationships into consideration. Parents. adolescents and children like having the opportunity to do something practical to alleviate a problem, rather than just sitting and talking about feelings. Through reductions in problems and increases in good times, whole relationships do change and this is very important. The therapist shares the agenda with the family, rather than making clever formulations hidden from them.

Outcome studies

There have been an enormous number (literally thousands) of well-conducted single-case studies, and hundreds of randomised controlled trials of behavioural treatments for children and adolescents. Bodily functions such as eating, sleeping, wetting and soiling have been successfully tackled, with effect sizes of 0.7–1.5 standard deviations. Antisocial behaviour in prepubertal children has repeatedly been shown to be improved, with typical effect sizes of 0.4–0.8 SD. Hyperactivity is helped in the short term for as long as the behavioural contingencies are applied, but the changes are not usually long-lasting and the effect size is only around 0.2–0.4 SD. Emotional disorders such as school refusal and psychogenic pain have responded, but usually with less dramatic improvements. However, some emotional disorders respond very well: cures of specific phobias in just a few sessions are common, and cures or substantial improvements in OCD occur in many cases after a course of about ten sessions of exposure therapy with response prevention.

Subject review

Scott S. (2008) Parenting programs. *In*: Rutter M *et al.* (eds) *Rutter's Child and Adolescent Psychiatry*, 5th edn. Wiley-Blackwell, Chichester, pp. 1046–1061.

Scott S, Yule W. (2008) Behavioral therapies. *In*: Rutter M *et al.* (eds) *Rutter's Child and Adolescent Psychiatry*, 5th edn. Wiley-Blackwell, Chichester, pp. 1009–1025.

Further reading

Ball T, Bush A, Emerson F. (2004) *Psychological Interventions for Severely Challenging Behaviours Shown by People with Learning Disabilities*. Leicester: British Psychological Society.

Beidel D *et al*. (2000) Behavioral treatment of childhood social phobia. *Journal of Consulting and Clinical Psychology* **68**: 1072–80.

Glazener CMA, Evans JHC, Peto RE. (2005) Alarm interventions for nocturnal enuresis in children. *Cochrane Database of Systematic Reviews* (1) CD01567.

CHAPTER 40

Cognitive, Interpersonal and Other Individual Therapies

We use the term individual therapies to refer to interventions based on a therapist seeing a child or adolescent on their own and working mainly via talking with them to change their beliefs, feelings and behaviour. Here we describe four varieties: cognitive therapy, social problem-solving skills therapy, interpersonal therapy, and counselling and psychotherapy. They differ from behavioural theories that chiefly address external contingencies, and family therapies that address how the family unit functions.

Cognitive therapy

A cognitive approach goes beyond externally observable behaviour and acknowledges the internal world of thoughts and mental schemas, if not feelings. Cognitions are recognised as having an independent effect on behaviour, and not being just epiphenomena secondary to external events and internal physiology. The mind is recognised as being able to direct behaviour as well as be aware of it.

Behavioural methods are especially useful in situations where:

1 External contingencies can be controlled, for example, in a family with parents present for several hours a day, or in a school class.
2 Individuals have cognitive abilities that are less well developed, for example, young children, those with low intellect.
3 Problems are easily identifiable by observable behaviours.

Cognitive methods can be especially useful for situations where:

1 The individual is less constrained by external contingencies and is relying more on self-direction and choosing their own immediate environment, for example, out on the street, in the school playground, or alone away from home.
2 Individuals have the capacity for independent thought, which can be translated into action.

Child and Adolescent Psychiatry, Third Edition. Robert Goodman and Stephen Scott.
© 2012 Robert Goodman and Stephen Scott. Published 2012 by John Wiley & Sons, Ltd.

3 Problems are primarily within the mind and not primarily observable behaviours, for example, anxiety, depression, traumatic memories.

Cognitive approaches draw upon the behaviourist tradition of precise measurement and objective empirical validation, and are often combined with behavioural interventions – when this is the case, the term cognitive-behavioural therapy (CBT) is often used. Such approaches are backed by a body of evidence demonstrating cognitive distortions or deficits in various disorders affecting children and adolescents, including aggression, ADHD, anxiety, PTSD and depression.

While cognitive approaches designed for specific disorders tend to focus on the content and structure of specific cognitions within the domain in question, interpersonal problem-solving approaches focus on enhancing the general processes required to generate solutions to everyday social problems. Rather than providing the 'right' way of thinking about the problem, this approach emphasises helping children generate their own, more useful, solutions.

Cognitive approaches for specific disorders

Depression

Distortions in thinking similar to those found in adults have also been demonstrated in children and adolescents. Their mental schemata will often be distorted so that negative events are experienced as internally caused (that is, their fault, rather than due, say, to bad luck), stable (that is, this is always what happens, rather than an unusual one-off event), and general (that is, this is typical of the whole of all areas of their life, rather than just this specific domain). They typically have pervasively negative view of the past, themselves now, and the future. Treatment programmes typically include:

1 Cognitive restructuring, involving confronting children and adolescents about their lack of evidence for their distorted perceptions.
2 Self-control skills promoting consequences for action (praise self more, punish self less), self-monitoring (paying attention to positive things they do), self-evaluation (setting less perfectionist standards for self) and assertiveness training.
3 Social skills, including methods to initiate interactions, maintain interactions, handle conflict and use relaxation and imagery.

A number of randomised controlled trials have shown that children and adolescents who receive CT for depression clearly do better than waiting list controls and those receiving traditional counselling. However, only about half respond, and even then the subsequent relapse rate is high, with a further 50% of these becoming depressed again; in adults, this relapse rate is similar for drug treatment. In adolescents, CT is useful since the evidence that antidepressants work is far less extensive than in adults. Refinements and adjunctive treatments in addition to basic CT packages are currently being developed, including relapse-prevention programmes and self-administered treatments (using DVDs, or online). However, two major trials in recent years, one in the USA ('TADS') and one in the UK ('ADAPT') showed that while CBT alone is effective for depression, medication (fluoxetine) is more so. Precise decision rules are still being researched for when CT should tried, when medication, and when both (see Chapter 10).

Anxiety and fear

Again, practice in children and adolescents has followed that in adults. Similar techniques are used, including correction of distortions in thinking; identification of physiological responses, body sensations and their interpretation; development of positive self-talk, guided imagery enabling mastery over fear-provoking situations; relaxation during exposure; and behavioural experiments whereby the child or adolescent puts themselves into the anxiety-provoking situation and monitors whether what happens is as bad as they feared. Randomised trials show good results, with over half of cases being returned to the normal range.

Aggression

Aggressive children and adolescents have been shown to do the following:

- Perceive far more hostile cues in social situations.
- Attend to fewer cues when interpreting the meaning of others' behaviour.
- Attribute hostile intentions to others in ambiguous situations.
- Underperceive their own level of aggressiveness.
- Generate fewer verbal, assertive solutions to conflict situations but more physically attacking ones.
- Believe this aggression will reduce aversive reactions from others and gain them tangible positive outcomes.

Aggressive children and adolescents additionally believe aggressive behaviour will increase their self-esteem, and value dominance and revenge more, and social affiliation less, than controls. Interventions usually target these cognitive anomalies, but also address general interpersonal social skills (see below), with a particular emphasis on slowing down automatic, immediate reactions to provocative situations in order to allow more deliberation about suitable responses. Trials have shown significant reductions in aggressive behaviour using social skills methods, persisting at one- and three-year follow-ups. Effects in prepubertal children are enhanced by the addition of parent-training programmes. However, purely cognitive approaches mostly fail to have any effect in real-life situations: aggressive adolescents can learn to stop, calm down and choose a negotiated settlement to a hypothetical dispute, but direct observation during encounters with peers, and self-reports of numbers of fights tend to show little impact. It may be that the fast physiological arousal that occurs in antisocial youths in confrontative situations leads to 'visceral' aggressive responding that over-rides thinking processes learned in calm contexts.

Attention deficit hyperactivity disorder

ADHD children and adolescents have short attention spans and difficulty in repressing immediate, often inappropriate, responses to stimuli rather than stopping and evaluating the best course of action. Cognitive therapy should, in theory, be well suited to address this kind of difficulty. Self-instructional programmes that attempt to slow down cognitive processing to permit examination of alternative courses of action have, however, not been especially effective. It is as if the very nature of the problem means the capacity to activate a different approach to information processing is absent. Behavioural programmes controlling immediate contingencies are more effective, but less so than medication, and with smaller effect sizes than in conduct disordered children and adolescents.

Social problem-solving skills programmes

Myrna Shure and George Spivack, in the USA, have developed perhaps the most comprehensive intervention programme, called Interpersonal Cognitive Problem Solving (ICPS). Many studies have shown that several groups of children and adolescents lack interpersonal skills, especially aggressive children and adolescents, rejected children and adolescents, isolated children and adolescents with few friends and some depressed children and adolescents. The ICPS programme concentrates on three core cognitive processes that have been shown to be impaired:

1 *Generation of alternatives*: the ability to come up with several different solutions to a problem situation.
2 *Consequential thinking*: the ability to see the immediate and longer-term consequences of each line of action proposed, and incorporate this in coming to a decision about the best response.
3 *Means–ends thinking*: the ability to distinguish the purpose of a plan of action from its content, so ways round an obstacle can be devised if the initial plan fails.

A variety of methods are used to foster these skills, including both individual and group processes with games, discussion and group interaction techniques. They can be applied even at preschool level, for example, the words 'or' and 'different' are taught to help children and adolescents think about alternative ways to tackle situations, for example, 'I can hit him or tell him I'm cross. Hitting is different from telling.' As these programmes have evolved, it has become evident that a number of core skills in perceiving the mental states of others need to be developed in many children and adolescents:

1 *Emotional awareness*. Becoming sensitive to the feelings and wishes of others. Some children and adolescents may even be unaware of their own basic feelings. As these are developed, they can be taught that not everyone feels the same way about things, and that children and

adolescents may feel differently at different times ('I can ask her later when she's feeling better').

2 *Social information gathering*. Games are played to develop skills in reading situations, listening for clues and asking others what they mean.

3 *Understanding motives*. Children and adolescents are taught to go beyond another person's behaviour to think why they might be acting that way, and to generate solutions appropriate to these motives.

Having developed these skills, most programmes go on to apply them, initially in hypothetical situations, and then in real situations. The cognitive steps may be spelt out to the child, for example, they are encouraged to count off on each finger as they go through the sequence of STOP-THINK-DO-REVIEW in generating and enacting solutions.

Outcome studies show strong effects in hypothetical situations, but more mixed results in real-life situations. These programmes are considerably enhanced if adults around the children and adolescents have also been taught the thinking, and thus can reinforce it in the heat of the moment. Under these circumstances short-term results are good, but long-term follow-ups have not yet been carried out.

Interpersonal psychotherapy (IPT)

This mode of therapy was developed for treating depression by Gerald Klerman and Myrna Weissman in New York, and then specifically modified for use with adolescents. IPT is a time-limited, brief psychotherapy based on the premise that depression occurs in the context of interpersonal relationships. The two main goals are to identify and treat, first, the patient's depressive symptoms and, second, the problem areas associated with the onset of the depression. Five specific areas are reviewed, and one or two worked on. Four are the same as in adult IPT: grief, interpersonal role disputes, role transitions and interpersonal deficits. A fifth area, single-parent families, was added because of its frequent occurrence and the conflicts it engenders for adolescents. The emphasis is on issues in current relationships rather than those in the past.

There are three phases of treatment. In the initial phase, depression as a clinical disorder is explained, and an effort is made to demystify the experience. The adolescent is encouraged to think of him or herself as in treatment and is assigned the sick role. Despite this, the adolescent is encouraged not to avoid the usual social expectations, but to see friends, attend school and behave in the family as normally as possible. Parents are seen and encouraged to be supportive rather than hostile or critical. The school is approached, and the effect of depression on school performance and behaviour explained.

In the middle phase the focus is on the problem area(s) selected:

1 *Grief* is not considered a problem unless it is prolonged or becomes abnormal. The therapist helps the adolescent discuss the loss of a loved

one, as well as identify and experience the associated feelings. As the patient begins to grieve appropriately and the symptoms dissipate, the loss should be better understood and accepted and the patient freed to pursue new relationships.

2 *Interpersonal role disputes* occur where one of the parties has different expectations to the other about the relationship. The therapist helps the young person to identify the dispute, to make choices about negotiations, to reassess expectations for the relationship, to clarify role changes, and to modify communication patterns to enable resolution of the dispute. Parents may be brought in to facilitate negotiations if they are a party to the dispute.

3 *Role transitions* occur when adolescents need to negotiate puberty, cope with sexual desires and the wish for intimate relationships, separate from parents and family, and achieve success in planning work or further education. There may be feelings of loss about letting go of old roles, or of fear or inadequacy about their ability to take on new roles. The therapist aims to help the young person to come to terms with these feelings and negotiate a viable future.

4 *Interpersonal deficits* are apparent when the individual appears to lack the social skills to establish and maintain appropriate relationships within and outside the family. As a result, the adolescent may be socially isolated or lacking close friends, which can lead to feelings of depression and inadequacy. The therapist reviews significant past relationships and identifies repetitive or inappropriate ways of behaving. New strategies are identified and discussed, and the young person is encouraged to apply these to current issues. Role-play may be used to identify problematic interpersonal situations and enable the adolescent to explore and practise new communication skills and interpersonal behaviours, for example, learning how to make friends. Practising within the session and in small increments at home can engender a sense of social competence in the young person that generalises to other situations.

5 *Single-parent families* may arise from divorce, separation, imprisonment of one parent, absence of a parent from the outset, or death of a parent by medical illness or violence. Each of these situations presents unique emotional conflicts for the adolescent and the custodial parent. Therapy aims to help the young person come to terms with the current situation and negotiate appropriate adaptations. There is often a need to grieve for the loss of the previous situation.

In the termination phase, progress is reviewed, often with other family members present. Symptoms and conflicts are presented in four categories: (1) those representing symptoms specific to the depressive episode; (2) those secondary to it; (3) more enduring conflict areas that represent personality style; and (4) those areas of conflict that are part of a normal developmental process. The adolescent will have already addressed feelings relating to termination of contact with the therapist, and a slight increase of depressive feelings following termination is predicted. Trials of IPT suggest it is as effective in treating depression in adolescents as in adults, and has an effect of the same order as cognitive-behavioural therapy.

Individual counselling and psychotherapy

There are differing levels, on a continuum from support and counselling at one end to psychodynamic psychotherapy at the other:

- *Support and counselling*. This includes unburdening of problems to a sympathetic listener, ventilation of feelings within a supportive relationship, and discussion of current problems with a non-judgemental helper. Advice may be given. The main aim is to relieve symptoms and restore the status quo prior to the difficulty, or come to terms with an event.
- *Intermediate levels of psychotherapy*. Interpersonal psychotherapy (IPT) as described above is an example of this.
- *Psychodynamic psychotherapy*. Here, a prolonged deep interpersonal relationship is fostered, during which both intra- and interpersonal processes are revealed and analysed. Disturbing early experiences may be relived, allowing conflicts that underlie symptoms to be explored and insight gained, and conflicts to be worked through and resolved without handicapping defences. Advice is not given. The aim is thus more than symptomatic relief: it is reintegration and change in personality functioning towards greater wholeness and maturity. Psychoanalytic interest in children's symptoms dates back to Sigmund Freud, who described the case of little Hans in 1909; in the 1920s his daughter Anna Freud elaborated child psychoanalysis, as did Melanie Klein in the 1930s. Later, Virginia Axline developed play therapy more formally. During sessions the therapist may feed back interpretations and formulations not only of material the child brings up, but also their immediate style of relating during the session.

A major issue in individual work at all levels is the quality of the interpersonal relationship between therapist and patient. Several adult studies show that irrespective of the particular form of personal therapy given, one of the major determinants of outcome is the warmth and empathy of the therapist. One way of addressing the need for this empirically would be to give the same (or as similar as possible) treatment by correspondence or in a manual. In the field of parent-training for child conduct disorder, studies show that these approaches are indeed effective, although less so than when a live therapist is involved.

In child and adolescent psychiatry, much work for the benefit of the child is done through the parents, and counselling and support for parents are part of many clinicians' basic repertoire irrespective of their child's disorder. It may be a major component in helping parents to come to terms with a diagnosis of intellectual disability, or in coping with their child's depression. Studies on counselling in these settings suggest parents find the apparent attitude of the clinician to them central ('likes me, likes my child'), and want an informal atmosphere where they can ask questions.

Direct work with children and adolescents differs in a number of ways from that with adults. First, the child may not have wanted to be seen alone; usually they do not have to give consent. Second, the method of working with younger children may need to be less talk-based initially, and focus on drawing or play to gain insight. Third, even when therapy can help children and adolescents come to terms with a difficult situation and offer them the opportunity to mature and change, children and adolescents are not masters of their own fate in the same way as adults, so they may well continue to be exposed to damaging or harmful influences, for example, harsh punishment and neglect within the family, or a mother who is an alcoholic. In these circumstances it is essential to try as hard as possible to ameliorate the conditions, and it may be unethical to give individual therapy without doing this.

There have been very few well-conducted evaluation trials of individual dynamic psychotherapy, so it is hard to judge its effectiveness at present.

Subject review

Fonagy P, Target M. (2008) Psychodynamic treatments. *In*: Rutter M *et al.* (eds) *Rutter's Child and Adolescent Psychiatry*, 5th edn. Wiley-Blackwell, Chichester, pp. 1079–1091.

Lochman JE, Pardini DA. (2008) Cognitive-behavioral therapies. *In*: Rutter M *et al.* (eds) *Rutter's Child and Adolescent Psychiatry*, 5th edn. Wiley-Blackwell, Chichester, pp. 1026–1045.

Further reading

Birmaher B *et al.* (2000) Clinical outcome after short-term psychotherapy for adolescents with major depressive disorder. *Archives of General Psychiatry* **57**, 29–36.

Dubicka B *et al.* (2010) Combined treatment with cognitive-behavioural therapy in adolescent depression: Meta-analysis. *British Journal of Psychiatry* **197**, 433–440.

Kennard B *et al.* (2009) Remission and recovery in the Treatment for Adolescents With Depression Study (TADS): Acute and long-term outcomes. *Journal of the American Academy of Child and Adolescent Psychiatry*. **48**, 186–195.

Mufson L *et al.* (2004) A randomized effectiveness trial of interpersonal psychotherapy for depressed adolescents. *Archives of General Psychiatry* **61**, 577–584.

Young J, Mufson L. (2009) Interpersonal psychotherapy for adolescents. *In*: Essau C (ed.) *Treatments for Adolescent Depression: Theory and Practice*. Oxford University Press, Oxford, pp. 261–282.

CHAPTER 41
Family and Systemic Therapies

Background

'No man is an island' wrote John Donne, and family therapy recognises this. Whereas psychodynamic therapy and biological psychiatry focus on the individual's internal mental processes and pathology as the root of problems, family therapy arose from the notion that the *family system* exerts a strong influence on all members, and that imbalances in the system can manifest themselves as problems in the *identified* patient who is presented as an expression of the family's *dysfunction* or *disequilibrium*. Children and adolescents are especially affected by these processes since so much of their lives take place within the family context. More recent developments in family therapy have acknowledged the influence of family belief systems and the attitudes prevalent in the current social and cultural climate. People's way of functioning is affected by their idea of how they should be. Gender, race and role expectations all influence people's beliefs and behaviour, as do a variety of personal and general experiences ranging from parental demands to TV advertisements. Indeed, because of the awareness of the interdependence with outside society and its systems, many practitioners now prefer to reflect their systems approach directly in their title and call themselves *systemic therapists*. A variety of methods have been developed to make use of these concepts in therapy.

Family systems theory began to develop in the late 1950s and in the 1960s. It recognised limitations in explanations of human behaviour based on *linear causality*, which focus on actions by individuals, and the content of what they say and do. As an alternative, Gregory Bateson, an anthropologist, introduced ideas from *cybernetics* into family therapy. He proposed that *reciprocal determinism* is at work, and that one needs to look at process rather than content. This will reveal the interdependence of family members: one event does not lead to another single event; rather, a change in one member affects all other members in differing ways, who then react and impinge upon the first person, and so on. Examination of the process reveals *circular causality*. Systems theory and thinking can be applied beyond the family to inform relations between the individual or the

Child and Adolescent Psychiatry, Third Edition. Robert Goodman and Stephen Scott.
© 2012 Robert Goodman and Stephen Scott. Published 2012 by John Wiley & Sons, Ltd.

family and wider networks and agencies such as other relatives and friends, school, and social services.

Example
- *Linear causality*: a depressed mother has produced a dependent son by failing to get him to leave home, and an uncontrolled daughter by supervising her inadequately.
- *Circular causality*: a mother is unhappy because her husband stays at work for much of the time. She turns to her 18-year-old son for companionship, so excluding her 15-year-old daughter. The son feels her loneliness and stays at home to be with her, and so puts off leaving home and going to college, and becomes increasingly withdrawn. The mother blames the father for being away so much and withholds sexual favours; she becomes depressed. The ensuing coldness between the parents leads the daughter into a series of superficial relationships, in which she seeks but never finds the comfort and warmth lacking at home.
- *Implication*: behaviour is as much determined by the interactional context in which it occurs as by the intrapsychic or emotional processes of any individual person. Failure to recognise this will impair the chances of improving the functioning of the referred individual, and may well pathologise them unnecessarily.

Terms used in family and systems therapy
- *Family system*. An entity whose component members influence each other, with relationships organised by family rules.
- *Subsystem*. For example, husband–wife dyad; mother–child, father–child; parents–children; males–females, etc.
- *Family rules*. These regulate and stabilise how the family functions as a unit. Many may be covert: 'If you complain to mother, it puts up her blood pressure', 'We never discuss money', 'Boys don't show feelings'. Dysfunctional families may follow dysfunctional rules, and helping them become aware of these during therapy may enable them to replace them with more useful ones.
- *Homeostasis*. This term has been brought to family functioning from physiology. It suggests that there are beliefs and behavioural mechanisms that keep relationships controlled within a relatively narrow range. For example, a threat to father's authority by a child's misbehaviour may trigger a look or counterthreat to bring the child into line, which in turn will lead to the child making a small adjustment of his or her behaviour, and so on. The codes to effect this *feedback loop* may be quite subtle and private. In times of transition due to changed circumstances or family life-cycle adjustments (see below) these old homeostatic responses may fail and get out of control; sterile, ineffectual patterns may become endlessly repeated. Recognising this can help families develop new, healthier patterns of communication and behaviour.
- *Family life-cycle framework*. This is a further way in which family and systems therapy recognises that external forces influence family and

individual well-being. The proposal is that there are *developmental tasks* that require mastery at each stage. Failure to come to terms with these changes and to make the necessary adjustments may then lead to strain or dysfunction in the family system and problems or symptoms in one or all family members. Successful negotiation of the transitions may require *first order changes* (defined as within the system but not affecting its structure) or *second order changes* (which require a fundamental alteration in the system's structure and function). Some of the life-cycle stages are shown in Box 41.1, though individual, socio-economic and cultural variations need to be considered, as do the impact of dislocations such as divorce, unemployment, severe illness, etc.

Box 41.1 Life-cycle stages

Stage		Tasks
1	Leaving home	**(a)** Develop own identity independent of family of origin
		(b) Form close peer relationships
		(c) Gain work and financial independence
2	Cohabitation	**(a)** Form marital system
		(b) Realign relationships with extended family, and friends
3	Family with young children	**(a)** Adjust marital system to make space for children
		(b) Join in child rearing, financial, and household tasks
		(c) Realign with extended family to incorporate parenting and grandparenting roles
4	Family with adolescents	**(a)** Adjust relationships so adolescent can move in and out of system
		(b) Refocus on midlife marital and career issues
		(c) Start joint caring for older generation
5	Children leaving home	**(a)** Renegotiate marital system as a dyad
		(b) Develop adult-to-adult relations with grown children
		(c) Accept in-laws and grandchildren into system
		(d) Cope with disability and death of parents
6	Late life	**(a)** Adjust couple functioning in face of physiological, financial and work-role decline
		(b) Dealing with loss of spouse, siblings and friends
		(c) Accepting assistance from children/outside agencies

Some working practices common to most types of family therapy

- *Seeing as many family members as possible*. This used to be very strongly recommended in order to assess the communication patterns and inter-relationships going on. The concern was that failure to see all members at least once would easily lead to erroneous conclusions being drawn, or to a lack of appreciation of important influences. Nowadays most family therapists will work with whoever can come, while recognising the importance of the family system. It is therefore possible to work in a systemic way with only one person.

- *Drawing a family genogram (family tree)*. This rapidly enables all the family members to be recognised for their influence, including grandparents, aunts and uncles, and deceased relatives. Intergenerational patterns may be revealed, and family stories (often called narratives) and expectations brought to light: 'He's the black sheep of the family'; 'I'm a Daddy's girl', 'All the men in our family die early or drink heavily.'
- *Use of colleagues to observe the therapy process*. This may be through a one-way mirror. The therapist then receives feedback on what is happening in the family and suggestions for interventions, which may be given through an ear bug, by a telephone, or by taking a break to talk to them.

Varieties of family therapy

There have been many varieties of family therapy, which have evolved over time within themselves and which have influenced each other. Whereas in the last century these were fairly clearly demarcated and distinct, nowadays many therapists draw on several approaches. Nonetheless it is helpful to know the varieties. *Structural* makes explicit the structure of a family in terms of who holds the power and what the communication patterns are. Therapy attempts to correct any distortions in this structure through practical manoeuvres. *Strategic* makes use of novel practical strategies to help families find a fresh way to break out of ingrained negative cycles of behaviour, without prescribing a 'correct' structure. *Milan* uses questioning to reveal to family members the forces and beliefs which constrain their behaviour towards each other, enabling them to change these if they are uncomfortable with what is revealed. *Solution focused therapy* concentrates on identifying the external events and contexts that are operating when the problem is *not* present or being expressed, and tries to work with the family to change the predominant circumstances to these. *Social constructionist systemic therapy* and *narrative therapy* build on the wider general currency of notions that there is no objective reality, rather, it is all construed. This conceptualisation then offers the opportunity to acknowledge the impact of social values, for example, relating to power inequalities due to gender, race or social class, and to reconstruct events, or retell a person's story, in a way that leads to helpful changes in their family and personal functioning. For example, a girl's predominant narrative that she has suffered as a victim of parental hostility could be 'rewritten' as the heroic survival of hard times, weaving in that despite this she achieved a number of notable specific successes, and is now ready to spread her wings and move on to be a successful young adult.

Irrespective of the particular type of family and systemic therapy, it offers a different way to think about personal difficulties. Prior to systems thinking, the dominant medical or psychodynamic models tended to locate pathology within the person, often as a constitutional or pathogenic characteristic; the cause was frequently seen as beyond the patient's conscious control. Therapy was likely to be targeted on the individual to alter the pathological process, whether by changing their mental processes through psychotherapy or their chemical processes through drugs.

From the mid-1960s to the mid-1980s, systems thinking and other developments led to a way of thinking that emphasised that people's behaviour was strongly influenced by their interaction and communication with those around them. Behavioural psychology had already described how the pattern of stimuli and responses could determine an individual's behaviour, but family systems thinkers focused on a more complex set of environmental determinants. The client was seen as a basically healthy person who was not functioning well because they were responding to unreasonable demands put on them by the outside system; anyone might reasonably respond that way in those circumstances. The therapist attempted to alter the family influences on the client, with the result that the whole system shifted, including the personal characteristics and problems of the client. Therapy was carried out in the 'here and now' working on current problems. It did not concern itself with past origins of difficulties, or with behaviour that the therapist, but not the client, perceived as a problem. The focus was on changing external contingencies rather than on the individual as a conscious agent.

The past two decades have seen further conceptual developments. The wider cultural context of people's lives has been more explicitly recognised, and there has been more focus on what people can do rather than what they cannot. The active, conscious processes through which a person shapes their sense of identity are more fully acknowledged, rather than their being seen as only reacting to events. People construct a story about themselves that has to be respected and worked with, using the person's own language rather than imposing professional jargon. The person is seen as having many strengths that may need mobilising to fight the difficulties outside themselves. The therapist focuses on helping the individual to deploy more of the effective strategies that are already part of their repertoire. This may be achieved by helping the person become aware of the narrative 'script' they are living, and enabling them to 'rewrite' a more positive story by which to live their life.

There are also other approaches to working with families which recognise the complexities of wider interrelationships, but which did not primarily evolve from cybernetic systems theory. These include psychodynamic family therapy and behavioural family therapy. The latter has had well-documented success in adult disorders improving the outcome for people with schizophrenia by reducing the number of critical comments by nearest relatives. In children and adolescents, behaviourally-based parent training is effective in improving disruptive behaviour. It is also totally systemic – in some versions of group parent training the child or adolescent is not even seen – yet perhaps ironically behaviourally-based parent training tends to not be seen by systemic therapists as part of their family of interventions.

Structural family therapy

Salvador Minuchin developed this approach in the 1960s, working with deprived ethnic minorities in the USA. It is geared to the present, and operates in the here and now. Thus, there is no discussion of past history, or the origins of dysfunctional relationships. Change occurs through action and not via gaining insight. Problems addressed are in the present day-to-day world, not unresolved past inner conflicts. It is based on a *normative family model* that is functioning well, in which there are *clear and well-marked boundaries in relationships*. This is especially true in:

1 The marital subsystem – protection of spouse privacy.
2 The sibling subsystem – a hierarchical organisation in which different tasks and privileges are consonant with the age and gender of the siblings, as determined by the family culture.
3 The boundary around the nuclear family, which is well demarcated, while recognising great cultural variations.

It is a fundamental principle that the symptom is the product of a dysfunctional family system, and that if the family organisation becomes more normal or functional, the symptom will disappear. Symptoms are not specific to dysfunctional structures.

Terms
- *Hierarchy*. The relative influence of each family member on the outcome of an activity. This needs to be defined in relation to specific circumstances, as it is not a permanent or invariable concept. For example, parents exercise responsibility and authority. A 'parentified' child or adolescent (who has taken on a parental role within the family) is an example of abnormality or dysfunction.
- *Boundary*. An invisible line that demarcates a system, subsystem or individual from its surroundings. It arises from the rules of who participates in an operation and how it is carried out, and from the roles each person takes towards others during a particular family function. The boundary preserves the integrity of the (sub)system so members can carry out tasks without interference, but should be permeable enough to allow interdependence. Thus, boundaries can be construed along a continuum, with one end too permeable and the other too rigid:
  - Enmeshment results from boundaries that are undifferentiated, permeable, or fluid. Individuals in the relationship are handicapped by not being able to be autonomous.
  - Clear boundaries promote healthy relationships.
  - Disengagement results from rigid, impermeable boundaries, and there is little interplay or communication between family members.
- *Alignments*. These occur through the joining or opposition of one member of a system to another in carrying out an operation; they can be positive or negative. Structures observed may include:
  - Coalitions of two family members against a third: for example, father and son against mother. Coalitions vary in how stable they are. Some

---

Box 41.2 An example of classical structural family therapy

Mr Jones is a maths teacher, and Mrs Jones is a former nurse who looks after their three children. Robert, 15, has incapacitating abdominal pain with no obvious organic cause and has missed most school for the last six months. Jane, 13, has no reported problems and is doing very well academically. John, 10, refuses to do what his mother asks and frequently swears at her.

During questioning it emerges that to make it easier for Mrs Jones to help Robert with his frequent bouts of pain in the night, he sleeps in the parents' bedroom in a camp bed. The repeated night disturbances led Mr Jones to suffer from lack of sleep, which was affecting his teaching, so he had moved into the spare room. Most evenings he spends correcting students' scripts in his study, and at weekends he goes fishing alone. He explains that he thinks Robert's problems derive from a delicate constitution worsened by appendicitis three years ago.

The therapist does not respond to this explanation for events rooted in the past, but she notices that Mr Jones and Jane sit together on one side of the room, John is in the middle, and Mrs Jones is at the other end sitting very close to Robert and whispering to him. After a while she decides that the boundary between Mr and Mrs Jones is rigid and they are disengaged, whereas that between Robert and Mrs Jones is too fluid and they are enmeshed. She therefore intervenes by altering the seating arrangements so Mr and Mrs Jones have to sit next to each other away from the children and are set the task of finding two practical steps to help Robert back to school for one hour a day. Meanwhile the three siblings are sat in the other corner of the room and instructed collectively to plan a treat for their parents.

These manoeuvres are designed to promote parental authority and strengthen the marital subsystem, and the sibling subsystem. For homework, the parents are instructed to go out one evening a week and to agree a joint implementation of their plan to get Robert back to school. Mr Jones, who hitherto hardly ever did anything with Robert, is instructed to take him fishing with him on Saturdays. In later sessions the sleeping arrangements are addressed, and Mrs Jones is asked what Robert does to get her to mollycoddle him so much. The therapist is thus reframing his behaviour as sympathy-seeking to avoid school rather than illness. Mrs Jones begins to see his role in organising her caring behaviour and gets quite angry at him, with the result that he moves out of the bedroom and Mr Jones moves back in. Both parents are supported in their programme to be consistent in accepting no excuses for not going to school. His abdominal pain ceases to be discussed much at all during sessions and gradually diminishes.

---

coalitions are based on detouring, for example, couple appear to get on, because they detour their problem via the child.

- ○ Triangulation, where each parent demands that the child is an ally in a conflict with the other.
- ○ Alliances when two share an interest not shared by a third. This is a healthy supportive structure, which is not detrimental to others.
- *Power* refers to relative influence.
- *Identified patient*. The person brought for help, although in fact the cause of the problem lies in the interaction patterns at a family-wide level

and will be affecting all members in different ways. The task of therapy includes revealing the way the symptoms of the identified patient are used by the family to support its functioning, and how they fit its transactions (Box 41.2).

Intervention techniques

The therapist is *active*, and *directive*. He or she challenges patterns of family interaction and reveals covert rules. This is done through *joining* the family system and *accommodating* to its style, getting to feel what it is like. He or she will acknowledge the painful situation, but absolve the individual from responsibility, for example, 'You are quite childish: how do the others manage to keep you that way?' He or she will *reframe* the symptom as part of the family structure and use the force of their personality, which should be powerful and empathetic, to help bring about change. To do this they may need to *unbalance* the system by exposing dysfunction, and destabilise it to encourage the emergence of a healthier structure. They may get the family to *enact* the problem within the room to see what is going on and provide alternatives, for example, if the daughter is anorexic, have a family meal.

Strategic family therapy

Here therapists use a range of *strategies* to get rid of the specific set of presenting symptoms. Unlike structural therapists, strategic therapists are not concerned about imposing some predetermined normative structure on the family.

This mode of working arises out of an interactional approach, where one communication is seen as arising in the context of another, not in isolation. In the case of children fighting, for instance, it is inappropriate to ask 'who started it'; since each party would say that they were only reacting to what the other did. Therefore, it is necessary to take the whole system as the unit of study.

Watzlawick stated that 'All behaviour is communication': just as it is impossible not to behave, so it is impossible not to communicate. For example, the husband who withdraws and 'refuses to communicate' with his wife is in fact speaking volumes about his resentment, anger and rejection of her. Paradoxical communication is confusing, typified by the double bind, where the first 'bind' is that the content and form of the message may contradict each other, and the second bind is the meta-communication that you are not allowed to notice the contradiction, for example, when a mother says to her daughter 'lovely to see you', while giving her a frozen stare.

The current pattern of communication and behaviour is held to maintain the presenting problem; its history and aetiology are seen as irrelevant. As a consequence, this can be a very optimistic therapy where, for example, years of rancorous feelings and despondent explanations can be bypassed in favour of concentrating on what can be done differently from now on.

Jay Haley and his wife, Cloe Madanes, were major developers of strategic therapy. Haley wrote a number of influential books, including *Problem-solving Therapy* in 1976. He argued that symptoms were not behaviours beyond one's control, but a strategy for controlling a relationship when all else failed. He cited the example of a woman who insisted her husband be home every night or she would have panic attacks. In this way she blamed her control of the situation on the panic attacks. Symptoms are used to control relationships when more up-front methods fail.

Strategic therapists concern themselves with current daily communication patterns as well as with repetitive sequences of interactions between family members. Communication defines the relationship; symptoms are tactics in this struggle. The therapist's goal is to manoeuvre the patient into developing other ways of defining the relationship so the use of symptoms as a method of exerting control will be abandoned.

Techniques

- The therapist has to design a strategy for each problem, and is responsible for change. The approach is pragmatic, concerned with what works. The therapists use their power to overcome 'resistance' of patients, and are 'manipulative', that is, keep the rationale for intervention hidden from patients.
- *Relabelling*. This is a tactic to emphasise the positive, making apparently dysfunctional behaviour seem reasonable. For example, Haley describes telling a wife whose husband chased her with an axe that he was trying to get close to her. Thus, both sides of a communication are examined, and the less obvious aspect is brought out, sometimes described as 'addressing the meta message', in this case that the husband cared desperately for his wife. Such relabelling can change the context of relationships and lead on to improvement.
- *Directives*. These are assignments set for families to perform outside the session. For example, a mother is told to stop interrupting when father and son are talking together. However, often these directives do not work as the families are resistant and have invested in the status quo.
- *Prescribing the symptom*. This may then be tried as a form of *paradoxical intervention*. The patient is told to keep on doing what they came to therapy to stop doing. This is designed to provoke defiance in the patient, who may come back next time and say they did it far less than previously. If they carry on, they are forced to recognise that they have some control over the behaviour, and confront its unreasonableness and the effect it has on others. The domineering mother may be instructed to carry on running absolutely all the small details of the family's lives and not to let anyone else have the slightest say about anything. A boy refusing school may be instructed never to go out of the house, and not even to look at a book. The issue then becomes one of control, as the patient is told they are in charge of the symptom. The domineering

wife no longer runs everything in the house if the therapist is telling her what to do; or if she resists the directive she will be less domineering. The assumption is that if the symptom was presented as a way of gaining an advantage, it will resolve once it puts the patient at a disadvantage (see Box 41.3).

- *Humour and metaphor*. These may be used to tap into a family's lighter side, release pressure, and sidestep logical thinking. To get families to break out of fixed patterns may require tangential, indirect 'uncommon solutions'.
- *Provision of alternatives*. Other activities are suggested to replace the problem behaviour.
- *Externalising the problem*. This technique attributes agency to the symptom in a light-hearted way to enable the family to unite against it, and has been well described by Michael White. This places less emphasis on failure, decreases conflict around the symptom, opens up new possibilities for action, and replaces pessimism with optimism. For example, rather than blame a boy for soiling, the trouble is ascribed to 'sneaky poos' who have to be taken on in a battle to beat them. Imaginative charts are drawn to show progress and to make it an epic game where the child is helped to devise creative strategies to win.

Box 41.3 An example of classical strategic family therapy using Haley's approach

The same family described in Box 41.2 is interviewed. However, this time no structural reorganisation of seating arrangements is made. The therapist notes that Robert's abdominal pain serves to keep his mother at home looking after him rather than return to nursing as she says she wants, but doesn't seem really to want. The therapist tells the family that the situation is serious and instructs Mrs Jones to increase her surveillance of Robert, checking his pain level every hour for the next fortnight, and under no circumstances is she to leave him unattended in the house. Robert is to report the slightest twinge of pain, being told that otherwise, if it is left too long, it is likely to get far worse. He must ask his mother to attend to him very closely, irrespective of her sacrifice.

   After two weeks of this, the family gradually become aware of how dominating Robert's pain is. Mrs Jones gets fed up with waiting on him hand and foot. Robert himself feels constrained as he now has to report sick all the time and isn't allowed out to see his friends in the evenings. A shift of attitude occurs and Mrs Jones responds less keenly to Robert's episodes of pain. He in turn reports less and starts going out more, eventually getting back to school.

Brief solution-focused therapy

This is a variety of strategic therapy developed by Steve de Shazer among others. This extends the approach that focuses on success, and typically involves no more than five to ten sessions. Questioning emphasises the exceptions: When was the symptom *not* present? What were you doing at the time? How could you do more of this? Differences are noticed in the severity of the symptom and attention is paid to what was happening at the time. The focus is on what happens when things are going right rather than on when things go wrong. The assumption is that people already know what they need to do to solve their complaints; the therapist has only to help them discover their own creative solutions for coming 'unstuck'. The solution may not be closely matched to the problem and may comprise quite different elements. De Shazer uses the metaphor of coming upon a locked door blocking progress to a more satisfactory life. Rather than spend a long time agonising about why the door is there and who locked it, all that is necessary is for the family to find a set of 'skeleton keys' that will open this door and others blocking their progress.

Techniques

- *Precise description* of the problem is requested: 'How would I know if her depression was getting better? What would I see?' Limited but achievable goals are aimed for, and by focusing on precise descriptions, the families are led to recognise improvements, however small. These then become reinforcing and provide the motivation for the family to keep doing things differently, and so lead on to further change.
- *Miracle question*: What would it look like if you woke up tomorrow and the problem was gone? What precisely would be different?
- *Miracle intervention*: X is to act tomorrow as if he had no problem, Y is to implicitly acknowledge this by her responses, X is to implicitly note these, but there is to be no discussion about it.
- *Focus on successes*: become aware of those occasions when the problem is absent. What is going on at the time? Notice these successes: how on earth did you manage not to do it (the symptom behaviour)? How are you managing not to do it now? So you managed the urge, let's develop your 'urge surfing'. If a strategy works, stick with it; if it doesn't, do something different.

Milan systemic family therapy

Developed by Selvini-Palazzoli, Prata, Boscolo and Cecchin in Milan, Italy, for chronic, resistant cases, this approach concerns itself with bringing out covert beliefs and meanings that constrain a family's behaviour. The model is to recognise and challenge the beliefs, so they can be re-examined and modified to fit what is going on more precisely, and the expectation is that behaviour will then be changed to fit in with the new set of beliefs or priorities. This is the opposite of structural family therapy, where the objective is to change behaviour through direct action rather than as a consequence of adjusting beliefs. According to Milan systemic therapy, there may be several conflicting sets of beliefs regarding a single action. Regarding a daughter who is staying out late, for example, a parent may feel she should come home earlier as she is at risk of being taken advantage of, but may also feel that if too much discipline is applied, she will run away from home like her older sister. As they are revealed, the beliefs can be tested against other family members' views and interests, and be developed accordingly. As with other modes of family therapy, the systemic approach has changed over time, with increasing emphasis on the role of language in shaping beliefs.

The central technique is one of circular questioning, in order to reveal how beliefs relate to the behaviour. Thus, each question follows on from the response to the last, aiming to reveal what meaning this has for other beliefs in the system, and to uncover their interrelationships. Whereas linear questioning proceeds convergently to clarify with increasing detail what the mental state or behaviour is, circular questioning aims to elicit the *connections* to other beliefs, and to other family members. Thus, one is aiming to see how experiences are connected to belief systems, rather than find out more and more about the experience. For example, if someone repeatedly brought anger to sessions, rather than continuing to explore the feeling, one would find out what it would mean to take the feeling away. One might discover they would be left believing they're worthless, impotent, a victim, and as this is even more unpleasant, they continue feeling angry.

Techniques

Hypothesising

- This is carried out before the session, before the family can impose its definition of the problem.
- It organises the questioning. It is an evolving process in which hypotheses are tested by gathering information.
- It clarifies the gains and losses the symptom brings to each family member, and how the symptom helps the family that is struggling with the prospect of change.
- In a family experiencing a chronic problem, each member moves to stop change, wishing to reinstate the status quo after the change has happened, and trying to retain old patterns even though they conflict with the new situation. This notion of 'resistance' to change was more characteristic of earlier systemic therapy; now there is a greater acceptance that families really do want to change.

Neutrality

- The therapist avoids getting drawn into the family system or taking sides; they may have a team on the other side of a one-way mirror to help them keep independent.
- Answers are not evaluated or agreed with: understanding is shown, and perhaps empathy, but no family member's view is accepted as right or definitive.
- The therapist remains allied with all family members.
- The therapist tries to understand and not to prescribe how the family should be, letting them generate their own solutions.

Circular questioning

- This means that one question leads on to the next in a different direction outwards, rather than linearly towards a definition of phenomena (see Box 41.4).

Box 41.4 An example of classical Milan systemic therapy

The same family described in Box 41.2 is interviewed. This time the therapist asks a series of questions eliciting the differences among family members, initially asking the daughter, Jane, 'Who is the most upset that Robert is not going to school?' She says her Daddy. Mrs Jones is asked what would happen if her husband got firm and insisted Robert went. Mr Jones interjects that he would never insist as this would be an authoritarian act, and his own father was a rigid disciplinarian who scarred him for life by his bullying – no son of his was going be treated the same way. Jane is now asked who would be most upset if Robert did go to school. She replies that her Mummy would be lonely. Mrs Jones is then asked again what would happen if her husband got firm and insisted Robert went to school. She replies that Robert is delicate and she is anxious that if he were pushed, he would have a nervous breakdown, just as Mr Jones did when he was 15. The younger brother John is asked what would happen if Robert went back to school. He replies that Jane would be triumphant, as she is clever but Robert failed his mock exams earlier in the year and would be made to look stupid. John says the whole family has had it drummed into them how important school success is – their father was a dustman's son but through academic success had become a middle-class teacher.

The therapist takes a break to consult her colleagues behind the one-way mirror. They suggest the family seem paralysed by two fear-provoking, conflicting beliefs: if you don't work hard enough you might fail academically; and if you work too hard you might have a breakdown. They recommend the therapist ask the family members how each of them sees the future in two years time. On her return to the family, she asks this. Robert says he would like to be free of pain and back to playing football, and grins as he says that by then he won't have to do maths any more. John says he hopes he'll be in the school football team at the secondary school he'll be attending by then. He adds that he wished that his father, Robert and he could play football together as they used to, stating proudly that his Dad used to be in the university team. Mother says she'd like to be nursing again, and Jane says she'd be impressed if her Mum did that. Father says he couldn't wish for any more than they have said, but hopes he won't have to wait two years for a football game with his sons: 'What about a game tonight?' The boys agree enthusiastically.

The therapist says she is impressed by the way the family work together to solve problems. She wonders whether Mr Jones' experience of having had a breakdown and then recovering could be used to help Robert. Mr Jones says it occurs to him that he could go back to helping Robert with maths. He had been anxious not to put pressure on his son but now thinks Robert probably doesn't know where to start, having been out of school for so long. Robert looks relieved. The family carry on discussing what they could do now, in order to get to where they want to be in two years time. At the follow-up visit two weeks later, Robert's pain is far less and he has begun a graded reintroduction to school.

- Individuals are asked to state the problem in behavioural terms, not in terms of mood states.
- The effect of the symptom on relationships is discussed: 'Who does what in response? Who is most affected? Who noticed first? Who is most worried?'
- Differences between people are considered: 'Who cares most that Lucy won't eat?'
- Hypothetical scenarios are considered, to define the effect of the symptom on relationships: 'If Jim didn't have the problem, who would be closest to him?'
- Timing is explored: 'What were relationships like before and after the "problem"?' Thinking about the future, 'What would happen if it never got better?'
- Questioning may be triadic, that is, asking a third person about the relations of the other two: 'How do your brother's tantrums affect your mother?'
- New alternatives are canvassed: 'What would have to happen to stop Jim misbehaving?' Meanings and actions are separated.
- Circular questioning of silent or 'mad' family members is used: 'If he were to speak, what would he say?'
- Emotions are treated descriptively, not sympathised with: 'Which of your children understands your depression best?' 'What would have to change to reduce your depression?'
- Information is shown to have different meanings for different family members, thus revealing family relationships.

Positive connotation
- This is more than a form of reframing or relabelling, because it tries to address the rules of the whole family 'game', rather than one individual's behaviour.
- Symptomatic behaviour is reframed as good because it helps maintain the system's balance, so facilitating family cohesion and well-being. Thus, volition is ascribed, and the symptom is seen as helping the family, not as a negative entity.
- The presumed intent is what is positively connoted, not the behaviour: 'Thank you for preventing the outbreak of family strife over your brother's bad behaviour by refusing to eat.' It was believed by early systemic therapists that because positive connotations express approval, families do not resist them. More recently therapists have taken the view that it is not change that is necessarily resisted, but approaches to treatment which do not match the families' beliefs.

After perhaps 30–40 minutes of a session, the systemic therapist often withdraws to confer with their team behind the one-way mirror for ten minutes or so. After this, they re-enter the room and give 'the message' which may be accompanied by a task for family members to carry out. An example of each follows.

Paradox and counterparadox

- A *paradox* is set up by the family's acceptance of the therapist's positive connotation: why does a good thing, family cohesion, require a symptom in its member? The therapist spells out the dilemma the family are in.

- A *counterparadox* may be presented by the therapist as a message designed to help the family find a way out. Rather than saying that the symptomatic patient should change and the rest of the family should not, the counterparadox is designed to break up the dysfunctional, paradoxical pattern, for example, by prescribing no change. The family is then left on their own to resolve the paradoxical absurdities after the session.

The invariant prescription

This task was developed by two of the four original Milan four, Selvini-Palazzoli and Prata. It aims to unhinge collusive parent–child patterns, in which a 'game' is played out by family members and keeps the child symptomatic. This is often achieved by the child or adolescent siding with the 'weaker' parent and defeating the 'winner' through illness behaviour. The parents are told to plan a few evenings out, departing before dinner without forewarning, leaving only a note saying 'We'll not be home tonight'. On return, they are not to give any explanations to their children, saying 'These things concern only the two of us'. Each parent is asked to keep a private notebook of the verbal and non-verbal behaviour that follows carrying out the prescription. This procedure is designed to strengthen the parental alliance and break pre-existing coalitions, blocking 'games' of control that had perpetuated abnormal behaviour.

Narrative approach

This approach to therapy is a recent development that has been adopted by some strategic and systemic therapists. It focuses on the stories people have which guide their lives. John Byng-Hall combines this with an emphasis on attachment theory in his variety of family therapy based on *Rewriting Family Scripts*, the title of his 1995 book. Adults and children in a secure enough setting can construct a new way of seeing their future and be helped to live it, liberated from past constraints and expectations. David Epston uses letter writing as part of the *Narrative Means to Therapeutic Ends*, the title of his 1990 book with Michael White. Often harrowing life stories and problems are rewritten using the person's terminology, but emphasising how all along they fought the incredible strains they were put under with heroism. Evidence is found of instances when they were not dominated by the problem, and they are encouraged to think about the future from the strong, competent person that has emerged from the interview so far. The person is encouraged to create or seek out a receptive social group from their immediate circle so as to be able to live out their new story and identity.

Evaluation of family therapy

Criticisms

Some family therapists have little knowledge of specific syndromes in child and adolescent psychiatry. Rather, all problems are seen as arising from abnormal patterns of relationships. They fail to recognise the contribution of partly or entirely constitutional disorders such as Asperger syndrome or ADHD. Even with a condition such as a disruptive behavioural disorder, where psychosocial factors are highly relevant, a family therapy approach might not pick up the specific reading disorder present in up to a third of cases, and so fail to address the causal contribution this may be making.

Some family therapists seldom see children or adolescents on their own. Yet an individual interview is often essential to reveal depression, bullying, or abuse. For fear or shame or other reasons, children and adolescents may not say what they mean in front of other family members.

Families come for help because they feel that their child's symptoms need addressing directly. However, they may be put off by what they perceive as irrelevant intrusion into their private relationships. Some forms, notably Milan systemic, may use a second team to observe the therapist, which is expensive. In Milan therapy, it is hard for a therapist to be neutral if they have statutory obligations to protect the child or adolescent from abusive practices. The lack of explanation of why the questioning is following this line, and the confusing nature of the intervention, can alienate some families who vote with their feet and don't come back.

Rejoinders

Many, if not all, of these concerns can be overcome through flexible working. For example, in a multidisciplinary team, it is often possible to have an initial general assessment before proceeding to family therapy, although in practice most family therapists do not work this way. Engaging the family is the art of the therapist, and a skilled one will not lose families by becoming too probing too soon, but will be sensitive to what the family can tolerate. One of the main advantages of having a background in family therapy is to be able to recognise and address intrafamilial influences on behaviour, which a linear 'diagnostic' approach fails to do.

Outcome studies

There have been several randomised controlled trials in the past decade for a restricted range of conditions, showing that: family therapy as practised at the Maudsley Hospital is an effective therapy for anorexia nervosa; Multisystemic Therapy (which, as its name suggests, includes several components, so that generalisation in the community is maximised) is helpful for juvenile delinquency, drug misuse and child abuse; Functional Family Therapy (a more classical approach but with a behavioural slant) is helpful for juvenile delinquency; and Brief Strategic Family Therapy is helpful for drug misuse. These are all notoriously hard conditions to treat, so the results are impressive, even if effect sizes are often modest, of the order 0.3–0.6 standard deviations.

Subject review

Carr A. (2009) The effectiveness of family therapy and systemic interventions for child-focused problems. *Journal of Family Therapy* **31**, 3–45. (An excellent, unbiased review of individual trials and meta-analyses.)

Eisler I, Lask J. (2008) Family interviewing and family therapy. *In*: Rutter M *et al.* (eds) *Rutter's Child and Adolescent Psychiatry*, 5th edn. Wiley-Blackwell, Chichester, pp. 1062–1078.

Further reading

Classic texts setting out theoretical and practical approaches:

Byng-Hall J. (1995) *Rewriting Family Scripts*. Guilford, London.

Haley J. (1976) *Problem-Solving Therapy*. Jossey-Bass, San Francisco.

Minuchin S. (1974) *Families and Family Therapy*. Harvard University Press, Cambridge, MA.

White M. (1995) *Re-authoring Lives*. Dulwich Centre, Adelaide.

More recent texts that include evidence of effectiveness:

Carr A (2006) *Family Therapy: Concepts, Process and Practice*, 2nd edn. Guilford, New York.

Henggeler S *et al.* (2009) *Multisystemic Therapy for Antisocial Behavior in Children and Adolescents*, 2nd edn. Guilford, New York.

Sexton T. (2011) *Functional Family Therapy in Clinical Practice: An Evidence-Based Treatment Model for Working with Troubled Adolescents*. Routledge, New York.

Vetere A, Dallos R (2003) *Working Systemically with Families*. Karnac Books, London. (A useful and relatively brief introduction.)

CHAPTER 42

Fostering and Adoption

When parents cannot look after their children, then it may be necessary for them to be fostered or adopted by another family. Evidence suggests that this is a more desirable option than placement in a residential children's home. Even where physical care is good and there is a suitable amount of stimulation, the number of staff and their rate of turnover in residential homes make it harder for children to make secure attachments to one or two people with whom they have an especially intimate relationship. This has led to a renewed emphasis on fostering and adoption, although it may not always be possible for particularly disruptive teenagers. The case for residential homes has not been helped by instances where the young people were found to have been abused by the very staff who were supposed to help them.

Fostering

In the UK, about 64,000 children are looked after by local authorities at any one time, most of whom are fostered (a few are in residential homes). That is around 1 in 1,000 citizens, or around 1 in 250 children under the age of 18. Thus, in a typical borough of 250,000 people, there might be 300 children who are fostered or looked after by the local authority. This figure is often doubled in more disadvantaged boroughs. The legal framework for children coming into the care of the local authority in England is determined by the Children Act (1989). The term 'looked after' by the local authority means it has gained parental authority, whereas if the parent voluntarily gives up care of their child, the term used is 'accommodated'. When a local authority gains parental responsibility, while this gives the authority controlling power, the birth parents are also still deemed to have some responsibility for the child – a complex situation.

More than half of foster care arrangements last less than six months, with the children then going back to their parents, for example, because parents were lone parents who had a serious physical or mental illness which has since got better. In addition to official arrangements made

Child and Adolescent Psychiatry, Third Edition. Robert Goodman and Stephen Scott.
© 2012 Robert Goodman and Stephen Scott. Published 2012 by John Wiley & Sons, Ltd.

through the local authority, some people may make private arrangements for others to bring up their children, and this is a more usual arrangement in some cultures, for example, in West African countries. In recent years, due to the lack of a dependable supply of suitable foster carers, there has been an increasing emphasis on holding extended family conferences, where a wide number of extended family members are brought together to see whether they might be able to look after a child where the birth parents cannot, a so-called 'kinship' fostering. This arrangement can have the advantage of preserving the child's identity within the family, and can have a more personal commitment from the relative looking after the child. However, it can be disadvantageous if the relative is unable to prevent access from an abusive or mentally disturbed birth parent who is, for example, his or her own brother or sister. Also, kinship carers often feel, and are, less supported by social services' departments than regular fosterers in the task of looking after children who are usually decidedly challenging, and may, for example, require the new carer to give up their job, or their bedroom.

Adoption

Until 50 years ago, the majority of children adopted in the UK and the USA were white, born to healthy single mothers, and were developing without developmental delays or major mental health problems. There were enough babies or infants to meet the demand for them. Most were placed in the first two years of life with married, white adoptive parents who were told very little about the birth families and had no contact with them. Now, in contrast, there are not enough infants to meet demand. The children come from ethnically diverse backgrounds, are older, and many have significant psychiatric problems or developmental delays. Most have experienced seriously inadequate parenting or frank abuse and often have complex needs. However, unlike fostered children, once the adoption process is complete, the local authority has no parental responsibility towards the child, who now is entirely the responsibility of his or her new parents. Sometimes this can lead to a withdrawal of support and services once legalities are completed, although in England now there is a legal duty on the local authority that arranged it to provide support for the first three years after adoption.

Nowadays the adopting parent will typically come from as close an ethnic match as possible, may or may not have a partner, and may be a same sex couple. Because of the shortage of typically developing younger children, there have been a number of inter-country adoptions from developing countries to developed countries. In particular, due to the very poor state of Romanian orphanages, a number of these children were adopted in the UK and the USA, which has provided the opportunity to examine the impact of providing good enough environment after initial severe deprivation – the English Romanian Adoptees study has been extremely informative. It found that intellectual catch-up was good, whereas social skill development was often substantially impaired, leaving the children seeming rather odd in social situations and unable to make friends. A further category of children who may be looked after or adopted is unaccompanied refugees, who often come from war-torn countries. Currently in England only about 3,000 children are adopted a year, whereas perhaps two or three times this number might benefit from it. The process is considered by many to be overly lengthy (typically taking almost two years from prospective adopters expressing an interest to their getting a child) and steps are being taken to try to speed this up and increase the number of children who are adopted.

Psychopathology

Many children being considered for fostering or adoption will have been subject to neglect and emotional abuse with scapegoating. Some will have been seriously physically and sexually abused by birth parents or other members of the family circle. Birth parents are likely to have a raised prevalence of a whole range of psychiatric disorders, which often have made it impossible for them to parent adequately; relevant problems include major psychoses and depression, drug abuse, personality disorders. Birth parents also have higher rates of intellectual disability which also makes the parenting task considerably harder. This means that the children are at risk of emotional and behavioural disturbances, psychiatric disorders and lower intellectual abilities from both genetic and environmental causes, and from the interaction of the two. It is often the case that the particular child who is being put up for fostering or adoption has a more difficult temperament or more problems than his or her siblings – sometimes older or younger siblings have stayed with the family, but the index child has had a particularly bad relationship with the parents, resulting in total rejection. This may be purely due to environmental reasons around at the time of the birth, which led the parent to be less able to cope with the child or scapegoat him or her, but quite often both the parent and independent observers will note that the child had a more difficult temperament from the outset.

Genetics and environmental inferences are likely to interact, so that children with more irritable temperaments and genetic risk factors may be more sensitive to adverse environments (see Box 33.2). This picture can lead to a relatively hopeful message, in that despite children with genetic risks being more vulnerable, if one can make the rearing environment benign at a suitably early stage, one can have a disproportionately beneficial effect in improving the outcomes for the children and adolescents.

The prevalence of psychiatric disorders in children looked after by local authorities is very high. The Office of National Statistics survey in England found that, of all looked-after children (therefore including short-term fostering), around 45% had a psychiatric disorder, compared with 10% of the total population (see Box 3.1). All psychiatric disorders are

commoner. Particularly raised is the prevalence of autistic spectrum disorders and ADHD-like syndromes, especially where there has been severe
deprivation. Attachment *disorders* are more prevalent than in the general
population but still uncommon, but insecure attachment *patterns* are
common. For example, one study of late-placed (mean age at removal
from family 7 years old) fostered adolescents found that 0% were securely
attached to their birth fathers, and only 10% to their birth mothers,
compared to 44% and 60% of controls to their fathers and mothers.

Long-term outcomes are poor, both in terms of presence of psychiatric
disorders, and psychosocial functioning. Among children looked after by
local authorities in England, only 12% obtain five or more grades A–C
GCSEs, compared with 56% in the nation as a whole; criminality rates
are 5–10 times higher. In contrast, studies of earlier adopted children
show only a slight increase in psychiatric disorders and good long-term
psychosocial outcomes.

Assessment

Mental health assessment needs to be comprehensive. Several informants
should be asked for information, not, for example, just the current foster
carers. It is important to get the original records and any medical information about both birth parents, including their psychiatric history, criminal
records, level of intellectual attainment and education, and drug and alcohol history. A thorough physical examination is essential as there are often
visual or hearing deficits that have previously not been uncovered, and not
infrequently dysmorphic syndromes. A thorough psychometric assessment
is essential as specific learning difficulties and intellectual disability are
common. The child or adolescent needs to be spoken to on their own for
some time to get a picture of their own mental state, their understanding
of their own story and their relationship with, or understanding of, their
birth parents and fosterers or prospective adopters. For children looked
after by the local authority, it is important to ensure that a social worker
is present at the assessment, and if possible, a senior manager too. This
is so that the results of the assessment can be put into action with the
understanding and resources of the management.

Issues in deciding placement

The best therapy for a child who cannot live with their birth parents is
a stable placement with loving parent figures who can meet the child's
needs by providing sensitive and encouraging care and treating them as
somebody really special. From this it follows that:

1 Residential placements to 'prepare' a particularly troubled child for
  a permanent placement later are not a good idea, although this is
  sometimes still practised. This merely prolongs the period of doubt for

the child or adolescent and prevents them from beginning to make secure and trusting relationships.

2 Frequent contact with a birth parent who makes unrealistic promises about how wonderful it would be to live with them, or is a sex offender or seriously abusive, is not advisable and can lead to ongoing disturbance in the child or adolescent.

3 After disruption of a foster placement, placing the child or adolescent with another set of foster carers who are of the same level of experience or skill, rather than specialist foster carers with a good back-up system is liable to lead to yet further disruptions.

4 Extensive efforts to try to offer parenting treatments with highly abusive parents who have little prospect of improving sufficiently to meet their child's needs will prolong stress and ambiguity for the child and may lose crucial time periods when they need to experience security and love consistently in order to develop healthily.

5 When a child or adolescent has to be moved, wherever possible, continuity of school placement and positive peer relationships should be encouraged, rather than moving the individual to a different area.

6 Placing the child or adolescent with several disruptive siblings so that they can be together in a multiple sibling placement is not indicated if the relationship between siblings is poor or if their behaviour is markedly aggressive or antisocial; such a placement is highly likely to lead to further disruption, as it is very difficult for any parents to take three or four disruptive children at once.

7 Placing a child in a family with two or three children who are around the same age is likely to lead to jealousies and reduce the attention that can be given to the newly placed child. In contrast, placing a child in a family that has a well-adjusted older child can work well, especially if the older child shows care and interest in the new child and provides a good role model.

8 Sometimes the birth parents may overcome the acute problems that that led to their child to come into care, for example, their mental health problem may improve. Under these circumstances, it is right to consider reunification. However, studies indicate that a high proportion of reunifications fail (typically over half), with the child needing to re-enter the care system and that even when children are deemed well enough cared for to remain in their birth families, their outcomes are worse than those who remain looked after.

Identity and contact issues

In addition to whatever treatment is indicated for psychiatric disorders, a number of issues may need to be addressed. These include: (1) helping young people to understand why their parents could not keep them, particularly if there are other siblings who are still living with them. Giving them a 'life-story book' with photos of their relatives can help this. (2) Deciding how much contact with birth parents should be allowed, especially where this is undermining or distressing; their divided loyalty as to whether they should be allowed to love both their foster parents and their birth parents (in practice, this is quite possible, but may mean, for example, making two sets of mothers day cards). Increasingly, court orders to unsuitable birth parents not to contact their children are being circumvented by the use of internet social sites such as Facebook, often with disturbing consequences for the young person. (3) Helping the young person understand their identity may include acknowledging which physical and personality characteristics they have inherited from their birth parents. Even where their birth parents have been very abusive, having a photograph of them or seeing them once when they are in their later teens can help the young person to understand where they got their physical appearance and various mannerisms.

Issues and therapeutic work with foster or adoptive parents

With looked-after children, there may be conflicts over issues such as education, which may not meet the child's needs in the view of professionals or the foster parents. However, the legal parent is the local authority, and the social worker who is *in loco parentis* for the child may be reluctant to pressurise or sue the local authority since it is the social worker's own employer. The child mental health team may need to work hard to encourage the local education department to carry out an adequate assessment, and even more, to provide adequate education to meet the special needs.

There can sometimes be ambiguity about whether the foster parents are to be treated like parents, or as co-professionals, and there may be issues about what is divulged to them. Adoptive parents may believe that 'love will conquer all', but it may become increasingly apparent that this is not the case as the child fails to improve, because of inherited difficulties or ineradicable scars of long-standing abuse. This may have been compounded by the adoptive parents not being told the true severity of the background, and being made to believe they should be grateful for being given a child; and may be further compounded by the allocating social worker not having a good grasp of the child psychopathology and the likely long-term prognosis. The adoptive parents may have difficulty growing to love the adoptive child and bonding with him or her, and they may need work helping them understand that these things may take a long time to develop. Guidance may be needed on helping foster or adoptive parents to explain the true state of affairs to the young person in age-appropriate terms, and create a storybook for the young person so they can complete the understanding of their identity.

Around 10% of late adoptive placements (that is, child over 5 years old on joining the family), and a higher proportion of late fostering placements, 'disrupt' when the foster or adoptive parents come to feel they cannot continue to look after the child. Research shows three factors are important in determining disruption: (1) lack of carer confidence about how to handle the child; (2) the presence of significant behaviour problems; and (3) the extent to which the carers 'click' with the child, that is, the extent to which the new parents feel the child is well matched to them and is loveable. Children who were scapegoated more than their siblings in their birth family are especially prone to disrupted placements. Parent training programmes offer a logical approach to help foster and adoptive carers since they have been shown to improve the two principal causes of disruption: parental confidence in managing the child, and the level of child behaviour problems.

Specific interventions

Behaviourally-based foster care trainings such as the programme *Fostering Changes* (http://fosteringchanges.com) can improve the skill with which foster carers and adoptive carers handle children, increase the stability of the placements, and lead to greater satisfaction for the foster and adoptive carers. There is a randomised controlled trial showing that this programme is effective in increasing carer confidence and reducing child behaviour problems.

It is particularly important to ensure that the child has adequate education. A relatively high proportion of looked-after children are out of school and not getting full-time schooling. When they are at school, the pressures on schools to be 'socially inclusive' may mean that they are put into a large class without special provision for the special teaching they need, and their self-esteem suffers as a result. As well as addressing the child's deficits, it is crucial that strengths are encouraged, be these, for example, prowess in sport, such as football, developing hobbies, such as interest in animals, singing, or whatever else. Such strengths can take on a particular importance when there is much less stability in the personal background and relationships of a child.

For children and young people who have a succession of disrupted placements because fosterers found them too challenging, specialist fostering may be indicated. There are various forms of therapeutic foster care. One of the best known, 'Multidimensional Treatment Foster Care', involves paying a salary to foster carers who take on just one child as a full-time job. The foster parents supervise the child very closely so they have little chance to engage in damaging or antisocial activities such as drug taking or unprotected sex. They are unremittingly encouraging about any and all achievements and closely responsive to the young person – this is likely to be in marked contrast to the negative feedback and criticism they have mostly experienced. But because social approval is often less effective in these young people (who have every reason to be mistrustful of adults), practical rewards in the form of points are also given. These are exchanged on a daily basis for privileges such as watching more TV, phoning friends and other rewards that motivate the particular child. Foster carers are supported with daily phone calls and weekly meetings with other foster carers and professionals. There is a separate individual therapist for the young person, a therapist who works with the birth family (even where there is no prospect of return home, there are inevitably issues to resolve, such as what happens during contact visits), and a skills trainer to help the young person learn to act appropriately when out in the community. In the USA, this approach has been proven effective with psychiatric in-patients being discharged, and with antisocial young people. It is being introduced for fostered young people in the UK, where a trial has shown that it is effective for very disruptive young people.

Because some fostered and adoptive children are very disturbed, their parents can get desperate, especially when sensible mental health services are lacking. Under these circumstances the fosterers or adopters may fall for plausible but non evidence-based approaches to assessment and treatment. Often these may take the form of so-called 'attachment' checklists which attribute almost all symptoms and behaviours to an attachment problem; at other times rare and exotic new syndromes are put forward as the answer. In both cases, inappropriate, sometimes harmful and sometimes very expensive treatments can be touted – as further elaborated in Chapter 17 on attachment disorders. In the USA, there have been six deaths from such 'treatments'. At a less severe but still worrying level, statements made in the Adoption and Fostering Clinic of one of the authors include:

If they have a tantrum, don't speak English to them, just gibberish.

Remove everything from their room while at school, replace with uncooked pasta, raw potato, cold baked beans in their slippers etc. and do not explain why.

Never let them out of your sight, even to the loo (or for a clinical assessment).

Baby her every night, no words just baby talk and re-enact the birth, push her out from between your legs – that she hates it proves it's important.

Never use time out or sanctions, think of all they've been through.

You can restrain them for hours – at the retreat, some kids may be restrained through the night in shifts.

Issues in selecting adoptive parents

These can be harder to select than foster parents, since in the majority of cases, there will be no evidence of the prospective adopters' skills in parenting because they have not been able to have children. Research suggests that if they are unresolved or unrealistic in their own view of relationships (as determined by the Adult Attachment Interview (AAI), see Chapter 32), this is predictive of doing less well once children are placed, with an increased chance of disruption. However, the current state of knowledge is insufficient to use the AAI to select adoptive parents. It is important to determine the extent of the support system and confiding relationships available to the adoptive parents, as the placement will inevitably be a considerable strain. Normal biological parents find having one child a strain, and yet adoptive parents may have no chance to learn 'on the job' and perhaps have two children in middle childhood placed with them, who may have considerable behaviour problems. While single parents can make good foster or adoptive parents, it will be essential that they have good, close support, as the job can be very demanding.

Subject review

Cohen N. (2008) Adoption. *In*: Rutter M *et al.* (eds) *Rutter's Child and Adolescent Psychiatry*, 5th edn. Wiley-Blackwell, Chichester, pp. 502–518.

Rushton A, Minnis H. (2008) Residential and foster family care. *In*: Rutter M *et al.* (eds) *Rutter's Child and Adolescent Psychiatry*, 5th edn. Wiley-Blackwell, Chichester, pp. 487–501.

Further reading

Meltzer H *et al.* (2003) *The Mental Health of Young People Looked After by Local Authorities in England*. Office of National Statistics, London.

Scott S, Lindsey C. (2003) Therapeutic approaches in adoption. *In*: Argent H (ed.) *Models of Adoption Support*. British Association for Adoption and Fostering, London, pp. 209–240.

Sinclair I. (2005) *Fostering Now: Messages from Research*. Department for Education, London. (An easy-to-read summary of several research projects on fostering in England.)

Wade J *et al.* (2010) *Maltreated Children in the Looked After System: A Comparison of Outcomes for Those Who Go Home and Those Who Do Not*. Department for Education, London.

CHAPTER 43

Organisation of Services

Imagine you are in charge of drawing up a plan for your area's child and adolescent mental health services (CAMHS). Depending on which country you come from, you might have been asked to do this on behalf of the government, a health maintenance organisation, or an international charity. This chapter cannot tell you exactly what to do, partly because the right answer will depend on local circumstances, and partly because there may be several good answers rather than one right answer. What this chapter does instead is introduce you to some of the key points you will need to consider in order to draw up your plan.

Why plan at all?

A good plan is better than a bad plan, but is it better than leaving the development of services to market forces? As far as the provision of consumer goods is concerned, free market economies have generally outperformed planned economies, at least in terms of quantity and choice. Could the 'invisible hand' of the free market do as well for child and adolescent mental health services? For some families who are well informed and wealthy, the free market can provide a good service. For society as a whole, though, it would probably be a mistake to leave child and adolescent mental health care to the free market without any planning or governmental involvement. Here are some of the reasons:

1 Families are good at shopping around for apples or shoes because they know what they want and they can judge what they are getting. By contrast, if an adolescent becomes depressed, how can the family know if they should be seeking psychoanalysis, cognitive-behavioural therapy, herbal remedies, inter-personal therapy, medication, family therapy or nothing at all? And even if they do know, how can they tell a good provider from a bad provider? Inadequate information can be a major barrier to the efficient operation of market forces. For example, private

Child and Adolescent Psychiatry, Third Edition. Robert Goodman and Stephen Scott.
© 2012 Robert Goodman and Stephen Scott. Published 2012 by John Wiley & Sons, Ltd.

hospitals might be able to sell expensive in-patient care to families who don't know that out-patient treatment would have been cheaper and more effective.

2 Except in large cities, specialist providers may have local monopolies. This could allow them to overcharge, thereby undermining the efficiency of a free market.

3 Private services are often unevenly distributed across a country, being concentrated in affluent areas, particularly in large cities. Exclusive reliance on free market forces will often leave some regions seriously underprovided.

4 For low-income families, the costs of prolonged treatment or in-patient admission will be prohibitively expensive, and even a brief out-patient consultation may be unaffordable. Since poverty is a powerful risk factor for psychiatric problems in many countries, exclusive reliance on the free market would cut off some of the most vulnerable children and adolescents from the help they need.

5 Even when parents are wealthy enough to afford private help for their children's mental health problems, they may prefer to spend their money on other things. Parental willingness to pay may be undermined by exactly those parental characteristics that contributed to their children developing problems in the first place. Imagine, for example, that Mr and Mrs Smith particularly dislike their son Joe and that their constant criticism of him has contributed to his developing behavioural problems. They may not be strongly motivated to get help for him even it is free, and they will probably be even less likely to do so if they have to pay.

6 Mental health is not just a private affair. You may be robbed or raped by Joe when he grows up – a disaster that could perhaps have been averted if only his family had been provided with help early on. Health care is what economists describe as a 'merit good' since it is not just the person who receives the health care who benefits – there are wider benefits for society as a whole. Merit goods are characteristically under-provided by a free market. The same often applies even more strongly to prevention.

7 'Joined up' working between health, social services and education is often an important part of the management of children and adolescents with psychiatric disorders, reflecting the complex interrelationship between mental health problems, social problems and learning difficulties. Free market forces may promote inter-professional and inter-agency rivalry rather than collaboration.

For these and other reasons, it is probably unwise for any society to rely exclusively on the 'invisible hand' of the free market to provide and allocate mental health provision and children and adolescents. To provide optimal care, the free market needs to be regulated, supplemented or replaced – but this will only improve matters if interventions are well planned.

Inclusiveness

Within health care, it is sometimes useful to distinguish between 'patient-centred' and 'population-centred' traditions. Most clinicians are firmly rooted in the patient-centred tradition – they focus on improving the health of the individual patients who present to their service. By contrast, the population-centred tradition focuses on the health of the population as a whole, including individuals who do not present to services. This sort of 'public health' perspective is often particularly relevant to planning. For example, a CAMHS might provide excellent treatment for children and adolescents with ADHD, and the clinicians working in the service might be rightly proud of how satisfied the families are. Unless the service also takes a population-centred view, they may not realise, for example, that they are providing this excellent service for just 100 individuals when the epidemiological data suggest that their catchment area probably contains around 1,000 children and adolescents with ADHD. What is happening to the other 900? Perhaps all is well: 600 are being well managed by family doctors and paediatricians, while the other 300 families have made a well-informed choice not to seek treatment. In most parts of the world, however, the reality is less satisfactory: many of the 'missing' children and adolescents are regarded as lazy, stupid or naughty; and even when parents and teachers suspect ADHD, they have not known how to access expert assessment and treatment. A British survey that followed up a large and representative sample of children and adolescents with psychiatric disorders (see Box 3.1) found that only a quarter of them were seen by specialist mental health professionals over the following three years, and although some of the remainder were seen by educational, social or paediatric services, that still left half of them receiving no help at all over the entire three-year period. This is unacceptable – there is no justification for neglecting the needs of individuals who have treatable chronic disorders that seriously undermine their present and future quality of life.

When planning services, it is important to aim for inclusiveness: meeting the mental health needs of all the children and adolescents in the catchment area whether or not they currently use these services. No one should be excluded because of their gender, ethnicity, social class, physical disability or intellectual level. Various barriers may make services seem inaccessible or unacceptable. For a service to be accessible, families and referrers have to know the service exists, they have to know what the service offers, and they have to be able to get there (so location is important, as is the availability of public transport). Accessibility is greater when services are open outside 9–5 hours and when there is a crèche for siblings. The wait for an appointment should not be excessive, and there needs to be some arrangement for responding rapidly to crises; some services aim to carry out the initial assessment rapidly in all cases, though there may then be a waiting list for non-urgent treatment. The acceptability of a service to families is also influenced by the attitudes of staff and the physical condition of the building.

Clearly defined boundaries

Many services are for a defined geographical catchment area. Within this area, it is important to decide which disorders should be the concern of mental health services. For example, will CAMHS be involved in the assessment and treatment of stuttering, obesity, enuresis, or dyslexia? Sometimes there will be pressure to do so, particularly if there is no other service for these problems. The price for doing this may be that the service then has to cut back on the assessment and treatment of 'core' mental health problems such as anorexia nervosa or obsessive-compulsive disorder. One area of controversy is how far mental health services should be involved in the assessment and treatment of disruptive behavioural disorders. These disorders are undoubtedly common, severe and costly to society, and there are evidence-based treatments (see Chapter 6). Clearly, these disorders need identification and treatment – the question is whether this should be done by health, education, social services, the voluntary sector, or some combination of these. At present, disruptive behavioural disorders account for over half of the work of many CAMHS. The advantage of this is that these children are getting help that might not otherwise have been available; the disadvantage may be the relative neglect of other disorders that require the sort of help provided by mental health services rather than education, social services or any other agency. Some hard-pressed CAMHS have responded to this pressure by dropping disruptive behavioural disorders from their remit in order to concentrate their resources on 'core' mental health problems – a potentially reasonable response provided someone takes responsibility for the management of behavioural problems.

Age boundaries may also be useful. At some point, child and adolescent services give way to adult services (hopefully with good transition arrangements). Should this transition happen at 14, 16 or 18, or according to clinical judgement? The advantage of the latter is that an immature 17-year-old who is still in school might best be seen by adolescent services, whereas a mature 16-year-old who has left school might best be seen by adult services. On the other hand, a fluid age limit may make it harder to allocate funding between services. Older teenagers are more likely than young children to have serious mental illnesses requiring lengthy or repeated hospital admissions – so extending a service from 0–15-year-olds to include substantial numbers of 16–18-year-olds could potentially double total costs. This is fine if the extra funding is made available, but could be a disaster if it diverts funding away from the treatment of under-16s.

Budgets that are fair to the young

Throughout the world, considerably more money is spent on mental health services for every million adults in the general population than on mental health services for every million children and adolescents in the general population. In Britain, the per capita spending on mental health is over five times greater for adults than children. It is true that some of the money spent by schools and social services is directed at the mental health of children and adolescents – but not enough to make up for a five-fold difference in mental health spending. It is not as if child and adolescent mental health problems are rare. As pointed out in Chapter 3 and elsewhere, these problems are very common and have a large immediate and delayed impact. In the short term, the problems distress the affected individual and may also place considerable stress on parents, siblings, teachers and classmates. In the longer term, failure to prevent or treat child and adolescent mental health problems leads to more crime, substance abuse, adult psychiatric disorder, school failure, unemployment and poor parenting. Rather than neglecting tomorrow's adults, there is a case for investing early in their present and future mental health.

At the same time, though, it is important to remember that increased mental health spending does not, by itself, guarantee improved mental health. Buying more of the wrong thing will not help. This is the main message of the Fort Bragg project, which cost $80 million and took five years to carry out. The evaluation compared ordinary child and adolescent mental health care with a more generously funded version that provided a better integrated and more accessible service, and where clinicians were effectively allowed to do what they thought best without having to worry about costs. The cost per case roughly doubled, and families were more satisfied, but there was no appreciable change in outcome, with children and adolescents getting better at the same rate regardless. The research team concluded that it had been a mistake to focus on the financing and organisation of services without first ensuring that the services were delivering effective treatments. More of what you don't need won't necessarily make you better.

High quality provision

The two mainstays of quality services are accurate assessment and evidence-based treatment. These key topics are covered in almost every chapter of this book. There is little to add here, other than noting that while there is growing evidence about which treatments work best, some CAMHS have been slow to adopt these. When there are proven treatments available, it makes no sense to neglect these in favour of treatments that have been shown to be largely or entirely ineffective, or treatments that have not been properly evaluated. It is not only wasteful but also unethical to deprive children and adolescents of effective treatments. Doing so results in unnecessary suffering in the short term and may cause lasting damage in the long term. Mechanisms need to be put in place to reward services for employing effective treatments and discourage services from continuing to use ineffective ones.

Providing value for money

Child and adolescent mental health needs are extensive but budgets are limited. Consequently, we need to find ways of doing more for less – without undermining quality. Here are some of the ways of providing value for money without compromising quality:

1 *Some help is free* or can be purchased at low cost by families themselves. It will often be appropriate to encourage families to use self-help books and websites (which can be located, for example, via www.youthinmind.info). Some self-help material is excellent, and for mild problems and resourceful families, this may be all that is needed. Telephone helplines, parents' organisations and other voluntary organisations can also be very helpful. Randomised controlled trials indicate that self-help by parents using books and manuals can be effective. Sometimes, this self-help is even more effective when parents are also provided with a little guidance and supervision from mental health professionals.

2 *Provide help in the most cost-effective setting.* Services to improve child mental health can sometimes be delivered more appropriately and economically outside specialist mental health settings. For example, it may be cheaper and more convenient for families if family doctors and paediatricians have the skills to prescribe stimulants for all but the most complicated or treatment-resistant cases of ADHD. Similarly, if high levels of bullying in local schools mean that child mental health services currently have to spend a lot of their time treating the resultant stress-related disorders, the cheapest and best solution may be greater investment in school-based programmes to reduce bullying. To facilitate this sort of work, child and adolescent mental health professionals can contribute to the training of teachers, paediatricians, social workers and other professionals, or work alongside them in schools, paediatric clinics, residential care homes and other settings. However, caution is needed since there is a growing literature on the need to use skilled and well-trained therapists to obtain a significant therapeutic effect. There are many innovative schemes to disseminate skills, but each of these should be evaluated in terms of both cost and effectiveness before they are widely adopted.

3 *Optimise the skill mix.* Specialisation and division of labour can greatly improve productivity. The scope for this depends on the size of the mental health team: the smaller the team, the less room there is for specialisation. If the team is potentially large enough to support specialisation, it is generally a waste of money not to do so. Imagine a team staffed entirely by child and adolescent psychiatrists – it would almost certainly be more expensive than a mixed team of psychiatrists and psychologists, and it might not provide as good a quality of psychological therapies either. Doctors are usually the most expensive team members and they should be used sparingly for delivering the things they can do best, for

example, medical assessment, pharmacotherapy, or integrated packages of pharmacotherapy and psychological therapy. It will rarely be a good use of resources to use doctors to deliver psychological therapies when there is no medical component. Similar considerations apply to all other professionals, including psychologists, nurses and family therapists: Are their unique skills being used appropriately? Could parts of their job be done as well (or better) by other people who cost less? Using highly qualified staff for simple tasks is likely to waste money that could be used to help more people. But don't forget that using under-qualified staff can do harm and reduce cost effectiveness if poorer quality treatment undermines successful outcomes. It may be a good idea to have simple cases treated by cheaper staff with less extensive training, but it is vital that they should be well supervised by more experienced staff.

4 *Use a graded approach.* Children and adolescents with mild problems do not usually need lengthy and complicated assessment and treatment – brief single-handed assessment and therapy may be all that is required. If a simple approach does not work, it may then be appropriate to move on to a more detailed multidisciplinary assessment and lengthier treatment packages. On the other hand, if the referrer makes it clear from the outset that a child has a complicated and puzzling disorder that is going to need a multidisciplinary assessment, it would be a waste of resources to do a single-handed assessment first. A flexible range of options is more efficient than a 'one size fits all' approach. It may be helpful to have a hierarchy of services:

1. For the majority of children with mild and moderate problems, the assessment and treatment can be delivered by single-handed child and adolescent mental health professionals working in schools and primary health centres. These professionals need a broad-based training that allows them to deliver relatively simple treatments for a wide range of problems.

2. Individuals who do not respond to simple approaches can be referred to the area's specialist CAMHS. Those with severe problems might best be referred directly to CAMHS at the outset. Since services are delivered by several professionals, there is room for specialisation and a flexible mixture of single-handed and team working.

3. An even smaller number of children and adolescents with rare and hard-to-treat disorders need to be seen by highly specialised regional or national services, whether as out-patients or in-patients.

A good example of a graded approach is the Triple P parenting programme. Level 1 is the provision of universally relevant parenting information through TV and radio programmes. Level 2 consists of two 20-minute consultations by a primary care worker using a manual to tackle isolated behavioural problems. Level 3 involves four 40-minute sessions for wider-ranging problems, delivered by a more experienced practitioner. Level 4 is a ten-week programme of two hours per week led by a qualified mental health practitioner. Those who do not respond well to this go on to level 5, which involves a further eight weeks of more intensive family work.

5 *Find the right balance between prevention and cure.* Prevention is such an attractive option that planners often assume that spending money on prevention is bound to be better value than spending money on a cure. This is not necessarily true. Some preventative approaches are not particularly effective (see Chapter 36). In some instances, it is cost-effective to invest money in prevention; in other instances, it is better to invest resources in early detection and effective treatment. Taking the example of the Triple P parenting intervention noted above, a universal prevention trial in several counties in North Carolina in the USA showed that it reduced the incidence of child abuse.

6 *Employ labour-saving devices.* Mental health assessments and treatments are very labour-intensive, and they probably always will be. There is room, though, for using computer technology to improve productivity while preserving quality. There are a growing number of options for computer-assisted assessment and treatment; the general aim is for the computer to take over the routine and repetitive parts of the job, leaving the professionals freer to do the interesting and innovative parts. For example, computer interviews can ask the routine questions, thereby identifying areas of concern to be explored in more detail by a mental health professional (for example, www.dawba.info/f1.html). In effect, computers can do much of the boring work that used to be done by underpaid junior staff – and do it cheaper!

7 *Prioritise the most cost-effective treatments.* If, despite the measures described above, it still is not possible to meet all child and adolescent mental health needs within the available budget, then provision will need to be rationed. The need for rationing is increasingly acknowledged in all areas of health care since there is widespread (but not universal) agreement that needs and wants are bound to outstrip the resources for meeting them. If rationing is necessary, one solution is to concentrate on the most cost-effective treatments, since doing so provides the greatest overall benefit for the available money. Others would argue, however, that this is not necessarily the fairest approach to rationing since it may result in individuals with mild but easily treated disorders getting more treatment than individuals with serious but hard-to-treat disorders.

Built-in improvement

It is important to design services so that they can improve with time. Two key ways to do this are 'continuing professional development' programmes for staff and routine outcome monitoring. All professionals need to commit themselves to lifelong learning, and services need to facilitate this. In addition, services need to monitor how much the people they treat improve as a result. This does not have to cost much – standard questionnaires completed by parents, teachers, children or adolescents are often sufficient. These 'customer' reports supplement clinician ratings of improvement and are arguably less prone to bias. Through routine outcome monitoring, services can see who they benefit most and least. This may lead to them concentrating more of their resources on what they do best, or it may lead to their trying new approaches for the sorts of problems that have not responded well in the past. Either way, changing practice in response to outcome monitoring increases the chance of the service doing more good this year than last year. It is this capacity for improvement that justifies investing scarce resources (time, money, energy) in monitoring outcome (see Box 43.1). A service can save money in the short term by ignoring outcome, but in the longer term it would thereby lose opportunities to change for the better.

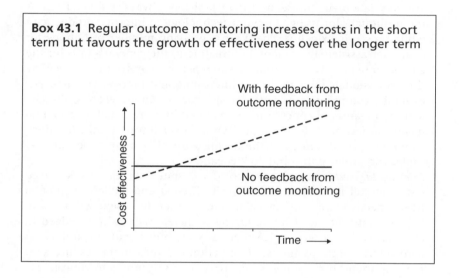

Box 43.1 Regular outcome monitoring increases costs in the short term but favours the growth of effectiveness over the longer term

Subject review

Wolpert M. (2008) Organization of services for children and adolescents with mental health problems. *In*: Rutter M *et al*. (eds) *Rutter's Child and Adolescent Psychiatry*, 5th edn. Wiley-Blackwell, Chichester, pp. 1156–1166.

Further reading

Bickman LA (1996) Continuum of care: More is not always better. *American Psychologist* **51**, 689–701.

Goodman R. (1997a) Child mental health: Who is responsible? An overextended remit. *BMJ* **314**, 813–814.

Goodman R. (1997b) Who needs child psychiatrists? *Child Psychology and Psychiatry Review* **2**, 15–19.

Prinz R *et al*. (2009) Population-based prevention of child maltreatment: The U.S. Triple P system population trial, *Prevention Science* **10**, 1–12.

Sanders MW *et al*. (2003) The Triple P – positive parenting program: A universal population-level approach to the prevention of child abuse. *Child Abuse Review* **12**, 155–171.

Index

Page numbers in *italics* indicate tables and boxes.

Child and Adolescent Psychiatry, Third Edition. Robert Goodman and Stephen Scott.
© 2012 Robert Goodman and Stephen Scott. Published 2012 by John Wiley & Sons, Ltd.